Diagnostic Imaging of
Infections and Inflammatory Diseases

Diagnostic Imaging of Infections and Inflammatory Diseases

A Multidisciplinary Approach

EDITED BY

Alberto Signore, MD, PhD

Professor of Nuclear Medicine, Nuclear Medicine Unit, Department of Medical-Surgical Sciences and of Translational Medicine, Faculty of Medicine and Psychology, "Sapienza" University, Rome, Italy

Ana María Quintero, MD

Radiologist, Department of Radiology, Clinica Reina Sofia, Clinica Colsanitas, Bogotá, Colombia

WILEY Blackwell

Library of Congress Cataloging-in-Publication Data
Diagnostic imaging of infections and inflammatory diseases : a multidisciplinary approach / edited by Alberto Signore, Ana Maria Quintero.
      p. ; cm.
   Includes bibliographical references and index.
   ISBN 978-1-118-48441-8 (alk. paper) – ISBN 978-1-118-48435-7 (print) –
ISBN 978-1-118-48438-8 (print) – ISBN 978-1-118-48439-5 (print) –
ISBN 978-1-118-48443-2 (print)
   I. Signore, A. (Alberto), 1959- editor of compilation.   II. Quintero, Ana Maria, editor of compilation.
   [DNLM: 1. Diagnostic Imaging–methods.   2. Communicable Diseases–radiography.
3. Communicable Diseases–radionuclide imaging.   4. Inflammation–radiography.
5. Inflammation–radionuclide imaging. WN 180]
   616.07'54–dc23
                        2013001677

Cover images: Main cover image © Baran Özdemir iStockphoto.com #17280971.
            Inset image courtesy of Professor Signore.
Cover design by Matt Kuhns

Printed in Singapore

10 9 8 7 6 5 4 3 2 1

Contents

List of Contributors

Mathieu Assal, MD
Department of Orthopedic Surgery, Geneva University
Hospitals *and* Faculty of Medicine, University of Geneva,
Geneva, Switzerland

Jenny T. Bencardino, MD
Associate Professor of Radiology, Department of Radiology,
NYU Hospital for Joint Diseases, New York, NY, USA

Nicolas Christian Buchs, MD
Department of Orthopedic Surgery, Geneva University
Hospitals *and* Faculty of Medicine, University of Geneva,
Geneva, Switzerland

Randall Bujan, MD
Assistant Radiologist, Don Bosco Radiologic Clinic, San Jose,
Costa Rica

Jorge Carrillo, MD
Professor of Radiology, Universidad Nacional de Colombia,
Bogotá, Colombia

Marco Chianelli, MD, PhD
Nuclear Medicine Physician and Endocrinologist,
Department of Endocrinology, Regina Apostolorum Hospital,
Albano, Rome, Italy

Josep Martín Comín, MD
Professor of Nuclear Medicine, Department of Nuclear
Medicine, Hospital Universitari de Bellvitge, L'Hospitalet de
Llobregat, Barcelona, Spain

Paola Anna Erba, MD
Nuclear Medicine Physician, Regional Center of Nuclear
Medicine, University of Pisa, Medical School, Pisa, Italy

Alba Rodríguez Gasén, MD
Nuclear Medicine Physician, Department of Nuclear
Medicine, Hospital Universitari de Bellvitge, L'Hospitalet de
Llobregat, Barcelona, Spain

Andor W.J.M. Glaudemans, MD
Nuclear Medicine Physician, Department of Nuclear
Medicine and Molecular Imaging, University Medical Center
Groningen, University of Groningen, Groningen, The
Netherlands

François-Xavier Hanin, MD
Nuclear Medicine Physician, Centre of Nuclear Medicine,
Molecular Imaging, Experimental Radiotherapy and
Oncology (MIRO) Unit, Université Catholique de Louvain,
Brussels, Belgium

Pierre Hoffmeyer, MD
Department of Orthopedic Surgery, Geneva University
Hospitals *and* Faculty of Medicine, University of Geneva,
Geneva, Switzerland

Ora Israel, MD
Professor of Nuclear Medicine, Department of Nuclear
Medicine, Rambam Health Care Campus, Haifa, Israel

François Jamar, MD, PhD
Professor of Nuclear Medicine, Centre of Nuclear Medicine,
Molecular Imaging, Experimental Radiotherapy and
Oncology (MIRO) Unit, Université Catholique de Louvain,
Brussels, Belgium

Diego Jaramillo, MD
Radiologist-in-Chief, Children's Hospital of Philadelphia,
Professor of Radiology, University of Pennsylvania,
Philadelphia, PA, USA

Bárbara Morales Klinkert, MD, MSc
Nuclear Medicine Physician, Nuclear Medicine and PET/CT
Center, Fundación López Perez (FALP), Santiago, Chile

Elena Lazzeri, MD, PhD
Nuclear Medicine Physician, Regional Center of Nuclear
Medicine, University of Pisa, Medical School, Pisa, Italy

Daniel Lew, MD
Department of Infectious Diseases, Geneva University
Hospitals *and* Faculty of Medicine, University of Geneva,
Geneva, Switzerland

Jorge Lopera, MD
Professor of Radiology, The University of Texas Health
Science Center, San Antonio, TX, USA

Francesca Maccioni, MD
Professor of Radiology, Department of Radiological Sciences, Faculty of Medicine and Dentistry, "Sapienza" University, Rome, Italy

Gaurav Malviya, PhD
Department of Nuclear Medicine and Molecular Imaging, University Medical Center Groningen, University of Groningen, Groningen, The Netherlands *and* Nuclear Medicine Unit, Department of Medical-Surgical Sciences and of Translational Medicine, Faculty of Medicine and Psychology, "Sapienza" University, Rome, Italy

Giuliano Mariani, MD
Professor of Nuclear Medicine, Regional Center of Nuclear Medicine, University of Pisa, Medical School, Pisa, Italy

Manuel Maynar, MD, PhD
Radiologist, Centro de Diagnóstico y Terapéutica Endoluminal CD y TE, Las Palmas de Gran Canaria University, Canary Islands, Spain

Christopher J. Palestro, MD
Professor of Radiology, Hofstra North Shore-LIJ School of Medicine, Hempstead, NY, USA *and* Chief, Division of Nuclear Medicine and Molecular Imaging, North Shore Long Island Jewish Health System, Manhasset & New Hyde Park, NY, USA

Nicola Petrosillo, MD
Director, 2nd Infectious Diseases Division, National Institute for Infectious Diseases, "L. Spallanzani", IRCCS, Rome, Italy

Ana María Quintero, MD
Radiologist, Department of Radiology, Clinica Reina Sofia, Clinica Colsanitas, Bogotá, Colombia

Sergi Quiroga, MD
Radiologist, Servicio de Radiodiagnóstico, Hospital Universitario Valle Hebrón, Barcelona, Spain

Zoraida Restrepo-Velez, MD
Research Fellow, NYU Medical Center, NYU Hospital for Joint Diseases, New York, NY, USA

Roy Riascos, MD
Associate Professor of Radiology, Department of Radiology, The University of Texas Medical Branch, Galveston, TX, USA

Alejandro Romero, MD
Radiologist, Servicio de Radiodiagnóstico, Hospital Universitario Valle Hebrón, Barcelona, Spain

Mike Sathekge, MBChB, MMed (Nucl Med), PhD, MASSAf
Professor & Head of Nuclear Medicine Department, University of Pretoria and Steve Biko Academic Hospital, Pretoria, South Africa

Giancarlo Schiappacasse, MD
Associate Professor of Radiology, Clínica Alemana, Facultad de Medicina, Universidad del Desarrollo, Santiago, Chile

Khalid Seghrouchni, MD
Department of Orthopedic Surgery, Geneva University Hospitals *and* Faculty of Medicine, University of Geneva, Geneva, Switzerland

Alberto Signore, MD, PhD
Professor of Nuclear Medicine, Nuclear Medicine Unit, Department of Medical-Surgical Sciences and of Translational Medicine, Faculty of Medicine and Psychology, "Sapienza" University, Rome, Italy

Martina Sollini, MD
Nuclear Medicine Physician, Regional Center of Nuclear Medicine, University of Pisa, Medical School, Pisa, Italy

Ilker Uçkay, MD
Department of Orthopedic Surgery, Department of Infectious Diseases, Geneva University Hospitals *and* Faculty of Medicine, University of Geneva, Geneva, Switzerland

Christophe Van de Wiele, MD, PhD
Professor and Head of Department of Nuclear Medicine, University Hospital Ghent, Ghent, Belgium

Carolina Whittle, MD
Professor of Radiology, Clínica Alemana, Facultad de Medicina, Universidad del Desarrollo, Santiago, Chile

Tobías Zander, MD, PhD
Radiologist, Centro de Diagnóstico y Terapéutica Endoluminal CD y TE, Las Palmas de Gran Canaria University, Canary Islands, Spain

Foreword

The care of patients presenting with signs of infectious or inflammatory diseases is often difficult because their symptoms are frequently non-specific; the diagnosis, differential diagnosis and decision about appropriate therapy is often a real challenge for the clinician. The implementation of the available diagnostic methods is complex and the evaluation of their results also complex and frequently contradictory. Many of these methods are not familiar to clinicians; therefore the decision about their role in the diagnostic process and the strategy to be adopted may be delayed. Most of the guidelines generally available still do not reflect consensual diagnostic strategies.

The editors of this book had the merit to involve clinicians, radiologists and nuclear physicians with the objective to review this difficult area disease by disease, to define the appropriate clinical questions that may arise in everyday practice and to compare the accuracy and diagnostic value of the available diagnostic methods. Their efforts have resulted in clear, didactic content that supports consultation in clinical practice, suggests solutions to the most frequently encountered pathological situations (osteomyelitis, spondylodiscitis, abdominal, soft tissue and vascular graft infections, HIV and chronic inflammatory diseases), and summarizes the consensual diagnostic strategies.

The book is an excellent illustration of the synergy that can be achieved between specialties and in the imaging specialties collaboration is of the utmost importance. Both radiology and nuclear medicine contribute, often in a complementary way, to obtaining the correct diagnosis and the timely evaluation of the therapeutic answer. The clear and objective comparison of the diagnostic value and performance of available methods in solving clinical problems allows us to define clear, precise, fast and less expensive diagnostic algorithms to assist clinicians for the benefit of our patients.

Representing our respective European professional–scientific communities (the European Association of Nuclear Medicine and the European Society of Radiology), we congratulate the editors and authors on their excellent work and recommend its exploitation by radiologists, nuclear physicians and clinicians.

Patrick Bourguet
Past President of the EANM
CRLCC Centre Eugène Marquis
Rennes, France

András Palkó
Past President of the ESR
University of Szeged
Szeged, Hungary

Preface

Having dedicated most of our scientific and clinical activity to the diagnosis of infections and inflammatory diseases we always had in mind to write a textbook on this topic. An initial book of this kind was published by one of us (AS) in early 2002, followed by a pictorial atlas and several chapters in other books dedicated to nuclear medicine and molecular imaging or to specific diseases. However, the multidisciplinary approach to diagnostic imaging of infections and inflammatory diseases has not been treated before in the systematic way that it is here.

We therefore combined our expertise and planned this multidisciplinary book by involving clinicians (infective disease specialists, endocrinologists, orthopedists and others), radiologists and nuclear medicine physicians. After initial enthusiasm we faced the difficulty of finding a common language among the contributors. Indeed, the way in which clinicians, radiologists and nuclear medicine physicians face and describe the same topic is very different, not only from a linguistic or medical point of view but, most importantly, in the way a patient is approached and images interpreted.

Clinicians tend to interpret images as "signs" and combine these with symptoms and other tests to reach the final diagnosis. Therefore, when describing images, they do it in the context of other tests, signs and symptoms, giving much less emphasis to the raw content of the image and all the possible functional–anatomical information that can be gained from images.

Radiologists usually prioritize a detailed anatomical description, some of which detail is irrelevant to the clinician, and aim to determine the diagnosis from identifying a multitude of anatomical features. When analyzing images, they carefully describe what they see and generally, will make a diagnosis only if anatomical abnormalities are found. But an anatomical abnormality is not always synonymous with disease and vice versa.

By contrast, in nuclear medicine, functional aspects and tissue characterization are more relevant, thus providing different information from radiology, often complementary. Nuclear medicine examinations are closer to physiology and histopathology, while radiological examinations are closer to anatomy. Again, in nuclear medicine a physiological/histopathological abnormality is not always associated with a disease state. It is therefore important to define the threshold of normality for most examinations and the qualitative and quantitative analysis of images is not always helpful in this.

As a consequence, clinicians, radiologists and nuclear medicine physicians have different ways of describing diseases and different ways of writing medical textbooks.

It was important for us to attempt to give uniformity to the way in which the clinical problems are described in the different chapters. All chapters have the same structure and authors were "forced" to adhere to a common way of approaching the disease. This was not just an editorial exercise. In our view, it reflects the merging of the different disciplines in clinical practice and emphasizes the collaboration within multidisciplinary teams to reach the correct diagnosis for fast and efficient cure of the disease.

In the past 10 years in particular, nuclear medicine and radiology have merged considerably with the introduction of hybrid imaging (SPECT/CT, PET/CT and, more recently, PET/MRI). Therefore, for most patients the diagnostic imaging work-up is completed by the fusion of the two specialties and physicians are becoming more and more used to interpreting images using a common language. Therefore, this textbook is also a milestone in the formulation of common diagnostic flow charts for the diagnosis of infections and inflammatory diseases. It is addressed to medical students as well as specialists in nuclear medicine and radiology, and also to all clinicians involved in infectious/inflammatory diseases who require an up-to-date view of integrated diagnostic imaging in this field.

At the end of each chapter, we asked the authors to include three to five clinical cases to better describe the diagnostic work-up of patients and to conclude these with the important teaching points that summarize the role of a particular imaging technique in a particular disease.

It has taken more than a year to thoroughly correct and edit, where necessary, all chapters in order to make the textbook the result of a team effort rather than a multiauthor collection; a concept that makes this book unique and undoubtedly useful.

Alberto Signore
Ana María Quintero

PART I

Infections and Host Response

CHAPTER 1

Epidemiology of Infections in the New Century

Nicola Petrosillo

National Institute for Infectious Diseases, "L. Spallanzani", IRCCS, Rome, Italy

Introduction

Over the past few decades, an alarming increase in infections caused by antibiotic-resistant pathogens, including methicillin-resistant *Staphylococcus aureus* (MRSA), vancomycin-resistant *Enterococcus* spp. (VRE), carbapenem-resistant *Pseudomonas aeruginosa*, extended-spectrum β-lactamase (ESBL)-producing *Escherichia coli* and *Klebsiella* spp., carbapenemase-producing Enterobacteriaceae and multidrug-resistant (MDR) *Acinetobacter* spp., has been observed in the hospital setting and healthcare-associated facilities [1–4].

The main mechanisms of antimicrobial resistance result from convergence of multiple and different factors, depending on the pathogen: expression of low-affinity penicillin-binding proteins; the alternative pathway for peptidoglycan synthesis; low outer membrane permeability; and presence of genes encoding extended-spectrum, OXA-type (oxacillin-hydrolyzing) or metallo-β-lactamases, carbapenemases, intrinsic or acquired efflux pumps, and aminoglycoside and fluoroquinolone modifying enzymes.

These resistance determinants, depending on their origin, can be chromosomally encoded or acquired from mobile genetic elements, and easily transferred among microbial strains, thus conferring extended drug resistance upon them [5–7].

Numerous factors are associated with high rates of antimicrobial resistance in the healthcare setting, including pressure on antibiotic use, severity of illness, numerosity of invasive devices, length of hospital stay, immunosuppression, malnutrition and ease of cross-transmission of antimicrobial-resistant pathogens [8,9].

Staphylococcal infections: healthcare-acquired MRSA and beyond

In 2003, 59.5% of *S. aureus* isolates in the US National Nosocomial Infection Surveillance (NNIS) intensive care units (ICUs) were MRSA [10]. Similarly, in some European countries, according to European Antimicrobial Resistance Surveillance System (EARSS) data, greater than 60% of isolates in 2007, mostly in critical care areas, were MRSA [11]. However, during recent years, although MRSA rates in most European countries are high, a significant downward trend has been reported in many ICUs [12–14].

MRSA is one of the main pathogens in hospital settings, including surgery and intensive care, and is becoming an alarming problem also in nursing home and other healthcare facilities. Patients colonized with MRSA can easily develop an infection when they undergo invasive procedures. Indeed, the role of *S. aureus* nasopharyngeal carriage as a

Diagnostic Imaging of Infections and Inflammatory Diseases: A Multidisciplinary Approach, First Edition. Edited by Alberto Signore and Ana María Quintero.
© 2014 John Wiley & Sons, Inc. Published 2014 by John Wiley & Sons, Inc.

risk factor for infection in the hospital setting has been widely documented [15]. Approximately 30% of colonized patients may develop an MRSA infection [16] and in nearly 20%, this is a bacteremia. In recent reports, carbapenem use has been related to MRSA colonization, with eight new cases of MRSA colonization per 1000 days of carbapenem therapy [17].

Despite the worldwide use of vancomycin, *S. aureus* resistance to this glycopeptide remains rare. Only nine cases of vancomycin-resistant *S. aureus* [VRSA; defined by a vancomycin minimum inhibitory concentration (MIC) of ≥1.6 mg/dL] have been identified to date and, as of 2007, approximately 100 vancomycin-intermediate *S. aureus* (VISA) isolates (defined by a vancomycin MIC of 0.4–0.8 mg/dL) have been reported worldwide [18].

Currently, the main concern is the shift in susceptibility to vancomycin, the so-called MIC "creep". This phenomenon is represented by small incremental increases in vancomycin MIC within the susceptibility range. One of the most controversial issues in the treatment of MRSA is the evidence for reduced vancomycin treatment efficacy in the management of bacteremia and pneumonia by MICs at the upper limit of susceptibility (i.e. MICs of 0.2 mg/dL compared with ≤0.1 mg/dL, which are still considered to be susceptible) [19–25]. The increase in treatment failure might be the result of higher frequencies of hetero-resistance to vancomycin among isolates with vancomycin MICs of 0.2 mg/dL [26]. Indeed, VISA isolates are those with a MIC between 0.4 and 0.8 mg/dL, whereas heterogeneous VISA (hVISA) strains appear to be sensitive to vancomycin with a susceptibility range of 0.1–0.2 mg/dL, even though they contain a subpopulation of vancomycin-intermediate daughter cells (MIC ≥0.4 mg/dL) [27].

Finally, although MRSA infections were traditionally limited to hospitals, reports of community-associated cases of MRSA (CA-MRSA) infections began to emerge in the late 1990s in the USA [28]. CA-MRSA are genetically and phenotypically distinct from the typical multidrug-resistant healthcare-associated MRSA. These strains are resistant to β-lactam antibiotics and typically susceptible to other antistaphylococcal agents; they often encode for Panton–Valentine leukocidin (PVL) and other exotoxins and virulence factors [29].

The vast majority of CA-MRSA carry one of two smaller SCC*mec* types, IV and V, without the additional resistance genes. In general, they are more susceptible to non-β-lactam antibiotics and appear to be associated with increased transmission and hospitalization, skin and soft tissue infection and, rarely, severe diseases including necrotizing pneumonia [30].

CA-MRSA strains have rapidly emerged worldwide and are now endemic in the USA where they are amongst the most commonly isolated pathogens in emergency departments. Furthermore, nosocomial transmission of CA-MRSA and hospital outbreaks have recently been observed in several countries [31].

Enterococcus spp.

Another emerging concern in surgery and intensive care areas is VRE diffusion [32]. Although the vast majority of clinical enterococcal infections are caused by *Enterococcus faecalis*, *Enterococcus faecium* has emerged in recent years as a major multiresistant nosocomial pathogen, with a great capacity for acquiring multiple antibiotic-resistance determinants, especially those encoding glycopeptide resistance (e.g. vanA- and vanB-resistance genotypes). Almost 100% of *E. faecium* isolates are now resistant to ampicillin, but high-level aminoglycoside resistance is also a major problem, as it is common in both *E. faecalis* and *E. faecium*, ranging from 25% to 50% in European countries.

Various risk factors for acquisition of VRE have been proposed, including environmental risk factors (extensive use of broad-spectrum antimicrobial agents; patient overcrowding in facilities; admission to an ICU, transplant ward or unit with high colonization pressure; contaminated surfaces and fomites where enterococci can survive for a long period even in dry conditions); patient risk factors (severity of illness; prolonged hospitalization; presence of indwelling catheters or invasive devices; prolonged mechanical ventilation; age; non-ambulatory status; immunosuppression as post-transplantation status; diarrhea; renal failure/chronic hemodialysis; and proximity to patients who are colonized by VRE); clinical risk factors (poor adherence to infection-control practices; unrecognized antimicrobial resistance in the facility; inappropriate treatment; and use of contaminated equipment) [33].

Multidrug-resistant Enterobacteriaceae: are we facing a new era?

Among Gram-negative agents, ESBL-producing Enterobacteriaceae are a great concern. The epidemiology of ESBLs has changed dramatically: until recently, most infections caused by ESBL-producing bacteria were described as being acquired nosocomially, often appearing in specialized units, but are now increasingly found in non-hospitalized patients, and the mode of transmission or source of this pathogen is still unknown [34,35].

More recently, the worldwide epidemic of Enterobacteriaceae resistant to carbapenems is also a major concern. Carbapenems have been widely used as the treatment of choice for serious infections caused by ESBL producers, exerting selection pressure for carbapenem resistance. *Klebsiella pneumoniae* carbapenemases (KPC)-type enzymes are emerging resistance determinants, especially for *K. pneumoniae* [36–38]. During the last decade, a rapidly evolving spread of KPC and β-lactamases has been documented worldwide, creating an endemic situation in many countries. KPC-associated infections are predominantly nosocomial and systemic infections, affecting patients with multiple risk factors [38,39]. Therapeutic failures and adverse impact on patient outcome, with high mortality rates ranging from 22% to 57%, have been reported [36].

Non-fermentative Gram-negative infections: a threat for critical patients

Multidrug-resistant non-fermentative organisms are a major concern in healthcare facilities worldwide. In more than 300 US hospitals surveyed by the Centers for Disease Control (CDC), rates of carbapenem resistance in *Actinobacter baumannii* isolates increased from 9% in 1995 to 40% in 2004 [40]. *A. baumannii* infections, mainly ventilator-associated pneumonia (VAP) and bloodstream infections, frequently affect critically ill patients in ICUs with major risk factors, including older age, presence of severe underlying diseases, immunosuppression, major trauma or burn injuries, a scheduled invasive procedure, as well as the presence of indwelling catheters, invasive mechanical ventilation, extended hospital stay and previous administration of antibiotics [41,42].

Carbapenem resistance to *P. aeruginosa* ranges between 10% and 48% in ICUs worldwide [43] and currently represents a major concern due to the lack of new drugs effective against these strains.

Prosthetic joint infections

The numbers of primary total hip and total knee arthroplasties has dramatically increased worldwide over the past decade. In 2006, about 800 000 hip and knee arthroplasties were performed in the USA [44] and 130 000 in England [45]. Kurtz *et al.* formulated projections for the number of primary and revision total hip and knee arthroplasties that will be performed in the USA through 2030 and estimated a 174% increase (572 000) in hip procedures per year and a 673% increase (3.48 million) in knee prosthesis per year [46]. While such procedures achieve great improvement in quality of life, the risk of infection represents a serious complication, occurring in 0.8–1.9% of knee arthroplasties and 0.3–1.7% of hip arthroplasties [47–49].

The incidence of joint prosthesis infection ranges between 1.5% and 2.5% for primary interventions and up to 20% for revision procedures; mortality ranges between 1% and nearly 3% [50]. The economic cost of this complication is up to $50 000 per patient and $250 000 million per year [51,52]. The increases in life expectancy and predicted number of joint replacement procedures are likely to register a significant increment in the number of prosthetic joint infections with a strong impact on countries' health economic balance in the next few years [53].

From an epidemiological point of view, joint prosthesis infections are classified in relation to the time of onset after surgery as "early" (first 3 months after surgery), "delayed" (between 3 months and 2 years after surgery) or "late" (>2 years after surgery). Table 1.1 shows the main risk factors for infection.

Microorganisms may reach the prosthesis at the time of implantation or later by hematogenous spread. The development of a biofilm has a strategic role in the pathogenesis of prosthetic joint infections. Foreign bodies remain devoid of a microcirculation that is crucial for host defense and the delivery of antibiotics. The biofilm represents a basic survival mechanism by which microbes resist external and internal environmental factors, such as antimicrobial agents and the host immune system [54].

Table 1.1 Risk factors for prosthetic joint infections

Patient-related risk factors
- Previous revision arthroplasty
- Previous infection associated with a prosthetic joint at the same site
- Tobacco abuse
- Obesity
- Rheumatoid arthritis
- Diabetes mellitus
- Neoplasm
- Immunosuppression

Surgical risk factors
- Simultaneous bilateral arthroplasty
- Long operative time (>2.5 hours)
- Allogeneic blood transfusion

Postoperative risk factors
- Wound healing complications
- Atrial fibrillation
- Myocardial infarction
- Urinary tract infection
- Prolonged hospital stay
- *S. aureus* bacteremia

Modified from Cataldo *et al.* [53] and Del Pozo and Patel [54].

Table 1.2 Rate of infection for prosthetic cardiovascular devices

Type	% Infection	
	First implant	*Revision*
Prosthetic heart valve	1–6	15
Pacemaker	1–2	3–30
Defibrillator	4	
Left ventricular assist device	50	
Vascular graft prosthesis	1–6	22
Hemodialysis tunneled catheter	12	
Hemodialysis arteriovenous graft	1–6	

Modified from Sampedro and Patel [64].

The most frequent etiological agents are staphylococci, accounting for more than 50% of prosthetic joint infections. *S. aureus* is usually isolated in early infections, whereas coagulase-negative staphylococci are isolated in late infections, as well as streptococci (9–10%), enterococci (3–7%) and anaerobes (2–4%) [55,56].

Gram-negative bacteria, mostly *P. aeruginosa*, *Enterobacter* spp., *Proteus* spp. and other relatively uncommon agents have an important clinical impact because they are difficult to treat [57,58]. Overall, about 20% of prosthetic joint infections are polymicrobial and 7–11% are culture negative [59,60]. Unusual pathogens, such as *Candida* spp., *Brucella* spp. and mycobacteria have also been reported [61].

In the last decade there has been an increase in reports of infections due to antibiotic-resistant bacteria; in a large surveillance study on surgical site infection after orthopedic interventions, 59% of the *S. aureus* isolates were methicillin resistant, with a higher risk of treatment failure than for infections caused by methicillin-susceptible *S. aureus* [62].

In conclusion, prosthetic joint infection represents a challenge for orthopedic surgeons, infectious diseases specialists, clinical microbiologists and all the other professionals involved in the care of patients receiving prosthetic joints. It is expected that the incidence of prosthetic joint infections will further increase due to better detection methods for microbial biofilms involved in prosthetic joint infections, the growing number of implanted prostheses in the aging population and the increasing residency time of prostheses, which are at continuous risk for infection during their implanted lifetime [63,64].

Prosthetic vascular infections

The medical device market in developed countries is exponentially growing [65] and represents a great health benefit and progress. However, infection is a challenging and growing problem associated with medical devices. In the USA, approximately 1 million nosocomial infections per year are related to indwelling medical devices [66]. In spite of the progress made in the prevention and treatment of device-associated infection, an increase in the number of patients with device-associated infections can be predicted from the increasing numbers of devices and the lifelong risk for bacterial seeding of devices (Table 1.2).

Prosthetic cardiovascular devices include heart valves, pacemakers, defibrillators, coronary artery stents, artificial arteries, aortic stents, central venous catheters and arterial catheters. The frequency of long-term prosthetic device infection varies with the type of implant and rates of infection are greater after revision, likely due to several factors, including longer operation times of surgery and poor circulation as a result of scars around the previous implant. Rates of infection in first implants and in revision surgery, respectively, are 1–6% and 15% for mechanical and prosthetic heart valves [67,68]; 1–2% and 3–10% for pacemakers [69]; and 1–6% and 22% for vascular graft prostheses [70,71]. Additionally, rates of infection for defibrillators [72], left ventricular assist devices [73], hemodialysis tunneled catheters [74] and hemodialysis arteriovenous grafts [75] are 4%, 50%, 12% and 1–6%, respectively. Along with the increasing number of implanted devices, the number of cardiac device-related infections has increased 124% between 1990 and 1999, and the rate of prosthetic valve infection has increased 50% over the same period (from 0.26 to 0.38 cases per 1000 Medicare beneficiaries) [76,77].

The microbiology of these infections is related to the ability of organisms to constitute the extracellular matrix of the biofilm. In the biofilm state, microorganisms are relatively immune to antibodies and phagocytes [78] and are also more resistant than free-living organisms to conventional antimicrobial agents [79].

Staphylococcus spp. are the most common microorganisms associated with device-related infections. Adherence of *S. aureus* to devices is dependent on the presence of microbial surface components recognizing adhesive matrix molecules [80]. However, biofilm formation is not limited to staphylococci; other Gram-positive organisms, including streptococci, *Enterococcus* spp., *Propionibacterium acnes*, *Corynebacterium* spp. Gram-negative organisms, including *P. aeruginosa* and Enterobacteriaceae; and fungi can produce biofilm.

In the pathogenesis of prosthetic vascular infections the host also plays an important role: the inflammatory response secondary to surgery and subsequent platelet aggregation and release of adhesins gives potential for microbial colonization [81].

All types of prosthetic vascular grafts are susceptible to infection via direct contamination during implantation or bacteremia after operation. Despite the use of perioperative systemic antibiotic prophylaxis, vascular graft infections still occur. To address this problem, antibiotic- and antimicrobial-impregnated grafts have been developed and their effectiveness assessed in experimental and clinical studies [82,83].

The gold standard for treatment of an infected prosthetic graft/device remains explantation and, for vascular grafts, subsequent reperfusion by placing a new graft, most commonly via an extra-anatomic uninfected route and less commonly via *in-situ* grafting using an autogenous (vein) conduit. Antimicrobial therapy is a vital adjunct to surgical management; in some cases it may be the only option if the patient is not fit for further operative intervention.

As the number of prosthetic vascular device increases, the development of new solutions for prevention and management of infections represents the challenge for the next decades.

Skin and soft tissue infections

Skin and soft tissue infections (SSTIs) reflect inflammatory microbial invasion of the epidermis, dermis and subcutaneous tissues, and can be considered to be the commonest infection in humans. SSTIs can be classified according to anatomical site, microbiological etiology, or severity. In 2003, an expert panel classified SSTIs according to the severity of local and systemic signs, thereby developing a system that guides the clinical management and treatment decisions for patients with SSTIs [84]. In 2005, the practice guidelines of the Infectious Diseases Society of America (IDSA) for the diagnosis and management of skin and soft tissue infections classified SSTIs into five categories: superficial, uncomplicated infection (includes impetigo, erysipelas and cellulitis); necrotizing infection; infections associated with bites and animal contact; surgical site infections; and infections in the immunocompromised host [85]. The Surgical Infection Society (SIS) has recently published new guidelines for the treatment of complicated SSTIs [86]. The guidelines deal exclusively with complicated SSTIs, including those that are deep or necrotizing, usually requiring surgical intervention (infected ulcers, infected burns and major abscesses) and occurring in patients with specific major co-morbidities that necessitate hospitalization.

The epidemiology of complicated SSTIs has changed somewhat in the last decade. The frequency of SSTIs has increased significantly since the late 1990s, predominately because of an increase in infections caused by CA-MRSA [87].

What has changed in *S. aureus* infections? Since its first appearance in 1961, in the past two decades the prevalence of MRSA has become widespread in hospitals, particularly in ICUs, representing a substantial burden in terms of morbidity, mortality and cost. It was estimated that deaths in patients with MRSA in the USA in 2005 surpassed those caused by human immunodeficiency virus (HIV) in the same year [88,89]. The increase in MRSA infections most likely reflects the growing impact of medical interventions, devices, older age and co-morbidities of patients. All of these represent risk factors for healthcare-associated (HA) MRSA infection, along with antibiotic use and overuse [90]. While the frequency of MRSA infections continues to grow in hospital settings [91], of rising concern is the emergence of MRSA in patients without apparent risk factors presenting from the community. Since 1998, several outbreaks of community-associated (CA)-MRSA in children, athletes, prisoners, military personnel, men who have sex with men, HIV-infected people, native Americans and aboriginal populations have been reported [89]. The prevalence of CA-MRSA infections varies widely according to region, reaching 20–50% of SSTIs in US cities [92]. Although initially thought to have spread from hospitals to the community, several studies have revealed a number of genetic and epidemiological differences between HA-MRSA and CA-MRSA [92]. CA-MRSA genetic features include the staphylococcal cassette chromosome *mec* (SCC*mec*) IV and V elements as the mechanism of methicillin resistance, and the gene encoding for the Panton–Valentine leukocidin (PVL) toxin.

Regarding the main pathogens isolated from SSTIs, data from the SENTRY Program, which includes 5800 consecutive patients admitted to hospitals in Canada and 32 states in the USA, show that *S. aureus* remains the most common pathogen isolated from complicated SSTIs, accounting for greater than 40% of all isolates, with *P. aeruginosa* being the second most common isolate (11%). Between 1998 and 2004, the number of SSTI pathogens resistant to at least one antibiotic increased for *S. aureus*, *Enterococcus* spp., *P. aeruginosa*, *E. coli*

and *Klebsiella* spp., with nearly 50% of the *S. aureus* isolates being resistant to methicillin [93]. Regarding surgical site infections (SSIs), which occur in more than 5% of patients undergoing surgery [94], the epidemiology is slightly different, with an even greater shift toward Gram-positive pathogens (*S. aureus*, coagulase-negative staphylococci and *Enterococcus* spp. in >50% of isolates) [95].

Management of complicated SSTIs is particularly challenging, because prompt recognition, timely surgical debridement or drainage, resuscitation if required and appropriate antibiotic therapy represent the cornerstones of clinical success. The mainstays of antimicrobial treatment are the penicillins, cephalosporins, clindamycin and co-trimoxazole. β-Lactam/β-lactamase inhibitor combinations are indicated for polymicrobial infection. A range of new agents for the treatment of MRSA infections has been compared with the glycopeptides; some of them, including daptomycin, linezolid and tygecicline, have distinct pharmacokinetic advantages.

Tuberculosis and human immunodeficiency virus in the new century

An ancient pathogen, *Mycobacterium tuberculosis*, and a new one, HIV, met about 30 years ago; their interaction resulted in an escalation of the burden of both diseases and also of their morbidity and mortality. This was more evident in those countries where HIV and tuberculosis (TB) were highly prevalent, and health and social conditions the poorest.

The history of dual TB/HIV infection has faced increasing challenges in the last decades, beginning with an exponential rise in TB case notifications in sub-Saharan Africa, a high case fatality rate [96], high rates of TB recurrence [97] and increased transmission in settings where people congregate. In industrialized countries, outbreaks of multidrug-resistant (MDR) TB have occurred since the 1990s in HIV-infected patients in healthcare facilities [98]. In 2005–2006 there was the dramatic outbreak of extensively drug-resistant (XDR) TB in HIV-infected individuals in a rural area in South Africa [99].

In the pre-HIV era, there was a marked improvement in TB management thanks to the expansion of directly observed therapy, short-course (DOTS) programs. When cases of HIV-associated TB dramatically rose, there was the clear demonstration that DOTS alone could not contain the epidemic [100]. Immediately in many African countries TB became the leading cause of death in adults with HIV infection [101] and TB was recognized worldwide as one of the commonest causes of morbidity in the course of HIV infection.

HIV is the strongest risk factor for developing TB disease in those with existing or newly acquired *M. tuberculosis* infection. The risk of developing TB is between 20 and 37 times greater in people living with HIV than amongst those who do not have HIV infection. In 2009, of an estimated 14 million TB cases globally, 1.6 million were HIV positive [102]. TB is responsible for more than a quarter of deaths in people living with HIV. In 2007, 456 000 deaths occurred in HIV-infected people with TB, representing 23% of the estimated 2 million deaths from HIV infection for that year [103]. These estimated numbers of HIV-related TB cases and deaths were nearly double those reported in previous years, although this is indicative of improved data collection rather than a real change in epidemiology.

The resistance of *M. tuberculosis* to specific drugs represents another challenge. MDR-TB emerged as a clinical entity in the early 1990s after a couple of decades of widespread use of rifampin. TB rates increased five-fold in sub-Saharan Africa during the 1990s because of HIV infection, and the lack of careful systems of treatment and prophylaxis led to the emergence of MDR-TB, the rate of which aggressively and exponentially increased in the Russian Federation and, later, in areas of sub-Saharan Africa with the highest burden of HIV infection [104,105]. The World Health Organization (WHO) detected an increase in the global caseload of MDR-TB from about 274 000 cases in 2000 to about 500 000 cases in 2007 (5% of the global case burden of TB) [102,106,107]. Most funding and resources for TB control are diverted to MDR-TB, since MDR-TB outcome is poorer than that of drug-sensitive TB [108].

Moreover, another threat has recently appeared with the emergence of XDR-TB, i.e. TB with resistance, at least, to rifampin and isoniazid, plus any fluoroquinolone and any of the injectable agents (amikacin, kanamycin or capreomycin). XDR-TB is more expensive to treat than MDR-TB and outcomes are poorer, particularly in patients who are HIV positive [109].

The dual HIV/TB epidemic represents a challenge for industrialized and developing countries and is a major problem for people living with HIV in resource-constrained settings. Therefore, the WHO has recommended 12 collaborative TB/HIV activities as part of core HIV and TB prevention, care and treatment services. They include interventions that reduce the morbidity and mortality from TB in people living with HIV, such as the provision of antiretroviral therapy and the "Three Is" for HIV/TB: intensified case finding of TB, isoniazid preventive therapy and infection control for TB [103, 110, 111] (Table 1.3).

Finally, providing good HIV care for HIV-infected people who develop TB represents a fundamental element in the management of TB/HIV patients. Provider-initiated HIV testing and counseling, co-trimoxazole preventive therapy and antiretrovirals should be regarded as the basic standard of care and yet gaps in implementation remain large. About 40% of all patients with TB are not tested for HIV and a large proportion with HIV infection and TB lack access to co-trimoxazole preventive therapy and antiretroviral therapy [102,112,113].

Table 1.3 WHO recommended collaborative activities against the dual epidemic of TB/HIV

1. Establish the mechanisms for collaboration:
   - Set up a coordinating body for TB/HIV activities that is effective at all levels of the health system
   - Conduct surveillance of HIV prevalence among TB patients
   - Carry out joint TB/HIV planning for resources, capacity building, communication, community participation and operational research
   - Conduct monitoring and evaluation
2. Decrease the burden of tuberculosis in people living with HIV/AIDS
   - Establish intensified tuberculosis case finding
   - Introduce isoniazid preventive therapy
   - Ensure TB infection control in the healthcare setting and in congregation settings
3. Decrease the burden of HIV in patients with TB
   - Provide HIV testing and counseling
   - Introduce methods to prevent HIV
   - Introduce co-trimoxazole prophylaxis
   - Ensure HIV/AIDS care and support
   - Introduce and provide antiretroviral treatment for HIV/TB individuals

Modified from Harries *et al.* [103] and WHO [111].

As the HIV-associated TB epidemic is continuing, bold but responsible action is needed in terms of better service provision, infection control and sound initiatives to minimize the impact of this dual infection in the new century.

References

1. Klevens RM, Edwards JR, Tenover FC, McDonald LC, Horan T, Gaynes R; National Nosocomial Infections Surveillance System. Changes in the epidemiology of methicillin-resistant *Staphylococcus aureus* in intensive care units in US hospitals, 1992–2003. *Clin Infect Dis* 2006;42:389–391.

2. Gaynes R, Edwards JR; National Nosocomial Infections Surveillance System. Overview of nosocomial infections caused by Gram-negative bacilli. *Clin Infect Dis* 2005;41:848–854.

3. Lockhart SR, Abramson MA, Beekmann SE *et al.* Antimicrobial resistance among Gram-negative bacilli causing infections in intensive care unit patients in the United States between 1993 and 2004. *J Clin Microbiol* 2007;45:3352–3359.

4. Cantón R, Novais A, Valverde A,*et al.* Prevalence and spread of extended-spectrum β-lactamase-producing Enterobacteriaceae in Europe. *Clin Microbiol Infect* 2008;14 (Suppl. 1):S144–S153.

5. Rice LB. The clinical consequences of antimicrobial resistance. *Curr Opin Microbiol* 2009;12:476–481.

6. Souli M, Galani I, Giamarellou H. Emergence of extensively drug-resistant and pandrug-resistant Gram-negative bacilli in Europe. *Euro Surveill* 2008; 13:ii, 19045.

7. Gholizadeh Y, Courvalin P. Acquired and intrinsic glycopeptide resistance in enterococci. *Int J Antimicrob Agents* 2000;16 (Suppl. 1):S11–S17.

8. Fish DN, Ohlinger MJ. Antimicrobial resistance: factors and outcomes. *Crit Care Clin* 2006;22: 291–311.

9. Barsanti MC, Woeltje KF. Infection prevention in the intensive care unit. *Infect Dis Clin North Am* 2009; 23:703–725.

10. NNIS System. National Nosocomial Infections Surveillance (NNIS) System Report, data summary from January 1992 through June 2003, issued August 2003. *Am J Infect Control* 2003;31:481–498.

11. EARSS Annual Report 2007. Available at: http://www.rivm.nl/earss/result/Monitoring_reports/Annual_reports.jsp/ (accessed August 22, 2011).

12. Thompson DS, Workman R, Strutt M. Decline in the rates of methicillin-resistant *Staphylococcus aureus* acquisition and bacteraemia in a general intensive care unit between 1996 and 2008. *J Hosp Infect* 2009;71:314–319.

13. Burton DC, Edwards JR, Horan TC, Jernigan JA, Fridkin SK. Methicillin-resistant *Staphylococcus aureus* central line-associated bloodstream infections in US intensive care units, 1997–2007. *JAMA* 2009;301:727–736.

14. Pagani L, Falciani M, Aschbacher R. Use of microbiologic findings to manage antimicrobials in the intensive care unit. *Infect Control Hosp Epidemiol* 2009;30:309–311.

15. Von Eiff C, Becker K, Machka K, Stammer H, Peters G. Nasal carriage as a source of *Staphylococcus aureus* bacteremia. Study group. *N Engl J Med* 2001; 344:11–16.

16. Mayhall CG. Methicillin-resistant *Staphylococcus aureus*/vancomycin-resistant Enterococci colonization and infection in the critical care unit. In: Cunha BA (ed). *Infectious Diseases in Critical Care Medicine*, 2nd edn. New York: Informa Healthcare, 2007.

17. Tacconelli E, De Angelis G, Cataldo MA *et al.* Antibiotic usage and risk of colonization and infection with antibiotic-resistant bacteria: a hospital population-based study. *Antimicrob Agents Chemother* 2009;53:4264–4269.

18. Morse PA, North N, Steenbergen JN, Sakoulas G. Susceptibility relationship between vancomycin and daptomycin in *Staphylococcus aureus*: facts and assumption. *Lancet Infect Dis* 2009;9:617–624.

19. Moise PA, Sakoulas G, Forrest A, Schentag JJ. Vancomycin *in vitro* bactericidal activity and its relationship to efficacy in clearance of methicillin-resistant *Staphylococcus aureus* bacteremia. *Antimicrob Agents Chemother* 2007;51:2582–2586.

20. Sakoulas G, Moise-Broder PA, Schentag J, Forrest A, Moellering RC Jr, Eliopoulos GM. Relationship of MIC and bactericidal activity to efficacy of vancomycin for treatment of methicillin-resistant *Staphylococcus aureus* bacteremia. *J Clin Microbiol* 2004,42: 2398–2402.

21. Moise-Broder PA, Sakoulas G, Eliopoulos GM, Schentag JJ, Forrest A, Moellering RC Jr. Accessory gene regulator group II polymorphism in methicillin-resistant *Staphylococcus aureus* is predictive of failure of vancomycin therapy. *Clin Infect Dis* 2004;38: 1700–1705.

22. Hidayat LK, Hsu DI, Quist R, Shriner KA, Wong-Beringer A. High-dose vancomycin therapy for methicillin-resistant *Staphylococcus aureus* infections: efficacy and toxicity. *Arch Intern Med* 2006; 166:2138–2144.

23. Maclayton DO, Suda KJ, Coval KA, York CB, Garey KW. Case–control study of the relationship between MRSA bacteremia with a vancomycin MIC of 2 μg/ml and risk factors, costs, and outcomes in inpatients undergoing hemodialysis. *Clin Ther* 2006;28: 1208–1216.

24. Soriano A, Marco F, Martínez JA et al. Influence of vancomycin minimum inhibitory concentration on the treatment of methicillin resistant *Staphylococcus aureus* bacteremia. *Clin Infect Dis* 2008;46: 193–200.

25. Lodise TP, Graves J, Evans A et al. Relationship between vancomycin MIC and failure among patients with methicillin resistant *Staphylococcus aureus* bacteremia treated with vancomycin. *Antimicrob Agents Chemother* 2008;52:3315–3320.

26. Howden BP, Ward PB, Charles PG et al. Treatment outcomes for serious infections caused by methicillin-resistant *Staphylococcus aureus* with reduced vancomycin susceptibility. *Clin Infect Dis* 2004;38:521–528.

27. Szabó J. hVISA/VISA: diagnostic and therapeutic problems. *Expert Rev Anti Infect Ther* 2009;7:1–3.

28. Moran GJ, Krishnadasan A, Gorwitz RJ et al.; EMERGEncy ID Net Study Group. Methicillin resistant *Staphylococcus aureus* infections among patients in the emergency department. *N Engl J Med* 2006;355: 666–674.

29. Yeung M, Balma-Mena A, Shear N et al. Identification of major clonal complexes and toxin producing strains among *Staphylococcus aureus* associated with atopic dermatitis. *Microbes Infect* 2011;13: 189–197.

30. Francis JS, Doherty MC, Lopatin U et al. Severe community-onset pneumonia in healthy adults caused by methicillin-resistant *Staphylococcus aureus* carrying the Panton-Valentine leukocidin genes. *Clin Infect Dis* 2005;40:100–107.

31. Otter JA, French GL. Nosocomial transmission of community-associated methicillin resistant *Staphylococcus aureus*: an emerging threat. *Lancet Infect Dis* 2006;6:753–755.

32. Fridkin SK, Edwards JR, Courval JM et al.; Intensive Care Antimicrobial Resistance Epidemiology (ICARE) Project and the National Nosocomial Infections Surveillance (NNIS) System Hospitals. The effect of vancomycin and third-generation cephalosporins on prevalence of vancomycin-resistant enterococci in 126 U.S. adult intensive care units. *Ann Intern Med* 2001;135:175–183.

33. Bryant S, Wilbeck J. Vancomycin-resistant enterococcus in critical care areas. *Crit Care Nurs Clin North Am* 2007;19:69–75.

34. Livermore DM, Canton R, Gniadkowski M et al. CTX-M: changing the face of ESBLs in Europe. *J Antimicrob Chemother* 2007;59:165–174.

35. Rodríguez-Baño J, Navarro MD, Romero L et al. Epidemiology and clinical features of infections caused by extended-spectrum β-lactamase-producing *Escherichia coli* in nonhospitalized patients. *J Clin Microbiol* 2004;42:1089–1094.

36. Carmeli Y, Akova M, Cornaglia G et al. Controlling the spread of carbapenemase-producing Gram-negatives: therapeutic approach and infection control. *Clin Microbiol Infect* 2010;16:102–111.

37. Cornaglia G, Rossolini GM. The emerging threat of acquired carbapenemases in Gram-negative bacteria. *Clin Microbiol Infect* 2010;16:99–101.

38. Nordmann P, Cuzon G, Naas T. The real threat of *Klebsiella pneumoniae* carbapenemase-producing bacteria. *Lancet Infect Dis* 2009;9:228–236.

39. Gasink LB, Edelstein PH, Lautenbach E, Synnestvedt M, Fishman NO. Risk factors and clinical impact of *Klebsiella pneumoniae* carbapenemase-producing *K. pneumoniae*. *Infect Control Hosp Epidemiol* 2009; 30:1180–1185.

40. Munoz-Price LS, Weinstein RA. Acinetobacter infection. *N Engl J Med* 2008;358:1271–1281.

41. Perez F, Hujer AM, Hujer KM, Decker BK, Rather PN, Bonomo RA. Global challenge of multidrug-resistant *Acinetobacter baumannii*. *Antimicrob Agents Chemother* 2007;51:3471–3484.

42. Maragakis LL, Perl TM. *Acinetobacter baumannii*: epidemiology, antimicrobial resistance, and treatment options. *Clin Infect Dis* 2008;46:1254–1263.

43. Petrosillo N, Capone A, Di Bella S, Taglietti F. Management of antibiotic resistance in the intensive care unit setting. *Expert Rev Anti Infect Ther* 2010;8:289–302.

44. National Hospital Discharge Survey. Survey results and products. Available at: Center for Disease Control and Prevention, http://www.cdc.gov/nchs/nhds_products.html (accessed September 14, 2010).

45. UK National Joint Registry. Available at: http://www.njrcentre.org.uk (accessed September 14, 2010).

46. Kurtz S, Ong K, Lau E, Mowat F, Halpern M. Projections of primary and revision hip and knee arthroplasty in the United States from 2005 to 2030. *J Bone Joint Surg Am* 2007;89:780–785.

47. Pulido L, Ghanem E, Joshi A, Purtill JJ, Parvizi J. Periprosthetic joint infection: the incidence, timing, and predisposing factors. *Clin Orthop Relat Res* 2008;466:1710–1715.

48. Choong PF, Dowsey MM, Carr D, Daffy J, Stanley P. Risk factors associated with acute hip prosthetic joint infections and outcome of treatment with a rifampin-based regimen. *Acta Orthop* 2007;78: 755–765.

49. Phillips JE, Crane TP, Noy M, Elliott TS, Grimer RJ. The incidence of deep prosthetic infections in a specialist orthopaedic hospital: a 15-year prospective survey. *J Bone Joint Surg Br* 2006;88:943–948.

50. Lentino JR. Prosthetic joint infections: bane of orthopedists, challenge for infectious disease specialists. *Clin Infect Dis* 2003;36:1157–1161.

51. Zimmerli W. Infection and musculoskeletal conditions: prosthetic-joint-associated infections. *Best Pract Res Clin Rheumatol* 2006;20:1045–1063.

52. Sculco TP. The economic impact of infected joint arthroplasty. *Orthopedics* 1995;18:871–873.

53. Cataldo MA, Petrosillo N, Cipriani M, Cauda R, Tacconelli E. Prosthetic joint infection: Recent developments in diagnosis and management. *J Infect* 2010;61:443–448.

54. Del Pozo JL, Patel R. Clinical practice. Infection associated with prosthetic joints. *N Engl J Med* 2009;361:787–794.

55. Zimmerli W, Trampuz A, Ochsner PE. Prosthetic-joint infections. *N Engl J Med* 2004;351:1645–1654.

56. Moran E, Masters S, Berendt AR, McLardy-Smith P, Byren I, Atkins BL. Guiding empirical antibiotic therapy in orthopaedics: the microbiology of prosthetic joint infection managed by debridement, irrigation and prosthesis retention. *J Infect* 2007;55:1–7.

57. Hsieh PH, Lee MS, Hsu KY, Chang YH, Shih HN, Ueng SW. Gram negative prosthetic joint infections: risk factors and outcome of treatment. *Clin Infect Dis* 2009;49:1036–1043.

58. Legout L, Senneville E, Stern R *et al*. Treatment of bone and joint infections caused by gram-negative bacilli with a cefepime-fluoroquinolone combination. *Clin Microbiol Infect* 2006;12:1030–1033.

59. Sia IG, Berbari EF, Karchmer AW. Prosthetic joint infections. *Infect Dis Clin North Am* 2005;19:885–914.

60. Berbari EF, Marculescu C, Sia I *et al*. Culture-negative prosthetic joint infection. *Clin Infect Dis* 2007;45:1113–1119.

61. Marculescu CE, Berbari EF, Cockerill FR 3rd, Osmon DR. Fungi, mycobacteria, zoonotic and other organisms in prosthetic joint infection. *Clin Orthop Relat Res* 2006;451:64–72.

62. Salgado CD, Dash S, Cantey JR, Marculescu CE. Higher risk of failure of methicillin-resistant *Staphylococcus aureus* prosthetic joint infections. *Clin Orthop Relat Res* 2007;461:48–53.

63. Trampuz A, Widmer AF. Infections associated with orthopedic implants. *Curr Opin Infect Dis* 2006;19:349–356.

64. Sampedro MF, Patel R. Infections associated with long-term prosthetic devices. *Infect Dis Clin North Am* 2007;21:785–819.

65. Darouiche RO. Treatment of infections associated with surgical implants. *N Engl J Med* 2004;350:1422–1429.

66. Truninger K, Attenhofer Jost CH, Seifert B *et al*. Long term follow up of prosthetic valve endocarditis: what characteristics identify patients who were treated successfully with antibiotics alone? *Heart* 1999;82:714–720.

67. Karchmer AW, Longworth DL. Infections of intracardiac devices. *Infect Dis Clin North Am* 2002;16:477–505.

68. Gandelman G, Frishman WH, Wiese C *et al*. Intravascular device infections: epidemiology, diagnosis, and management. *Cardiol Rev* 2007;15:13–23.

69. Harcombe AA, Newell SA, Ludman PF *et al*. Late complications following permanent pacemaker implantation or elective unit replacement. *Heart* 1998;80:240–244.

70. Seeger JM. Management of patients with prosthetic vascular graft infection. *Am Surg* 2000;66:166–177.

71. Young RM, Cherry KJ Jr, Davis PM *et al*. The results of in situ prosthetic replacement for infected aortic grafts. *Am J Surg* 1999;178:136–140.

72. Trappe HJ, Pfitzner P, Klein H, Wenzlaff P. Infections after cardioverter-defibrillator implantation: observations in 335 patients over 10 years. *Br Heart J* 1995;73:20–24.

73. Simon D, Fischer S, Grossman A *et al*. Left ventricular assist device-related infection: treatment and outcome. *Clin Infect Dis* 2005;40:1108–1115.

74. Palestro CJ, Swyer AJ, Kim CK, Goldsmith SJ. Infected knee prosthesis: diagnosis with In-111 leukocyte, Tc-99m sulfur colloid, and Tc-99m MDP imaging. *Radiology* 1991;179:645–648.

75. Baddour LM, Bettmann MA, Bolger AF *et al*.; AHA. Nonvalvular cardiovascular device-related infections. *Circulation* 2003;108:2015–2031.

76. Cabell CH, Heidenreich PA, Chu VH, Moore CM, Stryjewski ME, Corey GR, Fowler VG Jr. Increasing rates of cardiac device infections among Medicare beneficiaries: 1990–1999. *Am Heart J* 2004;147:582–586.

77. Baddour LM, Wilson WR. Infections of prosthetic valves and other cardiovascular devices. In: Livingstone EC (ed). *Mandell, Douglas and Benett's Principles and Practice of Infectious Diseases*, 6th edn, vol. 1. Philadelphia: Churchill Livingstone, 2005; pp. 1022–1144.

78. Donlan RM. New approaches for the characterization of prosthetic joint biofilms. *Clin Orthop Relat Res* 2005;347:12–19.

79. Costerton JW. Biofilm theory can guide the treatment of device-related orthopaedic infections. *Clin Orthop Relat Res* 2005;347:7–11.

80. Darouiche RO. Device-associated infections: a macroproblem that starts with microadherence. *Clin Infect Dis* 2001;33:1567–1572.

81. Donlan RM, Costerton JW. Biofilms: survival mechanisms of clinically relevant microorganisms. *Clin Microbiol Rev* 2002;15:167–193.

82. Giacometti A, Cirioni O, Ghiselli R et al. Efficacy of polycationic peptides in preventing vascular graft infection due to Staphylococcus epidermidis. J Antimicrob Chemother 2000;46:751–756.

83. Yasim A, Gul M, Atahan E. Efficacy of vancomycin, teicoplanin and fusidic acid as prophylactic agents in prevention of vascular graft infection: an experimental study in rat. Eur J Vasc Endovasc Surg 2006;31:274–279.

84. Eron LJ, Lipsky BA, Low DE, Nathwani D, Tice AD, Volturo GA; Expert panel on managing skin and soft tissue infections. Managing skin and soft tissue infections: expert panel recommendations on key decision points. J Antimicrob Chemother 2003;52 (Suppl 1):i3–17.

85. Stevens DL, Bisno AL, Chambers HF et al.; Infectious Diseases Society of America. Practice guidelines for the diagnosis and management of skin and soft-tissue infections. Clin Infect Dis 2005;41: 1373–1406.

86. May AK, Stafford RE, Bulger EM et al.; Surgical Infection Society. Treatment of complicated skin and soft tissue infections. Surg Infect (Larchmt) 2009;10:467–499.

87. Pallin DJ, Egan DJ, Pelletier AJ, Espinola JA, Hooper DC, Camargo CA Jr. Increased U.S. emergency department visits for skin and soft tissue infections, and changes in antibiotic choices, during the emergence of community-associated methicillin-resistant Staphylococcus aureus. Ann Emerg Med 2008;51:291–298.

88. Bancroft EA. Antimicrobial resistance: it's not just for hospitals. JAMA 2007;298:803–804.

89. Klevens RM, Morrison MA, Nadle J et al.; Active Bacterial Core surveillance (ABCs) MRSA Investigators. Invasive methicillin-resistant Staphylococcus aureus infections in the United States. JAMA 2007;298: 1763-1771.

90. Boucher HW, Corey GR. Epidemiology of methicillin-resistant Staphylococcus aureus. Clin Infect Dis 2008;46:S344–349.

91. Kluytmans J, Struelens M. Meticillin resistant Staphylococcus aureus in the hospital. Br Med J 2009;338:532–537.

92. Naimi TS, LeDell KH, Como-Sabetti K et al. Comparison of community- and health care-associated methicillin-resistant Staphylococcus aureus infection. JAMA 2003;290:2976–2984.

93. Moet GJ, Jones RN, Biedenbach DJ, Stilwell MG, Fritsche TR. Contemporary causes of skin and soft tissue infections in North America, Latin America, and Europe: Report from the SENTRY Antimicrobial Surveillance Program (1998–2004). Diagn Microbiol Infect Dis 2007;57:7–13.

94. Petrosillo N, Drapeau CM, Nicastri E, Martini L, Ippolito G, Moro ML; ANIPIO. Surgical site infections in Italian hospitals: a prospective multicenter study. BMC Infect Dis 2008;8:34.

95. Anderson DJ, Sexton DJ, Kanafani ZA, Auten G, Kaye KS. Severe surgical site infection in community hospitals: Epidemiology, key procedures, and the changing prevalence of methicillin-resistant Staphylococcus aureus. Infect Control Hosp Epidemiol 2007;28: 1047–1053.

96. Mukadi DY, Maher D, Harries AD. Tuberculosis case fatality rates in HIV prevalence populations in sub-Saharan Africa. AIDS 2001;15:143–152.

97. Korenromp EL, Scano F, Williams BG, Dye C, Nunn P. Effects of human immunodeficiency virus infection on recurrence of tuberculosis after rifampicin-based treatment: an analytic review. Clin Infect Dis 2003;37:101–112.

98. Edlin BR, Tokars JI, Grieco MH et al. An outbreak of multidrug-resistant tuberculosis among hospitalized patients with the acquired immunodeficiency syndrome. N Engl J Med 1992;326:1514–1521.

99. Gandhi NR, Moll A, Sturm AW et al. Extensively drug-resistant tuberculosis as a cause of death in patients co-infected with tuberculosis and HIV in a rural area of South Africa. Lancet 2006;368: 1575–1580.

100. De Cock KM, Chaisson RE. Will DOTS do it? A reappraisal of tuberculosis control in countries with high rates of HIV infection. Int J Tuberc Lung Dis 1999;3:457–465.

101. Corbett EL, Marston B, Churchyard GJ, De Cock KM. Tuberculosis in sub-Saharan Africa: opportunities, challenges, and change in the era of antiretroviral treatment. Lancet 2006;367:926–937.

102. World Health Organization. Global tuberculosis control 2010. Available at: http://www.who.int/tb/publications/global_report/2010/en/index.html (accessed August 1, 2011).

103. Harries AD, Zachariah R, Corbett EL et al. The HIV-associated tuberculosis epidemic – when will we act? Lancet 2010;375:1906–1919.

104. Gandhi NR, Nunn P, Dheda K et al. Multidrug-resistant and extensively drug-resistant tuberculosis: a threat to global control of tuberculosis. Lancet 2010;375:1830–1843.

105. Abdool Karim SS, Churchyard GJ, Abdool Karim Q, Lawn SD. HIV infection and tuberculosis in South Africa: an urgent need to escalate the public health response. Lancet 2009;374:921–933.

106. World Health Organization. Anti-Tuberculosis Drug Resistance in the World: The WHO/IUATLD Global Project on Anti-Tuberculosis Drug Resistance Surveillance. Geneva: WHO, 2008.

107. Wright A, Zignol M, Van Deun A *et al.* Epidemiology of antituberculosis drug resistance 2002–07: an updated analysis of the global project on anti-tuberculosis drug resistance surveillance. *Lancet* 2009;373:1861–1873.

108. Yew W, Leung C. Management of multidrug-resistant tuberculosis: update 2007. *Respirology* 2008;13:21–46.

109. Schaaf HS, Moll AP, Dheda K. Multidrug- and extensively drug-resistant tuberculosis in Africa and South America: epidemiology, diagnosis and management in adults and children. *Clin Chest Medr* 2009;30:667–683.

110. World Health Organization. Guidelines for intensified tuberculosis case-finding and isoniazid preventive therapy for people living with HIV in resource-constrained settings. Available at: http://whqlibdoc. who.int/publications/2011/9789241500708_eng.pdf (accessed August 1, 2011).

111. World Health Organization. *Interim Policy on Collaborative TB/HIV Activities.* Geneva: World Health Organization, 2004. Available at: http://whqlibdoc.who.int/hq/2004/WHO_HTM_TB_2004.330_eng.pdf (accessed August 1, 2011).

112. Stop TB Partnership. The Global Plan to Stop TB 2006–2015. Progress report 2006–2008. Available at: http://www.stoptb.org/assets/documents/global/plan/The_global_plan_progress_report1.pdf (accessed August 1, 2011).

113. World Health Organization. Global tuberculosis control: a short update to the 2009 report (December, 2009). Available at: http://www.who.int/tb/publications/global_report/2009/update/en/index.html (accessed August 1, 2011).

CHAPTER 2

Bacterial Osteomyelitis: The Clinician's Point of View

Ilker Uçkay[1,2], Nicolas Christian Buchs[1,2], Khalid Seghrouchni[1,2], Mathieu Assal[1,2], Pierre Hoffmeyer[1,2] and Daniel Lew[1,2]

[1]*Geneva University Hospitals, Geneva, Switzerland*
[2]*University of Geneva, Geneva, Switzerland*

Definition and microbiology

Osteomyelitis is an inflammatory process accompanied by bone destruction. The infection can be limited to a single portion of the bone or can involve several regions, such as the marrow, cortex, periosteum and surrounding soft tissue [1]. Osteomyelitis is a common term for bone infection, although non-infectious inflammation of bones and adherent structures exists [2]. For example, SAPHO syndrome is a rare immunological disorder that results in synovitis, *a*cne, *p*ustulosis, *h*yperostosis and *o*steitis [2,3]. Other immunological diseases, such as chronic recurrent multifocal osteomyelitis [2,4] or palmoplantar pustulosis [2], can also prevail with multifocal osteomyelitis [2]. Strictly speaking, osteomyelitis implicates inflammation of the bone and bone marrow. The term "osteitis" often would be more appropriate. In the literature, osteomyelitis sometimes refers to infections associated with bone implants. However, most authors use the expressions "implant" or "foreign body infections" when referring to such infections. All implant infections have an osteitis component, since the implant itself is inert to microorganisms.

Infection is almost exclusively of bacterial origin and rarely due to fungi (intravenous drug abusers [5] or in skull osteomyelitis [6] in immunosuppressed individuals) or parasites (e.g. echinococcosis). No case of viral bone infection has been described to the best of our knowledge. Among all bacteria and types of osteomyelitis, except those of the the jaw, *Staphylococcus aureus* dominates [7–10], followed by streptococci and Gram-negative pathogens [10] such as *Pseudomonas aeruginosa* [11]. Polymicrobial infection is frequent in trauma and long-lasting ulcerations [12,13], but not in hematogenous infection [7]. Anaerobes are seldom observed [10,14] and coagulase-negative staphylococci are retrieved almost exclusively in implant-related infections [8,15,16]. *Kingella kingae* is responsible for osteoarticular infections, including osteomyelitis, in young children under 4 years of age [17].

The literature lacks an internationally accepted definition of chronic osteomyelitis [18]. However, the diversity of pathogens, bones, origins and patients make any strict and consistent classification impossible. As for any infection, acute, subacute and chronic [1] are the headings of the main

Diagnostic Imaging of Infections and Inflammatory Diseases: A Multidisciplinary Approach, First Edition. Edited by Alberto Signore and Ana María Quintero.

groups [19], but these are not very useful in daily clinical practice. A commonly accepted definition of chronic osteomyelitis requires minimal symptom duration of 6 weeks to 3 months. However, this definition is also arbitrary [1]. Another classification is according to the presumed origin with hematogenous and continuity origin as the prevalent groups. In contrast to vertebral osteomyelitis, some arthroplasty infections, osteomyelitis accompanying septic arthritis or osteomyelitis in children with a known hematogenous acquisition [1,7], long bone, sacral and foot osteomyelitis is a chronic infection among adult patients [20] and is acquired *per continuitatem* during trauma, surgery or soft tissue ulceration [19] (e.g. in diabetic patients [21] or those with neurological disorders prone to decubitus). In rare cases, adult patients develop osteomyelitis after hematogenous seeding of long bones during bacteremia [1,22].

Several surgical classifications have been proposed. Among these, the Cierny–Mader classification [23] for long bone osteomyelitis or the PEDIS classification for diabetic foot osteomyelitis are the most frequently reported. The Cierny–Mader classification considers the quality of the host, the bone's anatomical nature, treatment and prognostic factors [24]. The terms acute and chronic are not used in this classification. Generally, surgeons understand a chronic osteomyelitis as infection requiring surgery, with established sequestra and bone deformities already present. Finally, infections associated with prosthetic joints can be classified as early (those that develop <3 months after surgery), subacute (3–24 months after surgery), or late (>24 months after surgery and often acquired by hematogenous seeding) [15,25].

Epidemiology

The epidemiology of osteomyelitis is heterogeneous with variability among involved bones, pathogens and settings. For example, resource-poor countries may reveal a higher proportion of tuberculous osteomyelitis or chronic osteomyelitis of traumatic origin [10] compared to resource-rich countries with a higher prevalence of foot osteomyelitis among elderly patients. For vertebral osteomyelitis, the incidence is estimated at 0.2–2 annual cases per 100 000 patients, and mostly middle-aged patients are affected with a male to female ratio of 2:1 for

which the reasons remain unclear [13,24]. The incidence of pediatric hematogenous osteomyelitis ranges from 3 to 76 annual cases per 100 000 children, also with a male predominance [20,26]. Osteomyelitis is seen in about 15–20% of all diabetic foot ulcer patients [1,27].

Many experts advocate that if the bone is infected, it may remain infected throughout life and even beyond unless amputation is performed. Recurrences of osteomyelitis after several years, if not decades, have been reported [28,29] and there is no internationally accepted minimal follow-up duration. Some authors suggest that "arrest" or "remission" is a more appropriate term than "cure" for defining outcome in chronic osteomyelitis [24]. In the literature, minimal follow-up times range from 3 months [30] to 1 or 2 years [18,31–34], while Tice *et al.* showed that 78% and 95% of all osteomyelitis recurrences occur within 6 and 12 months, respectively [35]. To date, remission is considered as complete clinical resolution of a former infection after a minimal follow-up of 2 years [36,37].

Pathogenesis

A large proportion of osteomyelitis is either trauma- or surgery-related [10] or due to ulcerations, e.g. in the diabetic patient. These infections occur *per continuitatem*. Most surgical site infections are believed to be acquired at the time of surgery and are caused by endogenous flora [38]. Arguments favoring this hypothesis are the efficacy of preoperative antibiotic prophylaxis together with the similarity of skin flora and pathogens. However, infection control issues are beyond the scope of this chapter and we will concentrate on mechanisms of osseous modification, biofilm formation and neutrophil defects.

Osseous modification

Numerous animal models exist for both acute and chronic osteomyelitis [39]. Chronic osteomyelitis has been shown to result from persistence of the acute hematogenous form in 4.4% of childhood bone infections [7,13]. Waldvogel *et al.* estimated chronicity in 15% of adult osteomyelitis cases [19].

Every chronic infection begins with an acute one. Bacteria adhere to the bone matrix and orthopedic implants via receptors to fibronectin and other structural proteins. They elude host defenses and antibiotics by hiding intracellularly [40] and by developing a biofilm [9]. Patchy ischemic bone necrosis occurs when the inflammation occludes the vascular tunnels. Segments of bone devoid of blood supply can become separated and are called sequestra [1]. This creates an ideal culture medium for bacteria and at 48 hours abscesses are formed [9]. At the infarction edge there is reactive hyperemia associated with increased osteoclastic activity [1]. This activity in turn causes bone loss. Meanwhile, osteoblastic activity occurs, in some cases exuberantly, causing periosteal apposition and new bone formation, called involucra [1]. There is much evidence that growth factors, cytokines, hormones and drugs regulate the proliferation and activity of osteoblasts and osteoclasts [1]. Exudate may also extend into the surrounding soft tissue through cloacae, which are holes in the involucrum. When sequestra or involucra become fibrotic, sclerosis may result. Bone sclerosis usually indicates infection present for more than 1 month [20] (Figure 2.1).

Biofilm

Biofilms are the hallmark of implant-related osteomyelitis, but are also important in the absence of a foreign body [21]. Approximately 60–80% of all microorganisms in nature exist in biofilms. Upon introduction into the human body, foreign bodies rapidly become coated by host components. Pathogen attachment is the second step [41]. Virulence factors such as adhesive proteins, enzymes and toxins play an important role [42,43]. Interactions involve non-specific physicochemical forces, such as van der Waal's forces, hydrophobic interactions and polarity [43,44]. Intercellular adhesion requires the synthesis of the polysaccharide intercellular adhesin (PIA) under the control of intercellular adhesion (*ica*) operon [44], which is considered to be one of the main genetic determinants involved in the accumulation phase of biofilm formation. Finally, the cells that attach irreversibly to surfaces form microcolonies and produce extracellular polymers. In this process, numerous molecules and components are involved such as fibronectin, fibrinogen, vitronectin, von Willebrand factor and cellular elements [9]. The structure of the biofilm is heterogeneous, both in space and over time, with channels that allow the transport of nutrients and oxygen [43]. A mature biofilm is composed of 25–30% pathogens and 70–75% amorphous matrix [15] (Figure 2.2).

Equally, pathogens undergo undefined and complex metabolic changes, and become less susceptible not only to the immune system, but also to antibiotics [42,45]. Chemotactic responsiveness is diminished and degranulation of specific granule

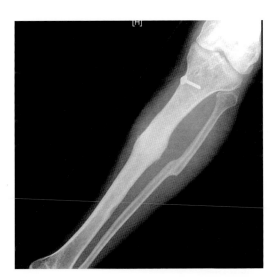

Figure 2.1 Standard X-ray of chronic osteomyelitis of the tibia. The bone is irregular in shape with involvement of the intramedullary canal and cortical extension. Proximal screw.

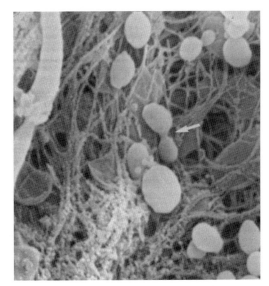

Figure 2.2 Biofilm of *Staphylococcus epidermidis* on a catheter surface with embedded staphylococci within the matrix. The arrow shows dividing bacteria. Scanning electron microscopy (magnification x 15 000). (Source: Uçkay *et al.* [15].)

content is increased. Additionally, the biofilm inhibits the genesis of mononuclear cells, T and B lymphocytes, thus adversely acting on both the cytotoxic and humoral defense responses [46]. Vandecasteele *et al.* observed an impressive decrease in bacterial metabolism and protein synthesis *in vitro* [47]. The authors measured the amount of 16S rRNA by quantitative polymerase chain reaction (PCR) as a surrogate marker of the actual metabolic activity of bacteria. A decrease in 16S rRNA content was reported as early as 2 hours after beginning the culture. The *ica* operon was mainly transcribed during early, but not late, infection [47]. Monzon *et al.* reported a dramatically decreased effect of vancomycin–rifampin therapy induced by staphylococcal biofilms in cultures older than 6 hours [48].

Biofilms provide significant resistance to antibiotics and innate host defenses. Antibiotics penetrate poorly into the thick, acidic matrix. Bacteria in deep layers are metabolically inactive and have an inherent lack of susceptibility to antibiotics [49], whereas planktonic cultures of the same organism do not [50]. This resistance is lost once the biofilm-attached bacteria revert to planktonic growth [49]. To date, no standardized antimicrobial susceptibility tests are available to evaluate drug activity on adherent bacteria [50]. Minimal inhibitory concentration (MIC) and minimal bactericidal concentration (MBC) evaluate only drug efficacy on planktonic bacteria in the logarithmic phases of growth [51]. For cell wall active antibiotics to be effective in biofilms, 100 to 1000 times the standard concentration is often required [50].

Group behavior is an important intercellular communication mechanism. Small signaling molecules are released into the natural environment and trigger specific responses in a coordinated manner in neighboring bacteria of the same species. This is known as "quorum sensing" and it plays an important role in biofilm formation [52,53].

Neutrophil defects

In the presence of a foreign body, neutrophils exhibit a decreased production of superoxide and have a lower content of enzymatic granules, an indication of impaired response to infection [9,54,55]. The interaction with the foreign material leads to a respiratory burst and exocytosis of enzymatic granules, leading to a neutrophil population composed of exhausted cells with low granule content and low killing capacity [9]. In this situation, the inoculum of staphylococci required to induce infection is reduced to as few as 100 colony-forming units [54]. Ultra-high molecular weight polyethylene wear particles released by prosthetic material may further compromise neutrophil antibacterial activity [56,57].

Diagnosis

Clinical signs and diagnostic imaging modalities (including radiological and nuclear medicine techniques) are suggestive for diagnosis, but cannot establish the nature of the pathogen [24], which is required for targeted therapy. Imaging aspects are discussed in greater detail in the later chapters.

In the diagnostic work-up of osteomyelitis, the ultimate proof requires growth of the same pathogens in several, at least two, bone samples [15]. Pathogens like *Propionibacterium acnes* may induce infection late after implant if empirical pretreatment with antimicrobial agents is used [13]. Small colony variants constitute a subpopulation of bacteria and have a slow growth rate, atypical colony morphology and unusual biochemical characteristics, making them a challenge for clinical microbiologists to identify [40]. Clinically, small colony variants are better able to persist in mammalian cells and are less susceptible to antibiotics than their wild-type counterparts, causing recurrent infections [58].

Eubacterial PCR testing has usually only low sensitivity and is still relatively expensive, thus making it unlikely to be used as routinely. In polymicrobial colonization or infection, its interpretation can be difficult. Moreover, it does not provide information about antibiotic resistance, except for genes coding for methicillin resistance. However, specific or multiplex PCR is beneficial in special circumstances when very slow growing or difficult to grow bacteria are suspected, such as *Kingella kingae* [17], *Brucella* spp. [59,60], *Coxiella burnetii* [61], *Bartonella henselae* [62], *Mycobacterium tuberculosis* [59], or *Mycobacterium ulcerans* [63].

In culture-negative osteomyelitis without microbial confirmation, diagnosis is established clinically using imaging techniques and, ultimately, histologically. Bacteremic disease is rare and the use of serum antistreptolysin-O titers for the diagnosis of invasive disease due to β-hemolytic streptococci is seldom reliable [64]. Of note, positive skin carriage for methicillin-resistant *S. aureus* (MRSA) does not predict an osteoarticular infection due to MRSA [65].

While bone probing has a sensitivity of 66% for osteomyelitis, a specificity of 85%, a positive predictive value of 89% and a negative predictive value of 56%, the value of pathogen identification with bone surface swabs is not clear [66]. In a study where sinus tract cultures were compared with cultures of operative specimens from patients with chronic osteomyelitis, only 44% of the sinus tract cultures contained the pathogen found in intraoperative cultures [67].

Treatment

The assessment of the patient's general condition and morbidities is of great importance. Not every osteomyelitis has to be treated. The key question is how much the patient will benefit from a long-lasting and maybe complicated treatment. Today, millions of individuals in resource-poor [7] and even rich countries have chronic osteomyelitis that discharges from time to time, but does not interfere substantially with daily activities of living.

A multidisciplinary team is necessary for optimal treatment [68,69]. In large centers, a team of orthopedic surgeons, infectious diseases specialists, diabetologists, nurses and specialized physiotherapists treats patients with osteomyelitis. For chronic osteomyelitis, antibiotics alone are very rarely successful because they cannot, or only to a limited extent, penetrate to the biofilm and sequestra. Without adequate debridement, chronic osteomyelitis does not respond to antibiotic regimens, no matter the choice of antibiotic or the duration of therapy [40]. Only in a few exceptions may antibiotic administration without surgery eradicate infection: childhood osteomyelitis, spondylodiscitis, tuberculous osteomyelitis and selected patients with diabetic toe osteomyelitis.

Surgical treatment

Optimal management includes sequestrectomy, resection of scarred and infected bone as well as soft tissue [1,23], obliteration of dead space, appropriate bone mechanical stability, adequate soft tissue coverage and restoration of an effective blood supply [18,22,70,71]. Adequate soft tissue coverage of the bone is considered necessary to arrest

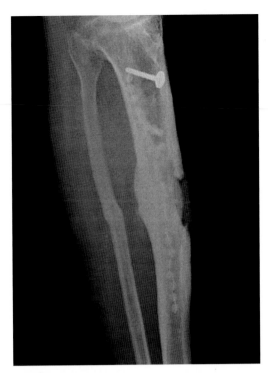

Figure 2.3 Lateral view of the same case as in Figure 2.2 showing cortical fenestration and insertion of gentamicin beads for treatment.

osteomyelitis [24]. Sometimes antibiotic-containing beads are also used (Figure 2.3). In the case of vascular insufficiency, a good blood flow is restored by vascular bypass or endovascular stenting. Coverage with a vacuum-assisted closure (VAC) dressing is discouraged by some surgeons or performed simply by others [72,73]. Amputation is infrequent for long bone osteomyelitis [7], in contrast to toe osteomyelitis of the diabetic foot. However, in certain patients, amputation may be preferable to multiple operations. For implant-related osteomyelitis, the implant is removed when the bone is stable. In the case of instability (recent implantation), debridement with antibiotic treatment is a temporary solution until bone stability is achieved and the implant becomes obsolete. Contrary to common belief, bone can heal even in the presence of infection.

Hyperbaric oxygen therapy

Hyperbaric oxygen therapy consumes very substantial resources [74]. It provides oxygen to promote collagen production, angiogenesis, osteogenesis and healing in the ischemic or infected wound [24,75]. Animals receiving hyperbaric oxygen showed an acceleration of all phases of fracture repair [75]. Several authors have suggested that adjunctive hyperbaric oxygen therapy might be useful in the treatment of human chronic osteomyelitis, even if the results are not consistent. The adjunctive role of hyperbaric oxygen in osteomyelitis is difficult to assess because of the multiple confounding variables of patient, surgery, organism, bone and antibiotic therapy [24].

Medical treatment

As a general principle, the duration of antibiotic administration does not depend on the pathogen. There are a few exceptions and long-lasting antibiotic treatment is documented in the literature for osteomyelitis with the following pathogens: tuberculosis [1,76], other mycobacteria such as *M. ulcerans* for Buruli ulcer [63], fungi [5,6], Q fever [61], cat scratch disease [62], brucellosis [59,60], or *Nocardia* spp. [77].

Whereas expert opinion and scientific evidence is rich for hematogenous childhood [1,26] or implant-related osteomyelitis [78], the optimal antibiotic duration post-debridement for implant-free osteomyelitis among adults remains unknown [1,16, 34,79]. Formerly, experts usually recommended intravenous (IV) therapy for 4 [22] to 6 weeks [1,71,79,80]. Today, opinion has rather switched to IV treatment during the initial 2 weeks [81]. Total duration of antibiotic treatment concomitant to surgery can be limited probably to 6 weeks for osteomyelitis with [82] or without [73] implant material. There are no clinical studies or documented records indicating the superiority of the 4–6-week course over shorter durations [24,73,79] (Table 2.1). Recent retrospective data suggest that regimens with an early switch to oral antibiotics are as effective as prolonged parenteral regimens, at least for osteomyelitis [11,83]. Several antibiotic agents have already proved their clinical efficacy when taken orally: quinolones [11,32], linezolid, clindamycin and fusidic acid combined with rifampin [71,84]. These drugs have an oral bioavailability of over 90% [85].

Special features of osteomyelitis

Spondylodiscitis with vertebral osteomyelitis

Unless a nosocomial infection occurs after spine surgery, hematogenous spread is generally the most common origin of vertebral osteomyelitis and/or spondylodiscitis [8]. In bacteremic disease, endocarditis should be excluded. No randomized controlled studies have evaluated antibiotic regimens for vertebral osteomyelitis. Practically, the choice of antibiotic agents is no different from any other osteoarticular infection, but a parenteral treatment of at least 3–4 weeks is usually suggested [8,86]. In an observational study comparing the outcomes in patients treated for various periods, remission rates and death were similar for 6 weeks or less as compared to more than 6 weeks of antibiotic therapy [87]. Prolonged antibiotic treatment is recommended in patients who have abscesses that have not been drained or who have spinal implants [8]. The role of antibiotics with good oral bioavailability has not been evaluated in spondylodiscitis and epidural abscesses [8,88]. Based on current expert opinion, a switch to oral treatment is feasible if a suitable drug with proven susceptibility to the pathogen is available and if compliance with oral therapy can be carefully monitored.

Surgical intervention is required in large abscesses, although drainage with a computed tomography (CT)-guided catheter is sufficient in many cases [8]. Surgery has to be considered in implant-associated infection, progressive neurological deficits associated with stenosis, instability, or severe deformity [8].

Diabetic foot osteomyelitis

Clinicians must recognize the main differential diagnoses of diabetic foot osteomyelitis: the Charcot foot [21,89], gout and inflammation due to ischemia itself [24,90,91]. In perforating ulcers, there is an underling osteomyelitis in about 15% [1] to 20% of cases [27,91,92], especially if the wound extends to the bone and joints [93]. Bone biopsy (with histology if there is sufficient material) [21,92] is valuable for establishing the diagnosis and for defining the pathogenic organism(s) [90]. Clinicians refer patients for diagnostic imaging (X-ray, magnetic resonance, bone scintigraphy or white blood cell scintigraphy) to obtain an answer to the following questions: Is there osteomyelitis and to what extent? Is the patient operable or is amputation required? Can bone biopsies be obtained from sites of interest? [70].

According to an international expert panel, no significant differences in outcome are associated with any particular treatment strategy [90]. There

Table 2.1 Antibiotic treatment of chronic osteomyelitis in adults

	Treatment of choice	Alternatives
Penicillin-sensitive *Staphylococcus aureus*	Benzylpenicillin (10–20 million U/day)	Cefazolin (1 g every 6 hours) Clindamycin (600 mg every 6 hours) Vancomycin (1 g every 12 hours)
Penicillin-resistant *S. aureus*	Nafcillin[a] (1 or 1.5 g every 4–6 hours) or cefazolin (2 g every 8 hours)	Second-generation cephalosporin (e.g. cefuroxime, cefamandole) Clindamycin (600 mg every 6 hours) Vancomycin (1 g every 12 hours) Ciprafloxacin (750 mg orally every 12 hours) or levofloxacin in combination with rifampin (600 mg/day) is also frequently used
Methicillin-resistant *S. aureus*[b]	Vancomycin (1 g every 12 hours)	Teicoplanin (400 g every 24 hours, first day every 12 hours)
Various streptococci (Group A or B β-hemolytic; *Streptococcus pneumoniae*)	Benzylpenicillin (10–20 million U/day)	Clindamycin (600 mg every 6 hours) Erythromycin (500 mg every 6 hours) Vancomycin (1 g every 12 hours)
Enteric Gram-negative bacilli	Quinolone (e.g. ciprofloxacin, 400–750 mg every 12 hours, with early switch to oral)	Third-generation cephalosporin (e.g. ceftriaxone 2 g every 24 hours; cefepime)
Serratia spp., *Pseudomonas aeruginosa*	Piperacillin (2–4 g every 4 hours) and aminoglycosides	Cefepime 2 g every 2 hours[c] or a quinolone and aminoglycosides (according to sensitivity; one daily dose)
Anaerobes	Clindamycin (600 mg every 6 hours)	Ampicillin–sulbactam (2 g every 8 hours) Metronidazole for Gram-negative anaerobes (500 mg every 8 hours)
Mixed infection (aerobic and anaerobic microorganisms)	Ampicillin–sulbactam (2–3 g every 6–8 hours)[d]	Imipenem (500 mg every 6 hours)[e]

All doses are given for normal renal/hepatic function and should be adjusted in renal or hepatic failure. Teicoplanin is not available in all countries.
[a]Flucloxacillin, oxacillin, or cloxacillin.
[b]Most coagulase-negative staphylococci are methicillin-resistant and treated with vancomycin or teicoplanin.
[c]Depends on sensitivities; a fourth-generation cephalosporin (cefepime), piperacillin/tazobactam, meropenem and imipenem are useful alternatives.
[d]Amoxicillin–clavulanate (1.1–2.2 g every 6–8 hours).
[e]In cases of Gram-negative aerobic microorganisms resistant to amoxicillin–clavulanate.
(Source: Lew *et al.* [1])

are no data to support the superiority of any particular route of delivery of systemic antibiotics or the optimal therapy duration [90]. Skin carriage of MRSA does not necessarily need anti-MRSA coverage [94]. Therapy aimed solely at aerobic Gram-positive cocci may be sufficient for mild-to-moderate infections in patients who have not recently received antibiotic therapy [90]. Broad-spectrum empirical therapy takes care of severe infections. Bioavailable oral antibiotics are sufficient in most cases of mild and moderate osteomyelitis. In severe diabetic foot infections, antibiotics are given initially IV to achieve maximal tissue concentrations in an area already compromised by arteriopathy, although no evidence for the superiority of IV medication exists [27,90]. Experts suggest 6 weeks of antibiotic therapy for acute osteomyelitis [21,27] and at least 12 weeks for chronic infection [27,91], if not up to 46 weeks [12,91]. No available evidence supports the use of hyperbaric oxygen or granulocyte-colony stimulating factors [90]. A diabetic foot problem always benefits from multidisciplinary diagnosis and therapy [12,21,27,36,68]. Concomitant treatment includes proper wound cleansing, debridement of callus and necrotic tissue [21] and off-loading of pathological pressure. Evaluation of interventions aimed at restoring blood perfusion is imperative before surgery [1,12].

Arthroplasty-related osteomyelitis

Antibiotics are initially administered IV for 2 weeks for arthroplasty-associated osteomyelitis, followed by oral therapy for a total treatment duration of 3 months in patients with hip prostheses and 3–6 months in those with knee prostheses [16,25,78]. However, recent retrospective data suggest that a 6-week course could be sufficient for all infections [82]. When lifelong suppressive oral treatment is an option, the overall success rate in prosthetic joint infection is 69% after a mean follow-up of 5 years [95].

Non-arthroplasty-related implant osteomyelitis

The goals of treating infection associated with internal fixation devices are consolidation of the fracture and prevention of chronic osteomyelitis. Thus, in contrast to prosthetic joint- associated infection, complete eradication of infection is not the primary goal, since the device can theoretically be removed after consolidation [96] or in the worst case scenario, temporary stabilization can be achieved with external fixation and removal of internal fixation.

The choice of antibiotic agents is the same as for all osteoarticular infections and the ideal duration of antibiotic treatment is unknown due to a lack of randomized trials. Some experts favor continuing antibiotics until implant removal and some weeks beyond [96]. Others prescribe the same antibiotics for 6 weeks only despite the presence of implant material. In chronic infections, defined by the onset of infectious symptoms after 10 weeks post-implant, the duration may be prolonged to 3 months [96]. Other experts treat for 3 months when the device is retained and 6 weeks when there is complete removal of all hardware [78]. In any case, the duration of therapy has to be decided on an individual basis. It is also unclear if rifampin should be added to the antibiotic regimen from the start, even if the implant is to be removed later. In our institution, we prefer to treat acute infections with combined rifampin for 6 weeks post-surgery, regardless of whether the device is expected to be removed or not. In the case of chronic infection, device retention

and good tolerability of the antibiotics, therapy can be prolonged to 3 months. If there is no documented bacteremia, the antibiotic regimen can be oral from the beginning.

Osteomyelitis associated with sickle cell disease

Sickle cell disease is an autosomal-recessive disorder that provokes anemia from childhood [97]. The disease also leads to bone necrosis caused by microvascular occlusion [98]. Its infectious hallmarks are Gram-negative pathogens [97], e.g. *Salmonella* spp. [1], although the association with *Salmonella* spp. is poorly defined [98]. The life-time incidence of osteoarticular infection in severe homozygotic disease is estimated at 3% [98]. Treatment is that of classical osteomyelitis.

Sacral osteomyelitis

This disease is chronic and related to decubitus in patients with multiple co-morbidities and/or neurological disorders. It is particularly difficult to treat, since there is no remission if the cause of chronic osteomyelitis cannot be treated. In these chronic decubitus patients, the infected sacral bone often cannot be excised and the patient cannot be improved neurologically. Prevention is of utmost importance. Thorough daily nursing care and debridement is the key to success. In ameliorated cases, plastic surgeons may graft onto the naked bone. The ideal duration of antibiotic administration is unknown. The aim is not to eradicate bone infection, but to control it. More data are needed in this field of osteomyelitis.

Jaw osteomyelitis

Chronic mandibular osteomyelitis occurs after dental procedures, trauma, or in very poor settings in patients with noma disease, but little research has been conducted so far regarding this condition. Causative pathogens are often polymicrobial and stem from the oral flora. *Actinomyces* spp. may mimic neoplasm. Treatment consists of maxillofacial surgery, often repeated, and long-lasting oral antibiotic therapy for which the choice of amoxicillin/clavulanate covers most oral flora.

Future options

Future research will probably improve knowledge of the metabolic properties of biofilm-grown bacteria. The high genetic variability of the bacterial genome and the discovery of specific genomic elements promoting its invasiveness [99] may offer the possibility to develop new drug targets [100]. Additional prospective trials need to be performed before this concept and other innovative approaches, such as urokinase [101], bacteriophages [102], ultrasonically enhanced antibiotic activity [103], or electric current treatment of biofilm [104], are proven to be superior to established combined antibiotic therapies. Finally, it is very difficult to evaluate osteomyelitis in small clinical studies or single centers. Sample size and international definitions need to be improved and more prospective and multicenter cohort studies performed to broaden and advance current knowledge.

Acknowledgements

We thank the teams of the Orthopaedic and Infectious Diseases Departments of Geneva University Hospitals.

References

1. Lew DP, Waldvogel FA. Osteomyelitis. *Lancet* 2004; 364:369–379.
2. Jansson A, Renner ED, Ramser J et al. Classification of non-bacterial osteitis: retrospective study of clinical, immunological and genetic aspects in 89 patients. *Rheumatology (Oxf)* 2007;46:154–160.
3. Karadag-Saygi E, Gunduz OH, Gumrukcu G, Akyuz G. SAPHO syndrome: misdiagnosed and operated. *Acta Reumatol Port* 2008;33:460–463.
4. Shimizu M, Tone Y, Toga A et al. Colchicine-responsive chronic recurrent multifocal osteomyelitis with MEFV mutations: a variant of familial Mediterranean fever? *Rheumatology (Oxf)* 2010;49: 2221–2223.
5. Legout L, Assal M, Rohner P, Lew D, Bernard L, Hoffmeyer P. Successful treatment of *Candida parapsilosis* (fluconazole-resistant) osteomyelitis with caspofungin in a HIV patient. *Scand J Infect Dis* 2006;38:728–730.
6. Blyth CC, Gomes L, Sorrell TC, da Cruz M, Sud A, Chen SC. Skull-base osteomyelitis: fungal vs. bacterial infection. *Clin Microbiol Infect* 2011;17: 306–311.
7. Beckles VL, Jones HW, Harrison WJ. Chronic haematogenous osteomyelitis in children: a retrospective review of 167 patients in Malawi. *J Bone Joint Surg Br* 2010;92:1138–1143.
8. Zimmerli W. Clinical practice. Vertebral osteomyelitis. *N Engl J Med* 2010;362:1022–1029.
9. Ciampolini J, Harding KG. Pathophysiology of chronic bacterial osteomyelitis. Why do antibiotics fail so often? *Postgrad Med J* 2000;76:479–483.
10. Beals RK, Bryant RE. The treatment of chronic open osteomyelitis of the tibia in adults. *Clin Orthop Rel Res* 2005:212–217.
11. Karamanis EM, Matthaiou DK, Moraitis LI, Falagas ME. Fluoroquinolones versus beta-lactam based regimens for the treatment of osteomyelitis: a meta-analysis of randomized controlled trials. *Spine* 2008;33:297–304.
12. Lipsky BA, Berendt AR, Deery HG et al. Diagnosis and treatment of diabetic foot infections. *Plast Reconstr Surg* 2006;117 (Suppl 7):212S–238S.
13. Craigen MA, Watters J, Hackett JS. The changing epidemiology of osteomyelitis in children. *J Bone Joint Surg Br* 1992;74:541–545.
14. Uçkay I, Dinh A, Vauthey L et al. Spondylodiscitis due to *Propionibacterium acnes*: report of twenty-nine cases and a review of the literature. *Clin Microbiol Infect* 2010;16:353–358.
15. Uçkay I, Pittet D, Vaudaux P, Sax H, Lew D, Waldvogel F. Foreign body infections due to *Staphylococcus epidermidis*. *Ann Med* 2009;41:109–119.
16. Leone S, Borre S, Monforte A et al. Consensus document on controversial issues in the diagnosis and treatment of prosthetic joint infections. *Int J Infect Dis* 2010;14:67–77.
17. Ceroni D, Cherkaoui A, Ferey S, Kaelin A, Schrenzel J. *Kingella kingae* osteoarticular infections in young children: clinical features and contribution of a new specific real-time PCR assay to the diagnosis. *J Pediatr Orthop* 2010;30:301–304.
18. Lazzarini L, Lipsky BA, Mader JT. Antibiotic treatment of osteomyelitis: what have we learned from 30 years of clinical trials? *Int J Infect Dis* 2005;9:127–138.
19. Waldvogel FA, Medoff G, Swartz MN. Treatment of osteomyelitis. *N Engl J Med* 1970;283:822.
20. Auh JS, Binns HJ, Katz BZ. Retrospective assessment of subacute or chronic osteomyelitis in children and young adults. *Clin Pediatr* 2004;43:549–555.
21. Hannan CM, Attinger CE. Special considerations in the management of osteomyelitis defects (diabetes, the ischemic or dysvascular bed, and irradiation). *Semin Plast Surg* 2009;23:132–140.
22. Parsons B, Strauss E. Surgical management of chronic osteomyelitis. *Am J Surg* 2004;188:57–66.
23. Cierny G, 3rd, Mader JT, Penninck JJ. A clinical staging system for adult osteomyelitis. *Clin Orthop Rel Res* 2003;414:7–24.
24. Calhoun JH, Manring MM. Adult osteomyelitis. *Infect Dis Clin North Am* 2005;19:765–786.

25. Zimmerli W, Trampuz A, Ochsner PE. Prosthetic-joint infections. *N Engl J Med* 2004;351:1645–1654.

26. Howard-Jones AR, Isaacs D. Systematic review of systemic antibiotic treatment for children with chronic and sub-acute pyogenic osteomyelitis. *J Paediatr Child Health* 2010;46:736–741.

27. Byren I, Peters EJ, Hoey C, Berendt A, Lipsky BA. Pharmacotherapy of diabetic foot osteomyelitis. *Expert Opin Pharmacother* 2009;10:3033–3047.

28. Darley ES, MacGowan AP. Antibiotic treatment of gram-positive bone and joint infections. *J Antimicrob Chemother* 2004;53:928–935.

29. Uçkay I, Assal M, Legout L et al. Recurrent osteomyelitis caused by infection with different bacterial strains without obvious source of reinfection. *J Clin Microbiol* 2006;44:1194–1196.

30. Panda M, Ntungila N, Kalunda M, Hinsenkamp M. Treatment of chronic osteomyelitis using the Papineau technique. *Int Orthop* 1998;22:37–40.

31. Cordero-Ampuero J, Esteban J, Garcia-Cimbrelo E. Oral antibiotics are effective for highly resistant hip arthroplasty infections. *Clin Orthop Rel Res* 2009;467:2335–2342.

32. Dellamonica P, Bernard E, Etesse H, Garraffo R, Drugeon HB. Evaluation of pefloxacin, ofloxacin and ciprofloxacin in the treatment of thirty-nine cases of chronic osteomyelitis. *Eur J Clin Microbiol Infect Dis* 1989;8:1024–1030.

33. Greenberg RN, Newman MT, Shariaty S, Pectol RW. Ciprofloxacin, lomefloxacin, or levofloxacin as treatment for chronic osteomyelitis. *Antimicrob Agents Chemother* 2000;44:164–166.

34. Conterno LO, da Silva Filho CR. Antibiotics for treating chronic osteomyelitis in adults. *Cochrane Database Syst Rev* 2009:CD004439.

35. Tice AD, Hoaglund PA, Shoultz DA. Risk factors and treatment outcomes in osteomyelitis. *J Antimicrob Chemother* 2003;51:1261–1268.

36. Venkatesan P, Lawn S, Macfarlane RM, Fletcher EM, Finch RG, Jeffcoate WJ. Conservative management of osteomyelitis in the feet of diabetic patients. *Diabet Med* 1997;14:487–490.

37. Boda A. Antibiotic irrigation-perfusion treatment for chronic osteomyelitis. *Arch Orthop Trauma Surg* 1979;95:31–35.

38. Uçkay I, Harbarth S, Peter R, Lew D, Hoffmeyer P, Pittet D. Preventing surgical site infections. *Expert Rev Anti Infect Ther* 2010;8:657–670.

39. Patel M, Rojavin Y, Jamali AA, Wasielewski SJ, Salgado CJ. Animal models for the study of osteomyelitis. *Semin Plast Surg* 2009;23:148–154.

40. Sendi P, Proctor RA. *Staphylococcus aureus* as an intracellular pathogen: the role of small colony variants. *Trends Microbiol* 2009;17:54–58.

41. Peters G. Pathogenesis of *S. epidermidis* foreign body infections. *Br J Clin Pract Suppl* 1988;57:62–65.

42. Costerton W, Veeh R, Shirtliff M, Pasmore M, Post C, Ehrlich G. The application of biofilm science to the study and control of chronic bacterial infections. *J Clin Invest* 2003;112:1466–1477.

43. Donlan RM. Biofilm formation: a clinically relevant microbiological process. *Clin Infect Dis* 2001;33:1387–1392.

44. von Eiff C, Peters G, Heilmann C. Pathogenesis of infections due to coagulase-negative staphylococci. *Lancet Infect Dis* 2002;2:677–685.

45. Vuong C, Otto M. *Staphylococcus epidermidis* infections. *Microbes Infect* 2002;4:481–489.

46. Lew D, Schrenzel J, Francois P, Vaudaux P. Pathogenesis, prevention, and therapy of staphylococcal prosthetic infections. *Curr Clinical Top Infect Dis* 2001;21:252–270.

47. Vandecasteele SJ, Peetermans WE, Carbonez A, Van Eldere J. Metabolic activity of *Staphylococcus epidermidis* is high during initial and low during late experimental foreign-body infection. *J Bacteriol* 2004;186:2236–2239.

48. Monzon M, Oteiza C, Leiva J, Amorena B. Synergy of different antibiotic combinations in biofilms of *Staphylococcus epidermidis*. *J Antimicrob Chemother* 2001;48:793–801.

49. Costerton JW, Lewandowski Z, Caldwell DE, Korber DR, Lappin-Scott HM. Microbial biofilms. *Ann Rev Microbiol* 1995;49:711–745.

50. Ceri H, Olson ME, Stremick C, Read RR, Morck D, Buret A. The Calgary Biofilm Device: new technology for rapid determination of antibiotic susceptibilities of bacterial biofilms. *J Clin Microbiol* 1999;37:1771–1776.

51. Widmer AF, Frei R, Rajacic Z, Zimmerli W. Correlation between *in vivo* and *in vitro* efficacy of antimicrobial agents against foreign body infections. *J Infect Dis* 1990;162:96–102.

52. Vadyvaloo V, Otto M. Molecular genetics of *Staphylococcus epidermidis* biofilms on indwelling medical devices. *Int J Artif Organs* 2005;28:1069–1078.

53. Mack D, Davies AP, Harris LG, Rohde H, Horstkotte MA, Knobloch JK. Microbial interactions in *Staphylococcus epidermidis* biofilms. *Anal Bioanal Chem* 2007;387:399–408.

54. Zimmerli W, Lew PD, Waldvogel FA. Pathogenesis of foreign body infection. Evidence for a local granulocyte defect. *J Clin Invest* 1984;73:1191–1200.

55. Johnson GM, Lee DA, Regelmann WE, Gray ED, Peters G, Quie PG. Interference with granulocyte function by *Staphylococcus epidermidis* slime. *Infect Immun* 1986;54:13–20.

56. Bernard L, Vaudaux P, Huggler E et al. Inactivation of a subpopulation of human neutrophils by expo-

sure to ultrahigh-molecular-weight polyethylene wear debris. *FEMS Immunol Medical Microbiol* 2007; 49:425–432.

57. Daou S, El Chemaly A, Christofilopoulos P, Bernard L, Hoffmeyer P, Demaurex N. The potential role of cobalt ions released from metal prosthesis on the inhibition of Hv1 proton channels and the decrease in *Staphyloccocus epidermidis* killing by human neutrophils. *Biomaterials* 2011;32: 1769–1777.

58. Proctor RA, von Eiff C, Kahl BC *et al*. Small colony variants: a pathogenic form of bacteria that facilitates persistent and recurrent infections. *Nature Rev* 2006;4:295–305.

59. Colmenero JD, Morata P, Ruiz-Mesa JD *et al*. Multiplex real-time polymerase chain reaction: a practical approach for rapid diagnosis of tuberculous and brucellar vertebral osteomyelitis. *Spine* 2010;35: E1392–1396.

60. Sürücüoğlu S, El S, Ural S *et al*. Evaluation of real-time PCR method for rapid diagnosis of brucellosis with different clinical manifestations. *Pol J Microbiol* 2009;58:15–19.

61. Landais C, Fenollar F, Constantin A *et al*. Q fever osteoarticular infection: four new cases and a review of the literature. *Eur J Clin Microbiol Infect Dis* 2007;26:341–347.

62. Hajjaji N, Hocqueloux L, Kerdraon R, Bret L. Bone infection in cat-scratch disease: a review of the literature. *J Infect* 2007;54:417–421.

63. Abgueguen P, Pichard E, Aubry J. Buruli ulcer or *Mycobacterium ulcerans* infection. *Med Mal Infect* 2010;40:60–69.

64. Uçkay I, Ferry T, Stern R *et al*. Use of serum antistreptolysin O titers in the microbial diagnosis of orthopedic infections. *Int J Infect Dis* 2009;13: 421–424.

65. Uçkay I, Teterycz D, Ferry T *et al*. Poor utility of MRSA screening to predict staphylococcal species in orthopaedic implant infections. *J Hosp Infect* 2009; 73:89–91.

66. Grayson ML, Gibbons GW, Balogh K, Levin E, Karchmer AW. Probing to bone in infected pedal ulcers. A clinical sign of underlying osteomyelitis in diabetic patients. *JAMA* 1995;273:721–723.

67. Mackowiak PA, Jones SR, Smith JW. Diagnostic value of sinus-tract cultures in chronic osteomyelitis. *JAMA* 1978;239:2772–2775.

68. Darbellay P, Uçkay I, Dominguez D *et al*. Diabetic foot infection: a multidisciplinary approach. *Rev Med Suisse* 2011;7:894–897.

69. Salvana J, Rodner C, Browner BD, Livingston K, Schreiber J, Pesanti E. Chronic osteomyelitis: results obtained by an integrated team approach to management. *Conn Med* 2005;69:195–202.

70. Carek PJ, Dickerson LM, Sack JL. Diagnosis and management of osteomyelitis. *Am Fam Phys* 2001; 63:2413–2420.

71. Mader JT, Shirtliff ME, Bergquist SC, Calhoun J. Antimicrobial treatment of chronic osteomyelitis. *Clin Orthop Rel Res* 1999;360:47–65.

72. Kumar S, O'Donnell ME, Khan K, Dunne G, Carey PD, Lee J. Successful treatment of perineal necrotising fasciitis and associated pubic bone osteomyelitis with the vacuum assisted closure system. *World J Surg Oncol* 2008;6:67.

73. Lack W, McKinley T. Marjolin's ulcer: incidental diagnosis of squamous cell carcinoma on hemipelvectomy for recalcitrant pelvic osteomyelitis. *Iowa Orthop J* 2010;30:174–176.

74. Berendt AR. Counterpoint: hyperbaric oxygen for diabetic foot wounds is not effective. *Clin Infect Dis* 2006;43:193–198.

75. Andel H, Felfernig M, Andel D, Blaicher W, Schramm W. Hyperbaric oxygen therapy in osteomyelitis. *Anaesthesia* 1998;53:68–69.

76. Martini M, Adjrad A, Boudjemaa A. Tuberculous osteomyelitis. A review of 125 cases. *Int Orthop* 1986;10:201–207.

77. Uçkay I, Bouchuiguir-Wafa K, Ninet B *et al*. Post-traumatic ankle arthritis due to a novel *Nocardia* species. *Infection* 2010;38:407–412.

78. Trampuz A, Zimmerli W. Antimicrobial agents in orthopaedic surgery: Prophylaxis and treatment. *Drugs* 2006;66:1089–1105.

79. Haidar R, Der Boghossian A, Atiyeh B. Duration of post-surgical antibiotics in chronic osteomyelitis: empiric or evidence-based? *Int J Infect Dis* 2010;14: e752–758.

80. Matthews PC, Conlon CP, Berendt AR *et al*. Outpatient parenteral antimicrobial therapy (OPAT): is it safe for selected patients to self-administer at home? A retrospective analysis of a large cohort over 13 years. *J Antimicrob Chemother* 2007;60:356–362.

81. Uçkay I, Lew DP. Infections in skeletal prostheses. In: Jarvis WR, Brachmann PS, Bennett JV (eds). *Bennett & Brachman's Hospital Infections*, 5th edn. Philadelphia: Lippincott, Williams & Wilkins, 2007, p. 39.

82. Bernard L, Legout L, Zurcher-Pfund L *et al*. Six weeks of antibiotic treatment is sufficient following surgery for septic arthroplasty. *J Infect* 2010;61:125–132.

83. Daver NG, Shelburne SA, Atmar RL *et al*. Oral step-down therapy is comparable to intravenous therapy for *Staphylococcus aureus* osteomyelitis. *J Infect* 2007; 54:539–544.

84. Uçkay I, Lustig S *et al*. *Hospital and community-acquired methicillin-resistant Staphylococcus aureus bone and joint infections. Methicillin-resistant Staphylococcus aureus.* New York: Nova Science Publishers, Inc, 2009.

85. Toma MB, Smith KM, Martin CA, Rapp RP. Pharmacokinetic considerations in the treatment of methicillin-resistant *Staphylococcus aureus* osteomyelitis. *Orthopedics* 2006;29:497–501.

86. Al-Nammari SS, Lucas JD, Lam KS. Hematogenous methicillin-resistant *Staphylococcus aureus* spondylodiscitis. *Spine* 2007;32:2480–2486.

87. Roblot F, Besnier JM, Juhel L *et al*. Optimal duration of antibiotic therapy in vertebral osteomyelitis. *Semin Arthritis Rheum* 2007;36:269–277.

88. Sendi P, Bregenzer T, Zimmerli W. Spinal epidural abscess in clinical practice. *QJM* 2008;101:1–12.

89. Vartanians VM, Karchmer AW, Giurini JM, Rosenthal DI. Is there a role for imaging in the management of patients with diabetic foot? *Skeletal Radiol* 2009;38:633–636.

90. Berendt AR, Peters EJ, Bakker K *et al*. Diabetic foot osteomyelitis: a progress report on diagnosis and a systematic review of treatment. *Diabetes Metab Res Rev* 2008;24 (Suppl 1):S145–S161.

91. Valabhji J, Oliver N, Samarasinghe D, Mali T, Gibbs RG, Gedroyc WM. Conservative management of diabetic forefoot ulceration complicated by underlying osteomyelitis: the benefits of magnetic resonance imaging. *Diabet Med* 2009;26:1127–1134.

92. Game FL, Jeffcoate WJ. Primarily non-surgical management of osteomyelitis of the foot in diabetes. *Diabetologia* 2008;51:962–967.

93. Lavery LA, Peters EJ, Armstrong DG, Wendel CS, Murdoch DP, Lipsky BA. Risk factors for developing osteomyelitis in patients with diabetic foot wounds. *Diabetes Res Clin Pract* 2009;83:347–352.

94. Lipsky BA. A report from the international consensus on diagnosing and treating the infected diabetic foot. *Diabetes Metab Res Rev* 2004;20 (Suppl):S68–S77.

95. Rao N, Crossett LS, Sinha RK, Le Frock JL. Long-term suppression of infection in total joint arthroplasty. *Clin Orthop Related Res* 2003;414:55–60.

96. Trampuz A, Zimmerli W. Diagnosis and treatment of infections associated with fracture-fixation devices. *Injury* 2006;37 (Suppl 2):S59–S66.

97. Al-Tawfiq JA. *Bacteroides fragilis* bacteremia associated with vertebral osteomyelitis in a sickle cell patient. *Intern Med* 2008;47:2183–2185.

98. Hernigou P, Daltro G, Flouzat-Lachaniette CH, Roussignol X, Poignard A. Septic arthritis in adults with sickle cell disease often is associated with osteomyelitis or osteonecrosis. *Clin Orthop Rel Res* 2010;468:1676–1681.

99. Yao Y, Sturdevant DE, Villaruz A, Xu L, Gao Q, Otto M. Factors characterizing *Staphylococcus epidermidis* invasiveness determined by comparative genomics. *Infect Immun* 2005;73:1856–1860.

100. Balaban N, Giacometti A, Cirioni O *et al*. Use of the quorum-sensing inhibitor RNAIII-inhibiting peptide to prevent biofilm formation in vivo by drug-resistant *Staphylococcus epidermidis*. *J Infect Dis* 2003;187:625–630.

101. Nakamoto DA, Rosenfield ML, Haaga JR *et al*. Young Investigator Award. *In vivo* treatment of infected prosthetic graft material with urokinase: an animal model. *J Vasc Interv Radiol* 1994;5:549–552.

102. Cerca N, Oliveira R, Azeredo J. Susceptibility of *Staphylococcus epidermidis* planktonic cells and biofilms to the lytic action of staphylococcus bacteriophage K. *Lett Appl Microbiol* 2007;45:313–317.

103. Carmen JC, Roeder BL, Nelson JL *et al*. Ultrasonically enhanced vancomycin activity against *Staphylococcus epidermidis* biofilms *in vivo*. *J Biomater Appl* 2004;18:237–245.

104. van der Borden AJ, van der Mei HC, Busscher HJ. Electric block current induced detachment from surgical stainless steel and decreased viability of *Staphylococcus epidermidis*. *Biomaterials* 2005;26:6731–6735.

PART II
Radiological Imaging

CHAPTER 3

Radiological Imaging of Osteomyelitis

Jenny T. Bencardino[1], Zoraida Restrepo-Velez[1], Randall Bujan[2] and Diego Jaramillo[3]

[1]NYU Hospital for Joint Diseases, New York, NY, USA
[2]Don Bosco Radiologic Clinic, San Jose, Costa Rica
[3]Children's Hospital of Philadelphia, University of Pennsylvania, Philadelphia, PA, USA

Introduction

The most common presentation of musculoskeletal infection is acute hematogenous osteomyelitis [1]. Its incidence has been calculated to be as high as 1 per 5000 [2]. More than 50% of cases of osteomyelitis involve children younger than 5 years of age, with 70% of these involving the lower extremities, predominantly the knee [2]. Methicillin-resistant *Staphylococcus aureus* (MRSA) is responsible for almost 30% of the cases in children [3]. The incidence of osteomyelitis appears to have nearly tripled over the past 20 years [4] whereas that of septic arthritis has remained stable.

Basic knowledge of the clinical problem

Hematogenous osteomyelitis classically results from seeding of bacteria in the metaphysis of a long bone or in the metaphyseal equivalents of the axial skeleton. *S. aureus* is usually involved. This microorganism travels through the bloodstream from the skin or mucosal membranes to areas of bone where blood is abundant and its flow slow. In immature skeletons, the metaphyses are richly vascularized and the sinusoidal loops of the metaphyseal venules have discontinuous epithelium, facilitating inva-

sion by microorganisms. *S. aureus*, in particular, has the capacity to adhere to the osseous matrix, releasing proteolytic enzymes that cause tissue destruction and allow further spread of the infection. From the medullary cavity, the infection extends into the subperiosteal space. In children, the periosteum is loosely attached to the bone, allowing accumulation of purulent collections. In cases where the elevation of the periosteum has been rapid, devascularization of the bone may occur, leading to associated septic osteonecrosis.

Metaphyseal equivalent locations are defined as portions of a flat or irregular bone that are adjacent to cartilage, including apophyseal growth plates, articular cartilage and fibrocartilage [5]. A metaphyseal type of vascularity is also seen in the periphery of round bones and secondary ossification centers. The most frequently involved metaphyseal equivalents are the ilium, vertebrae, greater trochanter and ischium. In the round bones, such as the talus and calcaneus, metaphyseal equivalents are located in the periphery of the bone. During infancy, the spread of infection from the metaphysis into the epiphysis is facilitated by the presence of transphyseal vessels [6]. Destruction of the epiphysis and damage to the adjacent joint are commonplace in infantile osteomyelitis.

Diagnostic Imaging of Infections and Inflammatory Diseases: A Multidisciplinary Approach, First Edition. Edited by Alberto Signore and Ana María Quintero.

Nevertheless, direct spread is not a common route of spread in septic arthritis. More frequently, the latter occurs as a result of hematogenous seeding of the synovium.

Trauma is a common predisposing factor for osteomyelitis as the formation of a hematoma may predispose to bacterial colonization. Other implied etiological factors include urinary tract infection, immunodeficiency and other pre-existing diseases [7].

Panton–Valentine leukocidin (PVL) gene-encoding organisms, primarily seen in MRSA infections, are associated with a higher erythrocyte sedimentation rate (ESR), C-reactive protein (CRP) concentration and frequency of positive blood cultures. Infections with PVL bacteria also have a greater prevalence of associated subperiosteal abscesses, myositis and pyomyositis [8]. It is important to remember that the high success rates of antimicrobial therapy depend on early diagnosis, including with bone sampling for microbiological and pathological examination [9].

In neonates, *Escherichia coli*, Enterobacteriaceae, Group B streptococci, other Gram-negative rods and *Candida albicans* can cause osteomyelitis, which is often multifocal and frequently extends into the epiphysis [10]. In Europe and Israel, *Kingella kingae*, an organism diagnosed primarily with polymerase chain reaction (PCR), is being detected with increasing frequency in children with osteomyelitis and is now the most prevalent bacteria in some series [11]. It is seen in children younger than 5 years of age, often involves the epiphyseal cartilage and is highly responsive to antibiotics. In recent years, a rise (up to 70%) has been reported in the association of community-acquired (CA) *S. aureus* osteomyelitis with subperiosteal abscess, pyomyositis, deep venous thrombosis and septic arthritis, all conditions that likely require surgical intervention [12]. A likely contributing factor is the simultaneous rise of CA-MRSA (see Chapter 1), which now accounts for 30–40% of cases of osteomyelitis. Browne and Arnold independently reported rates of surgery greater than 90% in patients with CA-MRSA [12,13]. A recent study suggests four clinical predictors for MRSA: temperature of greater than 38°C, hematocrit of less than 34%, white blood cell count of greater than 12 000 cells/µL and C-reactive protein level of greater than 1.3 mg/dL. The probability of MRSA osteomyelitis was 92% for

all four predictors, 45% for three, 10% for two and 1% for one [14].

The clinical questions

Recovery of the microorganism from a focus of osteomyelitis or a positive blood culture in a patient with clinical and radiographic findings consistent with infection often allows a definitive diagnosis of osteomyelitis [15]. Established osteomyelitis typically produces an elevated ESR in the range of 30–50 mm/h as well as a leukocytosis between 12 and 15 000/µL [16]. There is an increasing trend to rely on the CRP level, as its elevation precedes that of the ESR, usually within a day of the beginning of the infection [10]. CRP values may also help with the recognition of complications as thresholds of 3.6 mg/dL and 6 mg/dL have been established for the presence of subperiosteal abscesses and deep venous thrombosis, respectively [17,18].

Diagnostic imaging is a very important tool in the clinical armamentarium for the determination of the extent of disease. In a recent paper, a trend in patients with immature skeletons was noted for increased involvement of the non-ossified, cartilaginous, epiphyseal ossification centers [19]. More frequent extraosseous involvement and surgical indications are indicators that the diagnostic imaging of osteomyelitis should not be confined to the assessment of the bone, but should extend to the cartilaginous structures, surrounding soft tissues and adjacent vessels.

Pelvic osteomyelitis may be subtle. In children, it typically involves metaphyseal equivalents, which include the triradiate cartilage, pubic symphysis, ischiopubic synchondrosis, iliac apophysis and bone adjacent to the sacroiliac joints [20,21]. Magnetic resonance imaging (MRI) is particularly useful in this condition because of the complex pelvic geometry, which limits the detection of the disease on conventional radiographs. Also, the prevalence of associated soft tissue abnormalities is high [22]. In patients with acute hip pain and a clinical picture suggestive of infection, but negative joint fluid, pelvic MRI often yields the diagnosis of osteomyelitis or pyomyositis [23].

Postsurgical septic arthritis has been reported in as many as 3.9% of shoulder arthroplasties and less than 1% of unconstrained systems [24,25]. Infections may present any time from months to years after the surgery. In the last two decades, with improvements in operative technique and infection control, acute post-arthroplasty infection has significantly decreased; however, the rate of delayed infections has remained stubbornly constant. Diagnosing infected hardware may be difficult based on clinical findings [26]. An infected joint arthroplasty often requires surgical removal, with current options including a two-stage procedure, debridement and retention of the prosthesis, or a Girdlestone arthroplasty. In two-stage procedures, the use of beads and antibiotic-laden cement spacers has lowered infection rates [27]. Open debridement and retention of the prosthesis may be best suited to the treatment of an acute infection in the early postoperative period or of an acute hematogenous infection at the site of a secure and functional prosthesis [28]. Removal of a joint prosthesis because of infection with the Girdlestone procedure may leave a patient with a functional disability. Studies have shown a considerable rate of complications related to reimplantation after Girdlestone arthroplasty [29,30]. In a series of 44 patients undergoing reimplantation after a Girdlestone procedure, 98% were free of infection, but 11% had subsequent dislocations and 39% had a persistent limp [30]. Amputations may be necessary in cases of chronically infected total joint prosthesis, which may cause recalcitrant pain and a draining sinus tract.

Although hematogenous spread is the most common cause of osteomyelitis in most areas of the body, contiguous spread and direct implantation are more common in the ankle and foot [31]. The majority of osteomyelitis in diabetic feet occurs through contiguous soft tissue spread of infection from adjacent ulceration [31,32]. Foot-related complications requiring hospitalization have been reported in up to 15–20% of diabetics at some point in their lives [33]. The diabetic foot is the main reason for non-traumatic lower extremity amputations, which are 15–40 times more common in diabetics as compared to non-diabetics. After pedal amputation, the incidence of contralateral foot amputation within 2 years is as high as 50%. This reflects the systemic nature of the disease, but also appears to be related to the shift in weight bearing affecting the contralateral extremity. As a result, treatment of pedal osteomyelitis has switched over the past decade to ulcer prevention/care and revascularization procedures. Once infection is sus-

pected, aggressive medical and surgical management is instituted. Surgical care includes debridement of devascularized tissue and a partial, foot-sparing amputation intended to preserve functionality [34].

Methodological considerations

Recent imaging advances have changed the diagnostic approach to osteomyelitis. First, whole body MRI can now detect multifocal disease or abnormalities that are not well localized [25,35,36]. There is less of an advantage in using scintigraphy for those cases in whom there may be disseminated disease or in whom there are no focal symptoms. Growing concern about exposing children to radiation has led to the increasing substitution of MRI and sonography for scintigraphy and computed tomography (CT). Also, a significant percentage of cases of MRSA present with soft tissue findings and decreased vascularization, both of which are better depicted by MRI [16]. Finally, MRI has become more readily available, even on an emergency basis. In summary, there are increasing reasons to use MRI as the second imaging modality of choice after radiographs, using whole body MRI sequences when there is a suspicion of multifocal disease or in infants, when it is difficult to ascertain the location of the disease.

In peripheral and diabetic pedal infections, radiographs are insensitive to osteomyelitis in its early stages and cannot determine the extent of involvement of osseous or soft tissue disease. Radiographic findings are often delayed by as much as 2 weeks. Therefore, whether positive or negative, generally additional imaging is necessary. CT provides better definition than radiographs and can detect abscess formation (when contrast is used) as well as periostitis and cortical erosion, but it remains limited in determining the extent of involvement within the bone as well as in the soft tissues. Ultrasound may target areas for aspiration by detecting focal pockets of fluid collection in the subperiosteal space or soft tissue, as well as joint or tenosynovial effusion.

Multiple articles in the orthopedic and radiological literature have documented the use of MRI in the evaluation of osteomyelitis. Sensitivity ranges from 77% to 100% and specificity from 79% to 100% in large studies. Superimposed factors, such as prior surgery, neuropathic arthropathy and associated rheumatoid arthritis, may lower the specificity of

MRI. Regarding the use of gadolinium in MRI, some studies recommend intravenous contrast [37], whereas others consider it not to be necessary [38]. It remains controversial whether the addition of a contrast-enhanced sequence improves the accuracy of MRI for the diagnosis of osteomyelitis. However, it is not disputed that contrast enhancement improves detection of soft tissue infection [39]. It differentiates cellulitis from diabetic soft tissue edema and improves evaluation of the extent of the soft tissue disease. It helps detect sinus tracts and abscesses [39] and it is the only way to delineate areas of devitalization and necrosis [40].

Changes related to ischemia should be taken into account when interpreting MRI of the diabetic foot. Devitalized tissue typically presents as focal or regional lack of soft tissue contrast enhancement with sharp margins and increased enhancement in the surrounding soft tissues representing hypervascular tissue [41]. Only contrast-enhanced imaging allows reliable recognition of gangrene because the signal changes on T1- and T2-weighted images (T1WIs and T2WIs) are not characteristic. Soft tissue air, seen as small foci of signal void, is not specific as it may be identified within areas of devitalization without superimposed infection, typically related to overlying skin ulceration.

Normal findings and artifacts

Osteomyelitis typically spreads hematogenously in children and directly in the skeletally mature population without premorbid conditions. Radiographs are routinely used as a first-step imaging tool to rule out potential bone infection. Cortical and trabecular integrity can be evaluated using radiographs as established osteomyelitis will often have caused permeative bone destruction with associated periosteal reaction. Early osteomyelitis, however, can easily be missed on radiographs as reactive marrow edema and periostitis can easily go undetected. In patients with a clinical picture strongly suggestive of osteomyelitis with negative radiographic findings, MRI is indicated as a reliable imaging tool. The normal MR appearance of bone marrow has been extensively described in the radiological literature. Hematopoietic and fatty marrow are in dynamic relation to each other following an orderly progression from birth to advanced age with a wide range of normal. At birth, hematopoietic marrow predominates;

fatty marrow then progressively replaces the epiphysis and diaphysis of long bones, leaving the metaphysis with islands of hematopoietic marrow that may persist into adulthood.

Prominence of hematopoietic marrow deposits or diffuse hematopoietic marrow reconversion is characterized by the presence of hypercellular marrow in the axial skeleton and by expansion of hematopoietic marrow in the appendicular skeleton (marrow reconversion). It can be idiopathic, mainly occurring in middle-aged obese women, or can be seen in heavy smokers and athletes, mainly long distance runners. The process is similar to what occurs in response to forceful stimuli that elicit the production of red cells, including chemotherapy, chronic infection and chronic anemia. On T1WIs, hematopoietic marrow is associated with decreased signal intensity within the medullary cavity, similar to the muscle signal. On fluid-sensitive sequences, the hematopoietic marrow signal is of low-to-intermediate intensity. With contrast, signal intensity enhancement is moderate. It is important to keep in mind that marrow reconversion in the appendicular skeleton can present as ominous regenerating red marrow nodules that can simulate areas of marrow replacement as seen in osteomyelitis. This problem can be particularly challenging in patients with sickle cell anemia or thalassemia who are also prone to have osteomyelitis. The authors find it particularly useful to assess for an abnormal T2 bright signal in the setting of infection, as well as ring enhancement in subacute osteomyelitis and associated soft tissue findings such as soft tissue abscess and sinus tract.

Postoperative MRI presents unique challenges as fixation devices used in orthopedic surgery may contain metal and instruments used at the time of surgery can leave metal shavings behind. This metal can result in large areas of magnetic field inhomogeneity, local gradient-induced eddy currents on metal surfaces and radiofrequency (RF) shielding effects [42,43]. Of these factors, metal-induced field inhomogeneities result in the most severe artifacts. Knowledge of these artifacts and techniques used to reduce them have become essential. Factors to consider in MRI of patients with metallic fixation hardware or arthroplasty include the composition of the hardware, orientation of the hardware in relation to the direction of the main magnetic field (B_0), type of pulse sequence, strength of the magnetic field and MRI parameters (voxel size, field of view, image matrix and slice thickness). Ferromagnetic materials, which have high magnetic susceptibility, produce greater artifacts than titanium alloys. Magnetic field inhomogeneities change the phase and frequency of local spins. The result is mis-registration and loss of signal, resulting in distortion of the shape of the metallic object predominantly along the frequency axis. It is important, thus, to swap phase and frequency direction when required, so as not to obscure the area of pathology. The radiologist cannot control for the type of metal; however, certain changes in the imaging protocol can help reduce the degree of artifact. Whenever possible, the hardware should be positioned parallel to the main magnetic field. Turbo or fast spin echo (TSE or FSE) sequences should always be chosen and gradient echo sequences avoided. This is because the multiple 180° refocusing pulses help reduce the amount of field inhomogeneity and distortion. The lowest inter-echo spacing should be achieved so as to minimize the time between the 180° pulses. This can be achieved, at the expense of signal, by increasing (in most cases doubling) the bandwidth, which reduces the frequency sampling time and makes it possible to reduce the echo time (TE). Using longer echo trains, a high-resolution matrix and decreased sliced thickness can also help. If fat suppression is required, inversion recovery sequences are preferred to frequency selective fat saturation sequences which rely on field homogeneity.

Pathological findings and significance

Osteomyelitis

Conventional radiography
Conventional radiography is insensitive in the diagnosis of osteomyelitis, but it is often the first imaging modality performed in the assessment of this condition. Only 20% of cases have abnormal radiographic findings by the second week of disease [44]. Nevertheless, radiographs may help exclude other pathologies such as traumatic injuries and neoplasms [45]. If positive, however, radiographs can be a very useful tool in the follow-up of osteomyelitis. Focal areas of osteolysis are typically apparent only 7–10 days after the onset of symptoms. Earlier changes in the deep soft tissues may occasionally be radiographically apparent, as well as later find-

ings such as visible elevation of the periosteum (Figure 3.1).

MR imaging
MRI has become the principal imaging modality for bone infections. The main clinical questions concern the presence of bone involvement and soft tissue collections that may require drainage. MR fluid-sensitive sequences, such as fat-suppressed T2W and short tau inversion recovery (STIR), can easily detect early changes of inflammatory edema radiating from the focus of disease to the adjacent marrow, periosteum and soft tissues. In the appendicular skeleton, the preferred sites of bone involvement include the metaphysis of long bones, and in the axial skeleton, the metaphyseal equivalents [20]. Detection of an associated purulent collection or abscess as well as a draining sinus is facilitated by the use of contrast-enhanced MRI. These collections will typically appear with a non-enhancing T1 hypointense center surrounded by a halo of enhancing tissue (Figure 3.2). Small collections that are less than a few centimeters in size typically respond to antibiotic therapy, while large abscesses need to be drained. The decision to intervene is based on the clinical response as much as on the volume of the collection.

MRI is the most sensitive (approaching 100%) of all imaging methods for diagnosing osteomyelitis and has a high specificity (>81%) in most series. Fat-suppressed, contrast-enhanced MRI significantly increases the specificity (93%) in the diagnosis of osteomyelitis when compared with three-phase bone scintigraphy, and has a higher specificity than non-enhanced MRI, particularly in complicated cases [37]. It also increases the confidence in the diagnosis of drainable fluid collections. Despite the relatively high sensitivity and specificity of MRI, it may still be non-specific. The abnormal marrow signal may be seen in trauma or tumor. However, fluid-sensitive sequences have the highest sensitivity (96%) and negative predictive value, and thus can be used to screen patients suspected of having osteomyelitis. In subacute osteomyelitis, the lesions have a characteristic ring-like configuration (Brodie's abscess; see Figure 3.5); there is a peripheral rind of enhancing granulation tissue that is attempting to wall-off the infection and which is markedly contrast avid. The periphery of the abscess may demonstrate low signal intensity on T2WIs

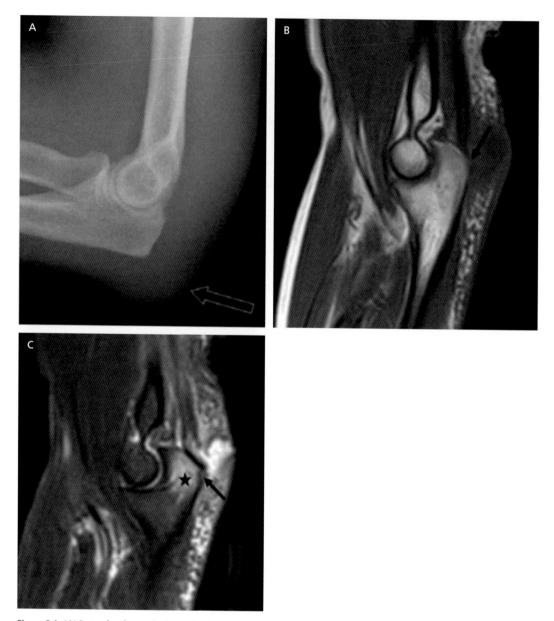

Figure 3.1 (A) Lateral radiograph shows focal cortical irregularity on the olecranon (arrow) and bursal soft tissue swelling. (B) Sagittal T1WI shows an infected olecranon bursitis. Note the early olecranon cortical erosion (arrow) without associated T1 hypointense marrow edema. (C) Sagittal fat-suppressed FSE T2WI shows focal cortical erosion (arrow) and reactive marrow edema (asterisk) connecting to the overlying infectious bursitis.

and the internal content tends to be homogeneously bright. In chronic osteomyelitis, dead infected tissue becomes sequestered within areas of lytic destruction of bone with a sclerotic margin, the so-called sequestrum within cloacae. The sequestered bone typically demonstrates low signal intensity on all pulse sequences if associated with infectious osteonecrosis, while the cloacae may be filled with bright fluid like the signal on T2WIs.

Osteomyelitis in children and young adults must be differentiated from normal hematopoietic marrow deposits typically located in the metaphyses of long bones and the metaphyseal equivalents of the axial skeleton. In general, the signal intensity

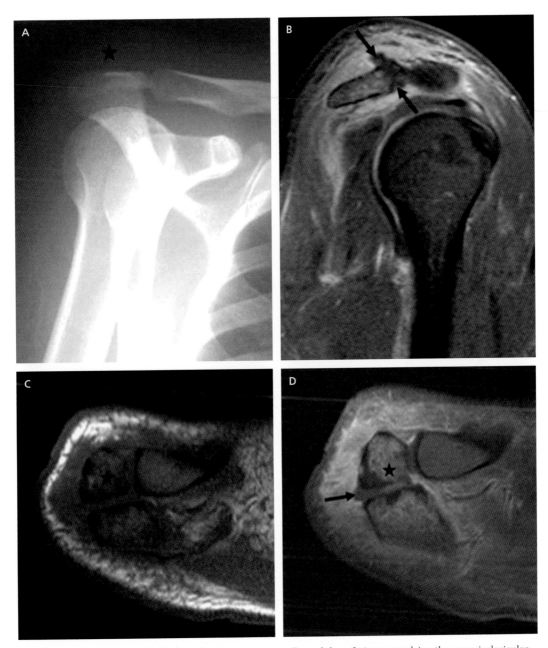

Figure 3.2 (A) Scapular view of the shoulder demonstrates swelling of the soft tissues overlying the acromioclavicular joint (asterisk). (B) Oblique sagittal fat-suppressed T1WI following intravenous contrast injection shows a discrete fluid collection with an enhancing thick wall (arrows) and marked periarticular inflammatory changes. (C,D) Axial pre-contrast T1 and axial post-contrast fat-suppressed T1 images show marrow replacement and cortical erosive changes at the interface between the secondary ossification center of the acromion (asterisk = os acromiale) and the acromial process with interposed non-enhancing purulent fluid (D, arrow).

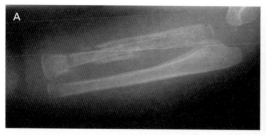
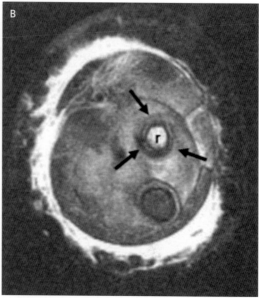

Figure 3.3 (A) Lateral view of the forearm in a 4-year-old boy with *Salmonella* osteomyelitis demonstrates extensive periosteal reaction along the radial shaft associated with obliteration of the soft tissue planes. (B) Axial FSE T2WI shows replacement of the marrow cavity of the radius (r) by intensely bright T2 signal associated with periosteal elevation (arrows), in keeping with acute osteomyelitis. Note the marked edema and swelling of all muscle compartments of the forearm as well as the deep subcutaneous fluid collection.

of normal hematopoietic marrow should be equal to or higher than that of muscle on T1WIs. The hematopoietic marrow deposits tend to be symmetrically distributed when compared to the contralateral side. Stress reaction and fractures may present as ill-defined areas of marrow edema without significant associated soft tissue changes. A helpful distinguishing feature of osteomyelitis is the extensive reactive inflammatory changes in the adjacent soft tissues (Figure 3.3). Bone neoplasms and osteomyelitis may also mimic each other. In general, a primary bone neoplasm manifests as a focal lesion with discrete margins replacing the bone marrow on T1W sequences. A very useful distinguishing feature between osteomyelitis and other bone marrow replacing processes is the presence of entrapped fat globules within the area of infection, whether in the medullary cavity, subperiosteal space or adjacent soft tissues. It is hypothesized that increased intramedullary pressure leads to fatty marrow necrosis with release of free fatty globules. Fat globules are more common in pubertal and post-pubertal children compared to prepubertal children [46]. Although not pathognomonic, the presence of fatty globules within the area of

suspected infection supports the diagnosis of osteomyelitis over neoplasm [47].

The controversy regarding intravenous gadolinium administration in the setting of osteomyelitis has led to the institution of protocols that involve contrast only after the MR study has been checked by a radiologist. If the water-sensitive sequences are normal, no contrast injection is required [48,49]. The exception to this rule would be a focal abscess involving the epiphyseal cartilage only. In this case, the abscess may be masked on fluid-sensitive sequences by the adjacent T2 bright cartilage [18]. In general, if the water-sensitive sequences are abnormal, contrast-enhanced MR images have been demonstrated to increase the diagnostic confidence of abscesses and sinus tracts, allowing a treatment decision with regards to aspiration and drainage procedures (Figure 3.4) [50].

Associated extraosseous complications, such as subperiosteal/soft tissue abscess formation, pyomyositis, deep venous thrombosis and septic arthritis, have become more prevalent in recent years [12]. This trend seems to be associated with the rise in CA-MRSA infections, which now account for 30–40% of cases of osteomyelitis [13]. The rate of

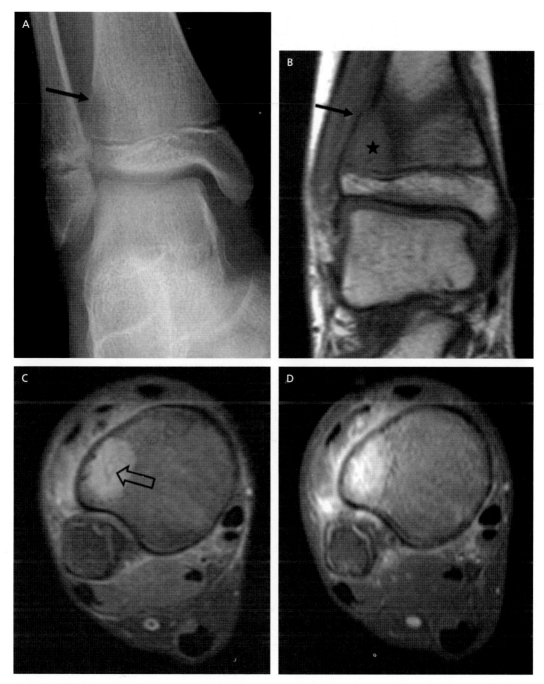

Figure 3.4 (A) Plain radiograph showing a subtle lucency (arrow) in the lateral aspect of the metaphysis in a child with right ankle pain of 2 weeks' duration. (B) Coronal T1WI shows focal cortical permeation of the distal lateral tibia (arrow) and a focus of abnormal marrow hypointensity abutting the physis (asterisk). (C,D) Axial fat-suppressed FSE T2WI and axial contrast-enhanced fat-suppressed T1WI demonstrate a discrete area of abnormal T2 hyperintensity and post-contrast enhancement in the right anterolateral distal tibial metaphysis, respectively. Note the central ring of hypointensity likely representing a Brodie's abscess (C, arrow). (E) Percutaneous fluoroscopically-guided needle aspiration of the abscess was performed with good clinical outcome.

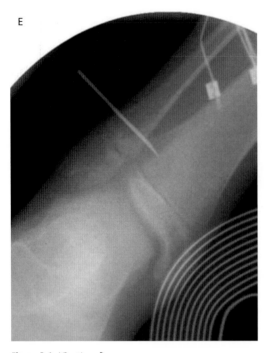

E

Figure 3.4 *(Continued)*

surgical intervention is greater than 90% in cases with CA-MRSA [12,13].

Another alarming trend is the increasing involvement of the cartilaginous epiphysis in younger patients [15]. Most of these complications require prompt surgical intervention in order to prevent spread of disease, permanent structural deformity and septicemia. MRI is the best radiological modality as it allows evaluation not only of the bone but also of the cartilaginous structures, surrounding soft tissues and adjacent vessels.

Chronic osteomyelitis is characterized by extensive peripheral reactive changes in an attempt to wall-off the area of infection. As described above, the hallmark presentation of chronic osteomyelitis is a Brodie's abscess, which is characterized by a focal area of central lysis surrounded by a well-defined, enhancing inner border, and a hazy, ill-defined and broader halo of marrow edema and sclerosis (Figure 3.5) [51]. A less well-contained focus of osteomyelitis can develop a central ossific necrotic focus or sequestrum, surrounded by pus and in turn walled off by reactive bone or involucrum (Figure 3.6). Sclerosing chronic osteomyelitis

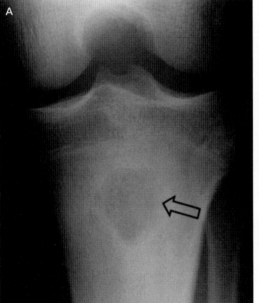
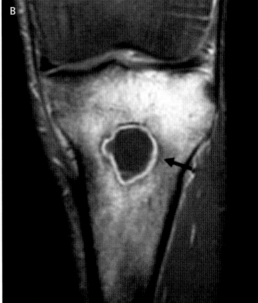

Figure 3.5 (A) Anteroposterior view of the knee in a 27-year-old male patient shows a lucent lesion with reactive sclerotic margins within the medullary cavity of the right proximal tibia (arrow). (B) Coronal fat-suppressed contrast-enhanced T1WI shows a central lesion with an enhanced rim and with extensive reactive marrow edema compatible with a Brodie's abscess (arrow).

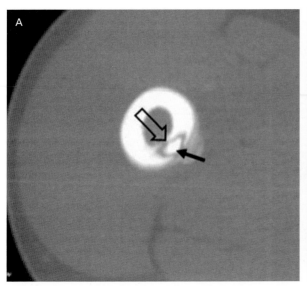 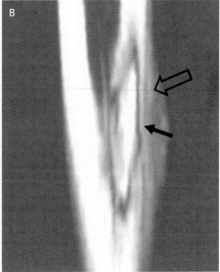

Figure 3.6 (A,B) Axial CT image and coronal 2D reformatted image of the right femur demonstrates a focal area of intracortical necrosis compatible with a sequestrum (black arrow) outlined by a lucent area in keeping with the involucrum (open arrow).

is a variant in which the bone is uniformly dense. *S. aureus* is the most common pathogen in chronic osteomyelitis with the tibia being the most commonly affected bone. Based on radiographs it is difficult to determine whether a chronic infection is active.

Ultrasound

Ultrasound (US) has been advocated as the imaging modality that may be able to resolve early changes of osteomyelitis that manifest as early periosteal thickening with associated juxtacortical soft tissue swelling. The sensitivity of US in the diagnosis of osteomyelitis has been reported to be between 46% and 53% and the specificity 63–100% [52,53]. Power and color Doppler imaging may help outline areas of hyperemia due to early inflammatory changes [54,55]. US may be particularly valuable in the diagnosis of early subperiosteal and soft tissue abscess formation (Figure 3.7). Elevation of the periosteum is easily identified on sonographic images as a distinct echogenic line displaced away from the underlying cortex by a complex fluid collection of mixed echogenicity [56]. The perichondrium is the site of attachment of the periosteum to the growth plate. A subperiosteal collection invariably elevates the periosteum to the level of its tight

perichondral attachment to the growth plate. In advanced cases, sonography may also show focal cortical destruction. However, this technique has poor sensitivity for the diagnosis of intraosseous pathology and thus is only of limited application.

CT imaging

CT is not considered a primary imaging modality in the diagnosis of osteomyelitis.

However, patients with pelvic osteomyelitis presenting clinically with pelvic pain may undergo a CT to exclude abdominopelvic pathology. In these cases, it is important to search for evidence of involvement of the soft tissue structures of the pelvic cavity and indirect clues to bone infection [20]. In addition, identification of the involucrum and sequestrum in patients with chronic osteomyelitis is facilitated by multiplanar CT reconstructions.

Imaging of complications

Most uncomplicated osteomyelitis responds to antibiotic therapy and less than 5% of patients develop chronic infections. Delays in the initiation of antibiotic therapy of more than 4 days lead to a significant increase in the likelihood of sequelae, which include deformity and reduced function [57]. In

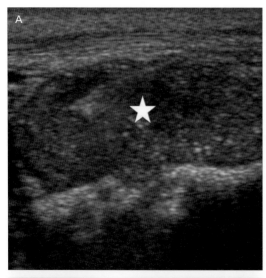

Figure 3.7 (A) Longitudinal sonographic image obtained along the dorsolateral aspect of the hindfoot at the site of palpable abnormality shows a complex fluid collection with posterior acoustic enhancement compatible with an abscess (asterisk). (B,C) Sagittal T1WI of the hindfoot demonstrating septic arthritis of the talonavicular joint with osteomyelitis of the talar head (t) and neck as well as navicular (n) associated with a focal soft tissue abscess.

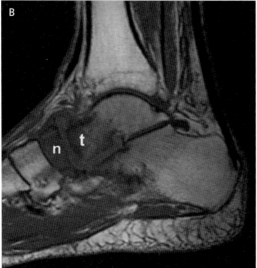

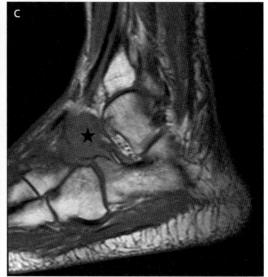

chronic osteomyelitis, a relatively small focus of disease may elicit a strong host bone reaction with a sclerotic zone attempting to wall-off the infection. Hence, a Brodie's abscess is defined by a necrotic center, a well-defined inner border and a rather ill-defined, hazy, broader outer halo of infection [58]. A less well-contained focus of osteomyelitis can undergo central necrosis (sequestrum), is surrounded by pus and, in turn, is walled off by reactive bone (involucrum). Lastly, chronic osteomyelitis may present as diffuse sclerosis of the affected bone which manifests as increased radiographic density.

Chronic infection is most commonly due to *S. aureus* and most frequently involves the tibia [59]. Determination of active infection in chronic osteomyelitis may be challenging. On MRI, persistence of reactive T2 hyperintense marrow edema and post-gadolinium enhancement are considered suggestive of infection (Figure 3.8). In children, positron emission tomography (PET)/CT appears to be superior to MRI in distinguishing between reparative activity and ongoing chronic infection [60].

Chronic bacterial osteomyelitis must be distinguished from chronic recurrent multifocal

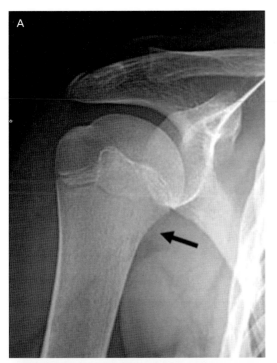

Figure 3.8 (A) Subtle area of periosteal elevation along the medial aspect of the right proximal humeral metaphysis (arrow). (B,C) Following intravenous therapy without adequate medical response, pre- and post-contrast fat-suppressed FSE T2WI and T1WI images demonstrate non-enhancing reactive marrow edema (B, asterisk) with focal lifting of the periosteum by a subperiosteal abscess (C, arrowhead) with reactive periostitis (C, open arrow). The abscess was drained percutaneously with a needle under fluoroscopic guidance. Note the attachment of the perichondrium (C, white arrow).

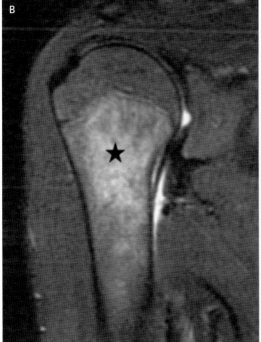

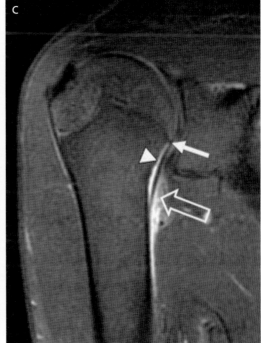

osteomyelitis (CRMO). The latter is a non-bacterial inflammatory multifocal disease that typically affects the metaphysis of long bones and the clavicle [61]. Whole-body MRI is useful in the evaluation of CRMO that demonstrates a pattern of symmetric involvement highly suggestive of this condition [62]. CRMO responds to anti-inflammatory agents rather than antibiotics. Chronic bacterial osteomyelitis should also be differentiated from osteomyelitis caused by atypical organisms such as tuberculosis and *Bartonella henselae* (cat scratch disease) [63].

Prosthetic joint infection

Infection is a painful, potentially fatal condition that can complicate hardware placement and joint replacements. Periprosthetic infections may necessitate removal of hardware if there are signs of septic loosening, component dissociation, or osteomyelitis. Radiographs are often unremarkable in the setting of periprosthetic soft tissue infections. Multidetector CT and the use of a hardware reconstruction algorithm helps to better assess for the presence of focal lytic areas adjacent to the prosthetic components in the setting of hardware-related osteomyelitis. Recently, new metal reduction artifact techniques in high-field MRI magnets have been introduced, including Slice Encoding for Metal Artifact Correction (SEMAC), view-angle tilting (VAT) and multiacquisition variable-resonance image combination (MAVRIC) [64–67]. The SEMAC technique, introduced by Lu and colleagues, is a modified spin echo sequence that uses VAT and slice-direction phase encoding to correct both in-plane and through-plane artifacts. Hargreaves *et al.* found that SEMAC imaging combined with standard echo-train imaging, parallel imaging, partial-Fourier imaging and inversion recovery techniques offered flexible image contrast with reduction of metal-induced artifact in scan times of under 11 minutes [68]. With the MAVRIC technique, multiple three-dimensional FSE image datasets are acquired at different frequency bands, offset from the dominant proton frequency and the images combined, resulting in decreased susceptibility artifact [64]. Chen *et al.* evaluated SEMAC and MAVRIC in 25 postoperative knees and found that both effectively reduced artifact extent compared to FSE [65]. A hybrid SEMAC–MAVRIC technique has also been proposed [68,69].

Diabetic foot infection

Radiographs are insensitive for osteomyelitis in the diabetic foot. MRI is highly sensitive for osteomyelitis and is very useful for determining precise extent of involvement for preoperative planning. It also provides very accurate evaluation of the soft tissues in the area of concern. Diabetic patients often have plantar calluses due to chronic friction. Callus is seen as a focal cutaneous and subcutaneous soft tissue prominence; the skin and subcutaneous signal often blends imperceptibly. Calluses often have low signal on T1WIs but show variable signal intensity on T2WIs based on the degree of granulation tissue and vascularity. Adventitial bursitis is also related to chronic friction manifest as a focus of fluid, usually thin and elongated or ovoid, in the subcutaneous soft tissues adjacent to a callus; if the focus is well defined without adjacent soft tissue inflammation, it can be confidently attributed to friction-related bursitis rather than abscess. In ulcerated callus, typically a large skin defect is seen with raised margins. Any form of skin disruption may serve as a route for soft tissue infection. It is particularly important to identify deep ulceration because there is a high association with underlying osteomyelitis. Soft tissue edema is very frequently observed in diabetic feet and should not be mistaken for cellulitis. The subcutaneous fat signal is not replaced in edema as it is in cellulitis. On contrast-enhanced images, subcutaneous edema shows minimal enhancement, unlike cellulitis, which enhances brightly. Gas can be seen within areas of cellulitis, particularly adjacent to skin defects (ulcers) or in devitalized areas. Abscesses appear as a focal collection of fluid-like signal with a thick enhancing rim on contrast-enhanced images. Sinus tracts are characterized by a thin, discrete line of fluid signal extending through the soft tissues.

On contrast-enhanced images, sinus tracts, like abscesses, stand out due to enhancement of the hyperemic margins. Septic joints often present with joint effusion. The infected fluid may decompress through a sinus tract or into a nearby tendon sheath (i.e. flexor hallucis longus). In septic tenosynovitis, there is a disproportionate amount of fluid within the affected tendon sheath as compared to other adjacent sheaths. The fluid often appears complex and a thick enhancing rim can also be seen around the tendon. Synovial thickening and enhancement is seen on contrast-enhanced images.

Marginal erosions and reactive edema are common. Osteomyelitis should be considered when the edema or enhancement relates to septic arthritis, extending deep into the medullary bone. Osteomyelitis is characterized by replacement of the normal fat marrow signal on T1W sequences and enhancement on contrast-enhanced images. Additional MR findings include cortical disruption and periostitis, the latter seen as a thin, linear pattern of edema and enhancement surrounding the outer cortical margin. A very important consideration is that over 90% of osteomyelitis of the foot and ankle is a result of contiguous spread through a skin ulcer; therefore, the majority of cases of diabetic foot osteomyelitis have associated soft tissue manifestation (skin ulceration, cellulitis, soft tissue abscess, sinus tract) [70].

Role for therapy follow-up and patient management

Once the diagnosis of osteomyelitis has been established, serial follow-up MRI studies appear of limited value in terms of affecting treatment [11]. Cases unresponsive to therapy or those with persistently elevated CRP levels may gain benefit from repeated MRI in order to assess for the potential development of an abscess.

References

1. Grimprel E, Cohen R. Epidemiology and physiopathology of osteoarticular infections in children (newborns except). *Arch Pediatr* 2077;14 (Suppl 2): S81–85.
2. Steer AC, Carapetis JR. Acute hematogenous osteomyelitis in children: Recognition and management. *Paediatr Drugs* 2004;6:333–346.
3. Dahl LB, Hoyland AL, Dramsdahl H *et al.* Acute osteomyelitis in children: a population-based retrospective study 1965 to 1994. *Scand J Infect Dis* 1998; 30:573–577.
4. Jaramillo D. Infection: Musculoskeletal. *Pediatr Radiol* 2011;41 (Suppl 1):S127–134.
5. Nixon GW. Hematogenous osteomyelitis of metaphyseal-equivalent locations. *AJR Am J Roentgenol* 1978;130:123–129.
6. Ogden JA, Lister G. The pathology of neonatal osteomyelitis. *Pediatrics* 1975;55:474–478.
7. Ranson M. Imaging of pediatric musculoskeletal infection. *Semin Musculoskelet Radiol* 2009;13: 277–299.
8. Bocchini CE, Hulten KG, Mason EO, Jr *et al.* Panton-Valentine leukocidin genes are associated with enhanced inflammatory response and local disease in acute hematogenous *Staphylococcus aureus* osteomyelitis in children. *Pediatrics* 2006;117:433–440.
9. Lew DP, Waldvogel FA. Osteomyelitis. *Lancet* 2004;364:369–379.
10. Offiah AC. Acute osteomyelitis, septic arthritis and discitis: Differences between neonates and older children. *Eur J Radiol* 2006;60:221–232.
11. Ceroni DD, Cherkaoui AA, Ferey SS *et al. Kingella kingae* osteoarticular infections in young children: clinical features and contribution of a new specific real-time PCR assay to the diagnosis. *J Pediatr Orthop* 2010;30:301–304.
12. Browne LP, Mason EO, Kaplan SL *et al.* Optimal imaging strategy for community-acquired *Staphylococcus aureus* musculoskeletal infections in children. *Pediatr Radiol* 2008;38:841–847.
13. Arnold SR, Elias D, Buckingham SC *et al.* Changing patterns of acute hematogenous osteomyelitis and septic arthritis: emergence of community-associated methicillin-resistant *Staphylococcus aureus. J Pediatr Orthop* 2006;26:703–708.
14. Ju KL, Zurakowski D, Kocher MS. Differentiating between methicillin-resistant and methicillin-sensitive *Staphylococcus aureus* osteomyelitis in children: an evidence-based clinical prediction algorithm. *J Bone Joint Surg Am* 2011;93:1693–1701.
15. Chen WL, Chang WN, Chen YS *et al.* Acute community-acquired osteoarticular infections in children: High incidence of concomitant bone and joint involvement. *J Microbiol Immunol Infect* 2010; 43:332–338.
16. Conrad DA. Acute hematogenous osteomyelitis. *Pediatr Rev* 2010;31:464–471.
17. Courtney PM, Flynn JM, Jaramillo D *et al.* Clinical indications for repeat MRI in children with acute hematogenous osteomyelitis. *J Pediatr Orthop* 2010; 30:883–887.
18. Hollmig ST, Copley LA, Browne RH *et al.* Deep venous thrombosis associated with osteomyelitis in children. *J Bone Joint Surg Am* 2007;89:1517–1523.
19. Johnson DP, Hernanz-Schulman M, Martus JE *et al.* Significance of epiphyseal cartilage enhancement defects in pediatric osteomyelitis identified by MRI with surgical correlation. *Pediatr Radiol* 2011;41: 355–361.
20. Connolly SA, Connolly LP, Drubach LA *et al.* MRI for detection of abscess in acute osteomyelitis of the pelvis in children. *AJR Am J Roengenol* 2007;189:867–872.
21. McPhee E, Eskander JP, Eskander MS *et al.* Imaging in pelvic osteomyelitis: support for early magnetic resonance imaging. *J Pediatr Orthop* 2007;27:903–909.

22. Connolly LP, Connolly SA, Drubach LA *et al.* Acute hematogenous osteomyelitis of children: assessment of skeletal scintigraphy-based diagnosis in the era of MRI. *J Nucl Med* 2002;43:1310–1316.

23. Karmazyn B, Loder RT, Kleiman MB *et al.* The role of pelvic magnetic resonance in evaluating non hip sources of infection in children with acute non traumatic hip pain. *J Pediatr Orthop* 2007;27:158–164.

24. Cofield RH, Edgerton BC. Total shoulder arthroplasty: complications and revision surgery. *Instr Course Lect* 1990;39:449–462.

25. Silliman JF, Hawkings RJ. Complications following shoulder arthroplasty. In: Friedman RJ (ed). *Arthroplasty of the Shoulder.* New York: Thieme, 1994, pp. 242–253.

26. Panousis K, Grigoris P, Butcher I *et al.* Poor predictive value of broad-range PCR for the detection of arthroplasty infection in 92 cases. *Acta Orthop* 2005;437: 83–88.

27. Ilyas I, Morgan DA. Massive structural allograft in revision of septic hip arthroplasty. *Int Orthop* 2001; 24:319–322.

28. Leone JM, Hanssen AD. Management of infection at the site of a total knee arthroplasty. *J Bone Joint Surg Am* 2005;87:2336–2348.

29. Rittmeister ME, Manthel I, Hailer NP. Prosthetic replacement in secondary Girdlestone arthroplasty has an unpredictable outcome. *Int Orthop* 2005;29: 145–148.

30. Charlton WP, Hozack WJ, Teloken MA *et al.* Complications associated with reimplantation after Girdlestone arthroplasty. *Clin Orthop Relat Res* 2003;407: 119–126.

31. Ledermann HP, Morrison WB, Schweitzer ME. MR image analysis of pedal osteomyelitis: distribution, patterns of spread, and frequency of associated ulceration and septic arthritis. *Radiology* 2002;223:747–755.

32. Morrison WB, Ledermann HP, Schweitzer ME. MR imaging of the diabetic foot. *Magn Reson Imaging Clin North Am* 2001;9:603–614.

33. Boulton AJ, Vileikyte I. The diabetic foot: the scope of the problem. *J Fam Pract* 2000;49 (11 Suppl):S3–S8.

34. Lavery I, Gazewood JD. Assessing the feet of patient with diabetes. *J Fam Pract* 2000;49 (Suppl):S9–S16.

35. Jaramillo D. Whole-body MR imaging, bone diffusion imaging: how and why? *Pediatr Radiol* 2010;40: 978–984.

36. Darge K, Jaramillo D, Siegel MJ. Whole-body MRI in children: current status and future applications. *Eur J Radiol* 2008;68:289–298.

37. Morrison WB, Schweitzer ME, Bock GW *et al.* Diagnosis of osteomyelitis: Utility of fat-suppressed contrast-enhanced MR imaging. *Radiology* 1993; 189:251–257.

38. Craig JG, Amin MB, Wu K *et al.* Osteomyelitis of the diabetic foot: MR imaging- pathologic correlation. *Radiology* 1997;203:849–855.

39. Morrison WB, Schweitzer ME, Wapner KL *et al.* Osteomyelitis in feet of diabetics: clinical accuracy, surgical utility and cost-effectiveness of MR imaging. *Radiology* 1995;196:557–564.

40. Ledermann HP, Morrison WB, Schweitzer ME. Pedal abscesses in patients suspected of having pedal osteomyelitis: analysis with MR imaging. *Radiology* 2002; 224:649–655.

41. Ledermann HP, Schweitzer ME, Morrison WB. Non-enhancing tissue on MR imaging of pedal infection: characterization of necrotic tissue and associated limitations for diagnosis of osteomyelitis and abscess. *AJR Am J Roentgenol* 2002;178:215–222

42. Lu W, Pauly KB, Gold GE, Pauly JM, Hargreaves BA. SEMAC: Slice Encoding for Metal Artifact Correction in MRI. *Magn Reson Med* 2009;62:66–76.

43. Lee MJ, Kim S, Lee SA *et al.* Overcoming artifacts from metallic orthopedic implants at high-field-strength MR imaging and multi-detector CT. *RadioGraphics* 2007;27:791–803.

44. Capitanio MA, Kirkpatrick JA. Early roentgen observations in acute osteomyelitis. *Am J Roentgenol Radium The Nucl Med* 1970;108:488–496.

45. Jaramillo D, Treves ST, Kasser JR *et al.* Osteomyelitis and septic arthritis in children: appropriate use of imaging to guide treatment. *AJR Am J Roentgenol* 1995;165:399–403.

46. Mattis TA, Borders HL, Ellinger DM, Junewick JJ. Relationship between the clinical characteristics of osteomyelitis and the finding of extraosseous fat on MRI in pediatric patients. *Pediatr Radiol* 2011;41: 1293–1297.

47. Davies AM, Hughes DE, Grimer RJ. Intramedullary and extramedullary fat globules on magnetic resonance imaging as a diagnostic sign for osteomyelitis. *Eur Radiol* 2005;15:2194–2199.

48. Averill LW, Hernandez A, Gonzalez L *et al.* Diagnosis of osteomyelitis in children: utility of fat-suppressed contrast-enhanced MRI. *AJR Am J Roentgenol* 2009; 192:1232–1238.

49. Kan JH, Young RS, Yu C *et al.* Clinical impact of gadolinium in the MRI diagnosis of musculoskeletal infection in children. *Pediatr Radiol* 2010;40: 1197–1205.

50. McCarthy JJ, Dormans JP, Kozin SH *et al.* Musculoskeletal infections in children: basic treatment principles and recent advancements. *Instr Course Lect* 2005; 54:515–528.

51. Jones HW, Harrison JW, Bates J *et al.* Radiologic classification of chronic hematogenous osteomyelitis in children. *J Pediatr Orthop* 2009;29:822–827.

52. Buckles VL, Jones HW, Harrison WJ. Chronic hematogenous osteomyelitis in children: a retrospective review of 167 patients in Malawi. *J Bone Joint Surgery Br* 2010;92:1138–1143

53. Boaz K. Imaging approach to acute hematogenous osteomyelitis in children: An update. *Semin Ultrasound CT MR* 2010;31:100–106.

54. Collado P, Nardo E, Calvo C et al. Role of power Doppler sonography in early diagnosis of osteomyelitis in children. *J Clin Ultrasound* 2008;36:251–253.

55. Keller MS. Musculoskeletal sonography in the neonate and infant. *Pediatr Radiol* 2005;35:1167–1173.

56. Chua CL, Griffith JF. Musculoskeletal infections: ultrasound appearances. *Clin Radiol* 2005;60:149–159.

57. McCarthy JJ, Dormans JP, Kozin SH et al. Musculoskeletal infections in children: basic treatment principles and recent advancements. *Instr Course Lect* 2005; 54:515–528.

58. Jones HW, Harrison JW, Bates J et al. Radiologic classification of chronic Hematogenous osteomyelitis in children. *J Pediatr Orthop* 2009;29:822–827.

59. Buckles VL, Jones HW, Harrison WJ. Chronic hematogenous osteomyelitis in children: a retrospective review of 167 patients in Malawi. *J Bone Joint Surg Br* 2010;92:1138–1143.

60. Warmann SW, Dittmann H, Seitz G, Bares R, Fuchs J, Schäfer JF. Follow-up of acute osteomyelitis in children: the possible role of PET/CT in selected cases. *J Pediatr Surg* 2011;46:1550–1556.

61. Girschick HJ, Zimmer C, Klaus G et al. Chronic recurrent multifocal osteomyelitis: what is it and how should it be treated? *Nat Clin Pract Rheumatol* 2007; 3:733–738.

62. Fritz J, Tzaribatchev N, Claussen CD et al. Chronic recurrent multifocal osteomyelitis: comparison of whole-body MR imaging with radiography and correlation with clinical and laboratory data. *Radiology* 2009;252:842–851.

63. de Kort JG, Robben SG, Schrander JJ et al. Multifocal osteomyelitis in a child: a rare manifestation of cat scratch disease: a case report and systematic review of the literature. *J Pediatr Orthop B* 2006;15: 285–288.

64. Hayter CL, Koff MF, Shah P, Koch KM, Miller TT, Potter HG. MRI after arthroplasty: Comparison of MAVRIC and conventional fast spin-echo techniques. *AJR Am J Roentgenol* 2011;197:W405–411.

65. Chen CA, Chen W, Goodman SB et al. New MR imaging methods for metallic implants in the knee: artifact correction and clinical impact. *J Magn Reson Imaging* 2011;33:1121–1127.

66. Toms AP, Smith-Bateman C, Malcolm PN, Cahir J, Graves M. Optimization of metal artefact reduction (MAR) sequences for MRI of total hip prostheses. *Clin Radiol* 2010;65:447–452.

67. Kolind SH, MacKay AL, Munk PL, Xiang QS. Quantitative evaluation of metal artifact reduction techniques. *J Magn Reson Imaging* 2004;20:487–495.

68. Hargreaves BA, Chen W, Lu W et al. Accelerated slice encoding for metal artifact correction. *J Magn Reson Imaging* 2010;31:987–996.

69. La Rocca Vieira R, Rybak LR, Recht M. Technical update on magnetic resonance imaging of the shoulder. *Magn Reson Imaging Clin N Am* 2012;20: 149–161.

70. Morrison W, Ledermann HP. Diabetic pedal infection. In: Pope T, Bloem HL, Beltran J, Morrison WB, Wilson DB (eds). *Imaging of the Musculoskeletal System*. Philadelphia: Saunders Elsevier, 2008, pp. 1291–1309.

Clinical cases

Case 1

A 27-year-old female evaluated for chronic osteo-myelitis of the tibia (Figure 3.9).

Teaching points
• Diffuse sclerosis and cortical thickening in the setting of prior hardware fixation of fractures with an associated island of intramedullary necrotic bone and non-healing, enlarging pin tracks should raise suspicion for chronic osteomyelitis.
• CT provides great visualization of intramedullary sequestrate while contrast-enhanced MRI can reliably pinpoint enhancing sinus tracks and abscesses

that need to be drained and resected in order to achieve control of the infectious process.

Case 2

A 3-month-old male with pain in his thigh (Figure 3.10).

Teaching points
• A periosteal reaction in a non-ambulating neonate or infant should raise clinical suspicion for osteomyelitis.
• MRI is particularly useful in detecting associated soft tissue infection in order to support the diagnosis.

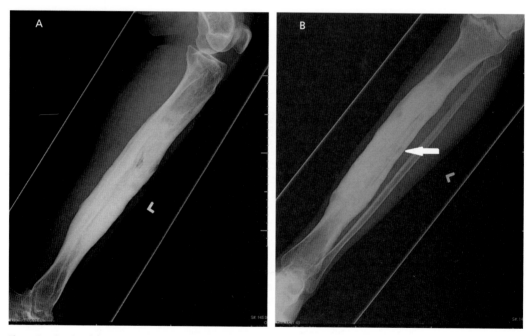

Figure 3.9 (A,B) Left knee anteroposterior and lateral views show lucent tracks within the tibia indicative of prior hardware removal (B, arrow) as well as deformity of the tibia due to a healed fracture deformity. There is diffuse sclerosis of the proximal to distal tibial diaphysis compatible with the clinical history of chronic osteomyelitis. (C–H) Multislice helical sections were obtained through the leg, including sagittal and coronal reformatted images. Diffuse circumferential cortical thickening of the tibial diaphysis (C,G, asterisk), most prominent within the mid shaft, is consistent with chronic osteomyelitis. There are linear/curvilinear foci of sclerotic ossification within the medullary space consistent with sequestrae (G, arrow). Well corticated tracts are noted extending through the tibial diaphysis and relate to removal of hardware (H, arrow). (I–O) T1WIs of the left tibia/fibula before and after contrast demonstrate findings compatible with chronic osteomyelitis involving most of the left tibial diaphysis with extensive cortical thickening (J, asterisk). Note the intracortical tracts representing cloacae. There is enhancing intramedullary granulation tissue with central non-enhancing sequestrum. There is no evidence of intramedullary or soft tissue fluid collection.

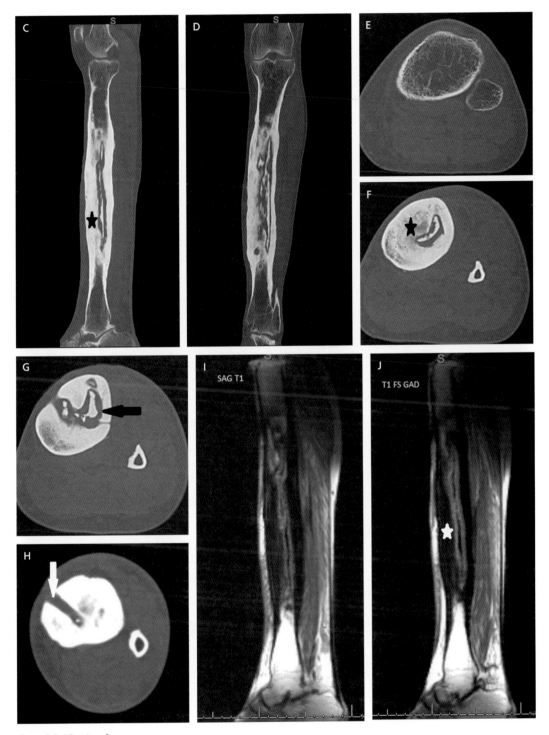

Figure 3.9 (*Continued*)

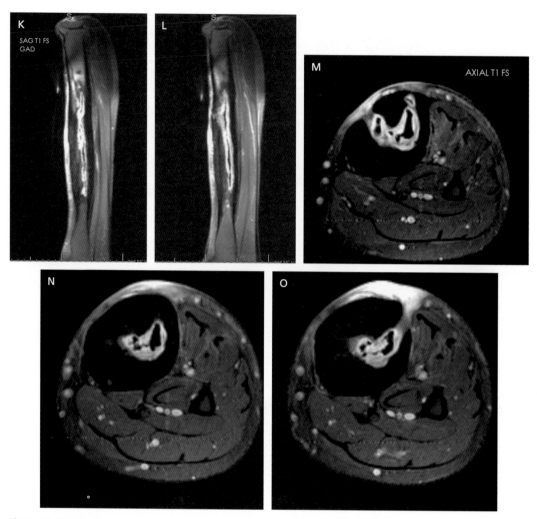

Figure 3.9 *(Continued)*

Case 3

A 46-year-old female with a Charcot foot and questionable mid-foot septic arthritis and osteomyelitis (Figure 3.11).

Teaching points
• Differentiating Charcot arthropathy and osteomyelitis can present a diagnostic challenge.
• In the diabetic foot, almost invariably, osteomyelitis develops as a result of direct spread of infection from a skin ulcer with associated draining sinus tract.
• Although the changes in the marrow as well as the presence of sclerosis, fragmentation and erosions in bone are seen in both Charcot arthropathy

and osteomyelitis, a ring-enhancing soft tissue abscess and sinus tract adjacent to the area of cortical/marrow abnormality will support infection over neuroarthropathy in the differential diagnosis.

Case 4

A 70-year-old male with diabetic foot and know Charcot arthropathy, evaluated for osteomyelitis (Figure 3.12).

Teaching points
• Rocker-bottom deformity leads to abnormal biomechanics of the foot with pressure-related breakdown of the skin, secondary ulceration and sinus

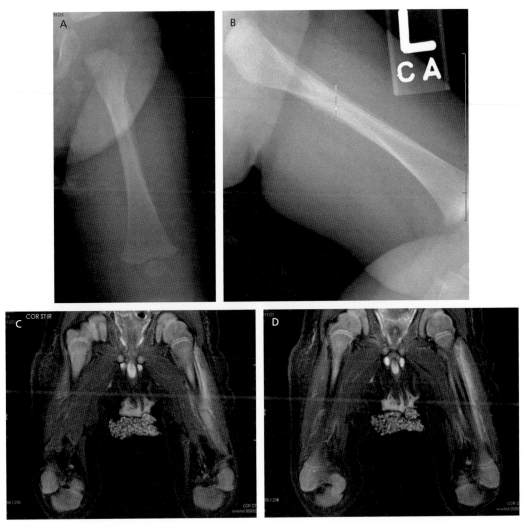

Figure 3.10 (A,B) Anteroposterior and lateral views of the left femur demonstrate concentric lamellar periosteal reaction in the left proximal femoral diaphysis likely related to osteomyelitis. Fracture cannot be definitely excluded, nor can the possibility that findings may be secondary to fracture complicated by infection. (C–H) Enhancing periostitis along the left femoral diaphysis with periosseous edema predominantly within the vastus musculature. The muscle edema may reflect myositis, given that it enhances. No discrete walled-off soft tissue or intramedullary fluid collection was identified to indicate the presence of an abscess. There was no evidence of associated cortical destruction. The findings are highly suggestive of early manifestations of osteomyelitis.

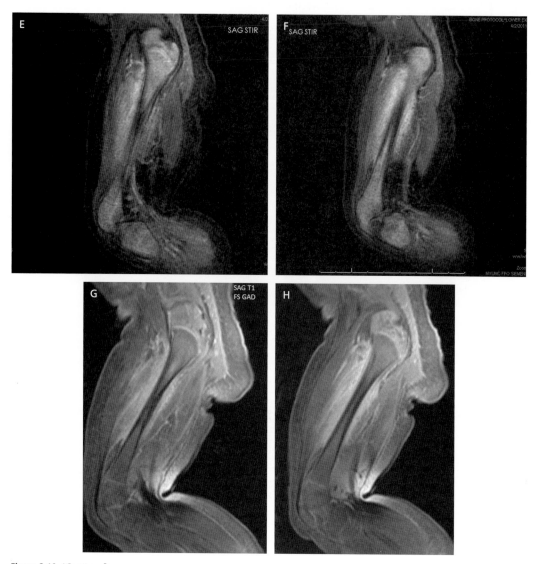

Figure 3.10 (*Continued*)

tract formation, which provide skin microorganisms with access to the bone.

• Osteomyelitis of the cuboid, calcaneus, first metatarsal sesamoids and fifth metatarsal head is frequently due to this pathophysiology.

Case 5

A 48-year-old male with an infected left hip prosthesis requiring hardware removal for phlegmon/ abscess formation about the left hip with sinus tract and ulceration, and suspected left hip septic arthritis/osteomyelitis (Figure 3.13).

Teaching points

• Areas of osteolysis adjacent to hardware material can be due to particle disease or infection.

• The presence of skin ulceration and a draining sinus tract leading into the area of osteolysis help distinguish between these two processes.

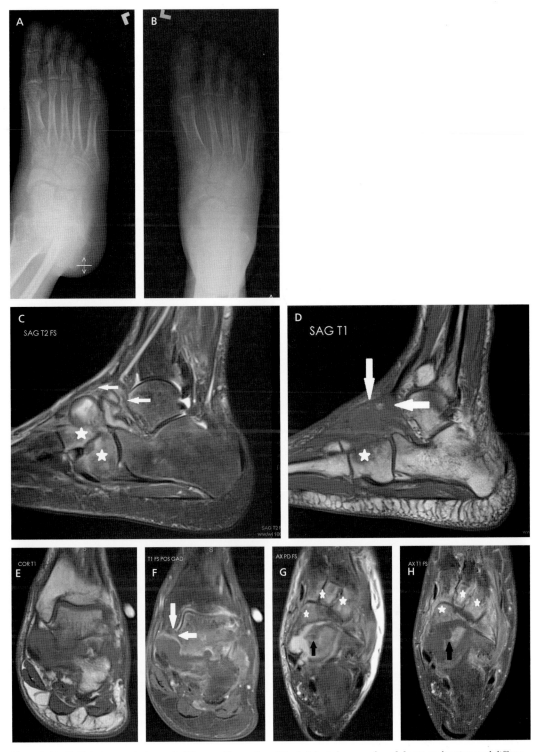

Figure 3.11 (A,B) Anteroposterior and oblique radiographs of the left foot show profound demineralization and diffuse soft tissue swelling. Disruption of the articulating surfaces in the proximal surface of the navicular and talar head is seen associated with fragmentation of the navicular bone. (C–H) Charcot arthropathy. A large talonavicular joint effusion with thin peripheral enhancement is noted extending medially and laterally along the dorsum of the midfoot and forefoot (C,D,F, white arrows). T1W and T2W bone marrow signal abnormality is associated with enhancement compatible with reactive marrow edema involving the talar head, navicular and anterior calcaneus with extension into the cuneiforms, cuboid and the second and third metatarsal bases (C,D,G,H, asterisks). Erosions along the talonavicular articulation and metatarsal bases are also noted (G,H, arrows). Note the absence of a soft tissue sinus tract or ulceration compatible with non-infected Charcot arthropathy.

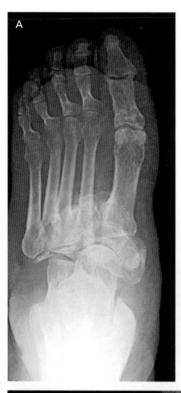

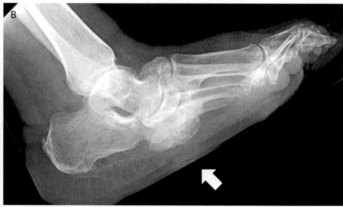

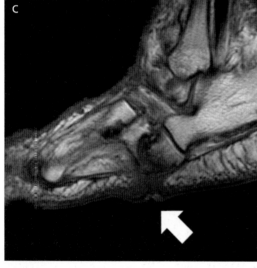

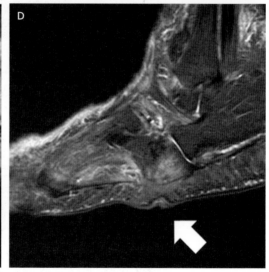

Figure 3.12 (A,B) Anteroposterior and lateral views of the left foot demonstrate typical radiographic manifestations of Charcot arthropathy, including subluxation of the Lisfranc joint with associated subchondral sclerosis and slight fragmentation. Note the focal skin defect along the plantar aspect of the cuboid bone compatible with ulcer and draining sinus tract (B, arrow). (C,D) Sagittal T1WI and STIR image demonstrate abnormal marrow signal in the cuboid bone in continuity with the skin ulcer and subcutaneous sinus tract compatible with diabetic foot and superimposed osteomyelitis. Note the rocker-bottom deformity of the foot, which likely contributes to abnormal weight bearing and break down of the skin at the pressure site (C,D, arrow).

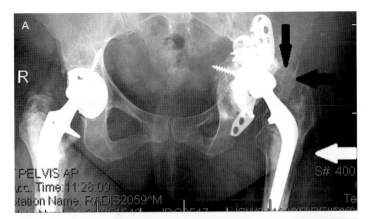

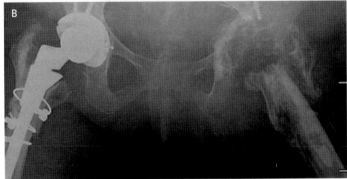

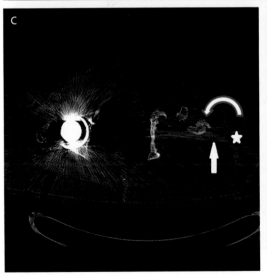

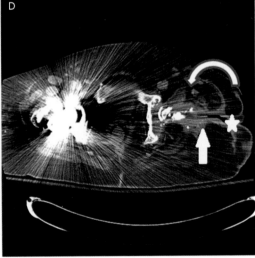

Figure 3.13 (A) Anteroposterior (AP) radiograph of the pelvis demonstrates findings compatible with loosening of the left acetabular component, which is vertically tilted. Note the erosive changes of the greater trochanter and left lateral acetabular roof (black arrows), as well as the discrete cortical destruction with periosteal reaction along the lateral margin of the left proximal femoral shaft (white arrow). (B) AP radiograph shows status post left hip prosthesis removal due to infected draining sinus and periarticular abscess formation with secondary osteomyelitis. (C,D) Axial CT bone and soft tissue images of the hips demonstrate large skin ulceration (asterisk) with deep sinus tract formation (straight arrow) as well as sclerosis, erosions and fragmentation of the greater trochanter (curved arrow) in keeping with septic arthritis and osteomyelitis.

CHAPTER 4

Radiological Imaging of Spine Infection

Ana María Quintero[1] and Roy Riascos[2]

[1]*Clinica Reina Sofia, Clinica Colsanitas, Bogotá, Colombia*
[2]*The University of Texas Medical Branch, Galveston, TX, USA*

Introduction

This chapter discusses the radiological imaging of the most common infections of the spine and focuses on pyogenic, non-pyogenic and post-procedural infections.

Spine infections have different anatomical and etiological classifications. Here the term spondylodiscitis is used to describe the different presentations of vertebral osteomyelitis, spondylitis and discitis, which are all the result of the same pathological process; epidural abscess and facet joint arthropathy [1].

Although there have been improvements in therapy (both antimicrobial and surgical), morbidity from spine infections remains significant.

Basic knowledge of the clinical problem

Spondylodiscitis is the main manifestation of hematogenous osteomyelitis, representing 3–5% of all cases of osteomyelitis [2–4] and identified in about 1 in 250 000. Its incidence is increasing, likely due to a combination of factors: increase in susceptible population [increase in average age, immunodeficiency, drug abuse, diabetes mellitus, human immunodeficiency virus (HIV) and chronic use of steroids], increase in spinal surgery, increase in healthcare-associated infections and better diagnostic capabilities. Age of presentation has a bimodal distribution: a first peak is seen in childhood and a second during the fifth–sixth decades of life [3,4]. It has a male preponderance with a male to female ratio of 3:1 [4].

The clinical questions

Diagnosis is often delayed due to the insidious onset of symptoms and high frequency of low back pain in the general population; the literature refers to a delay of 2–6 months from onset of clinical signs to diagnosis [3,4]. The diagnosis of spondylodiscitis is based on clinical, laboratory and radiological features, and can be difficult. Clinicians need radiological support to establish early and appropriate treatment.

Methodological considerations

Plain radiographs are usually the initial imaging modality used in patients with back pain; however, they are not useful in the early phases of spondylodiscitis when no skeletal changes are seen.

Computed tomography (CT) is less sensitive and specific than magnetic resonance imaging (MRI) in the detection of spondylodiscitis, but provides better planar detail of bony abnormalities than plain radiographs.

MRI with contrast is the modality of choice in patients with suspected spine infection. The advantages of MRI include: multiplanar imaging

Diagnostic Imaging of Infections and Inflammatory Diseases: A Multidisciplinary Approach, First Edition. Edited by Alberto Signore and Ana María Quintero.

capability and direct evaluation of bone marrow, intervertebral disc, neural structures (including spinal cord), epidural space and peripheral soft tissues.

Normal findings and artifacts

It is very important to be able to differentiate degenerative changes in the intervertebral disc and endplate from infection, and thus avoid confusion. Modic's classification [5] describes three types of endplate degenerative changes. In Modic type I changes, the endplates may be hyperintense on T2-weighted images (T2WIs) and hypointense on T1-weighted images (T1WIs), should not enhance with contrast medium and should not be confused with infectious disease. In degenerative disc disease, the disc may calcify and the hydrated calcium may be represented by increased T1 intensity within the disc.

Pathological findings and significance

Pyogenic spondylitis

Two main patterns of presentation have been described, one for adults and another for children, due to their different vascular supply to the spine. In children, intraosseous arteries display extensive anastomoses and vascular channels penetrate the disc. Therefore, a septic embolus is unlikely to produce a substantial osseous infarct and the infection is often limited to the disc. In adults, the disc is avascular and the intraosseous anastomoses involute by the third decade of life, creating end peripheral periosteal arteries and allowing septic emboli to develop into large wedge-shaped subdiscal infarcts [2,6].

Pyogenic osteomyelitis usually does not compromise the posterior vertebral elements. It affects primarily the lumbar spine, followed by the thoracic and cervical spines. It can involve one or more spinal levels [2,7].

Pathogens can infect the spine by three routes: hematogenous spread from an infected microembolus, direct inoculation, or from contiguous tissues. The hematogenous arterial route is predominant; the infected microembolus lodges in a metaphyseal artery, resulting in infarction and subsequent infection. Infection is more frequently located at the endplates due to the increased number of arteries at this location. Infection can then extend to the opposite vertebral endplate via primary periosteal arteries or across the interspace to the adjacent endplate via intermetaphyseal arteries [6].

The site for the primary focus of infection may originate in the genitourinary tract, skin/superficial soft tissues, intravascular devices, gastrointestinal tract, respiratory tract, heart or oral cavity [8].

A wide variety of pathogens have been described as the cause of spondylodiscitis, with *Staphylococcal aureus* being responsible for almost half of the non-tuberculous cases. In patients older than 50 years, the infection is acquired in the community, with no obvious portal of entry of infection. Recently, methicillin-resistant *S. aureus* has been increasingly reported in these cases. Other pathogens that cause spondylodiscitis include Enterobacteriaceae. Of these, those that most frequently infect the spine are: *Escherichia coli*, *Proteus*, *Klebsiella* and *Enterobacter* spp., which are usually associated with urinary tract infections. Other less common pathogens include *Pseudomonas aeruginosa*, coagulase-negative staphylococci and streptococci [2].

Symptoms of spondylodiscitis are often non-specific and may vary widely. Back or neck pain is the most common symptom, but up to 15% of patients may present without pain. Patients usually describe the pain as insidious and constant, being worse at night. Fever is less common and is experienced in only half of patients. Neurological deficits can be present in a third of cases. Spinal deformities can be seen especially as a late complication and are most common in tuberculous spondylitis [2]. Prognosis depends on the timing of diagnosis and early use of antimicrobial therapy. Mortality ranges from 2% to 17%. The disease can relapse and present with neurological deficits and pain [3].

Patients with spondylodiscitis can have an abnormal leukocyte count, C-reactive protein (CRP) and erythrocyte sedimentation rate (ESR). In patients with acute disease there is an increase in ESR, but in the chronic stages the leukocyte count and ESR parameters can be normal; typically there is an increase in CRP [3].

Differential diagnoses include degenerative and inflammatory diseases (Modic type 1) and acute cartilaginous node.

Conventional radiography

Changes on plain radiographs start to become evident 2–8 weeks after the onset of symptoms.

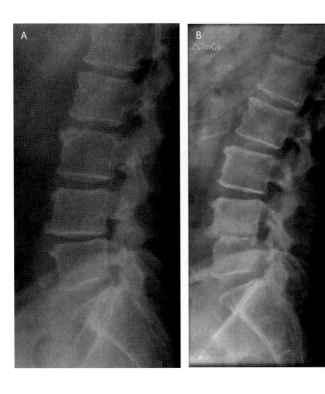

Figure 4.1 Patient with lumbar pain and clinical suspicion of infection. (A) Initial lateral plain film shows loss of height of the intervertebral space L4–L5, with small anterior spurs, consistent with degenerative disc space disease. (B) Persistence of clinical infection symptoms and follow-up images with MRI and radiography. The lateral plain film 3 months later shows total loss of height of the interverterbral space with vertebral endplate cortical erosion and sclerosis.

Plain radiographs have a reported sensitivity of 82%, specificity of 57% and accuracy of 73% [9]. Typical findings include loss of definition of adjacent endplate margins, decreased vertebral height, narrowing of the intervertebral space and, eventually, destructive changes in vertebral endplates and vertebral bodies [2,6]. These changes may be slight and difficult to differentiate from degenerative disease (Figure 4.1).

CT imaging

In the early stages of disease, osteolytic and osteosclerotic changes in the endplates, and spinal deformities, are best seen on coronal and sagittal reconstructions (Figure 4.2). CT improves the visualization of para-vertebral abscesses, especially after intravenous injection of contrast. It provides a valuable tool to diagnose patients who are contraindicated for MRI [3,10].

MR imaging

MRI has a reported sensitivity of 96%, specificity of 93% and accuracy of 94% for the diagnosis of spondylodiscitis [4,9]. Spine infection usually involves two consecutive vertebrae and the intervening disc. To optimize the diagnosis, the protocol should include sagittal T1WIs and T2WIs, a sagittal T2W fat-suppressed sequence and contrast-enhanced sagittal and axial T1W sequences (Figure 4.3). The most frequent findings include decreased disc height (52.3%), disc hypointensity on T1WIs compared with adjacent normal discs (29.5%), hyperintensity of the disc on T2WIs (93.2%), contrast enhancement of the disc (95.4%), presence of a nuclear cleft sign (83.3%), erosion or destruction of at least one vertebral endplate (84.1%) and presence of inflammatory para-spinal or epidural tissue (97.7%) [7]. Ledermann *et al.* [7] compared their findings with the literature and concluded that criteria with good to excellent sensitivity include evidence of para-spinal or epidural inflammatory tissue, contrast enhancement of the disc, hyperintensity or fluid equivalent signal on T2WIs and erosion or destruction of vertebral endplates on T1WIs. Criteria with low sensitivity include hypointensity of the disc on T1WIs and decreased height of the intervertebral space [6,7,11].

Biopsy and pathogen detection

Identification of the specific pathogen involved in the infection and its sensitivity to antibiotics is very important for therapy. The least invasive means of

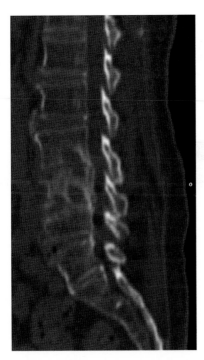

Figure 4.2 Sagittal multiplanar reconstruction CT image shows diffuse decreased bone marrow density due to osteopenia, with higher density of bone marrow at L3. The loss of height of the L2–L3 and L3–L4 intervertebral spaces, sclerosis and irregularities of vertebral plates, with rounded lytic lesions, confirm osteomyelitis and discitis within these two intervertebral spaces. The intervertebral space L4–L5 shows degenerative disease.

identification is through blood cultures. Other possible ways to sample the pathogen are percutaneous CT-guided needle puncture (Figure 4.4) and surgery [3]. A percutaneous biopsy has an accuracy of 70–100% [4].

Granulomatous diseases: spinal tuberculosis

The first description of tuberculous infection of the spine in 1779 was by Percival Pott, a British orthopedic surgeon. Hence, spinal tuberculosis (TB) is also known as Pott's disease. Spinal TB can be the initial manifestation of disease; however, it is typically secondary to involvement of the lung or abdomen [12].

A tenth of cases of extrapulmonary TB occur in the musculoskeletal system and around a half of these affect the spine [13]. The spine is the most serious of all the skeletal complications of this

disease [14]. Spinal disease occurs mainly in the infant population in developing countries where it affects the thoracic spine; in countries where the incidence is lower, such as in Europe and North America, it is more common in the adult population and most commonly affects the lumbar spine [15–17].

New techniques, such as the introduction of polymerase chain reaction (PCR) for the detection of *Mycobacterium tuberculosis*, introduced in 1994, have improved the identification of early disease [18].

Spinal disease can be divided into vertebrodiscal disease and spinal canal disease.

Vertebrodiscal disease

TB affecting the vertebra and the disc is much more common than spinal canal disease.

TB can spread to the spine through hematogenous spread and most commonly affects the anterior aspect of the vertebral bodies. Lymphatic spread is rare. The initial stage of the disease is a pre-pus inflammatory reaction with Langerhans and epitheloid cells [19]. This granulation tissue can cause vascular thrombosis. Later in the disease, tissue necrosis and inflammatory cell breakdown cause an abscess that does cause pain or show increased temperature, commonly known as a "cold abscess". Around 80% of the patients have a soft tissue component that usually affects the psoas musculature.

The infection can spread through the anterior longitudinal ligament to the adjacent vertebral bodies without affecting the disc (skipped lesions). The involvement of more than two vertebral bodies favors the diagnosis of tuberculous spondylosis [20].

As the disease advances, it can affect the intervertebral disc and erode the endplates adjacent to the disc. The disease, if left untreated, can cause an anterior compression deformity of the vertebral body known as a gibbous deformity. It can also extend into the epidural space and cause thecal sac compression.

Spinal TB is generally classified as early or late, but renewed effort has been made to better classify the disease and improve treatment. The Gulhane Military Medical Academy (GATA) [21] has proposed a new classification based on clinical and imaging criteria:

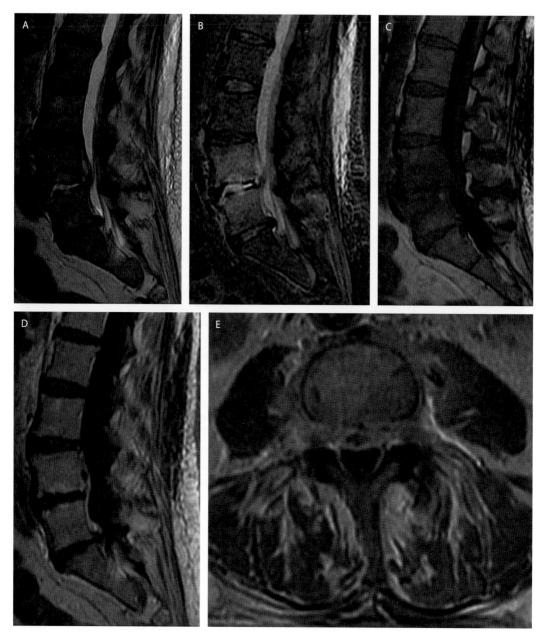

Figure 4.3 *S. aureus* spondylodiscitis in a 67-year-old female. Recommended MR protocol. (A) Sagittal T2WI shows: diminished height of the L4–L5 intervertebral space and irregularity in the cortical endplates. The disc shows hyperintensity and this continues posteriorly with a hyperintense epidural collection that compresses the dural sac. (B) Sagittal fat-suppressed T2WI shows hyperintensity of the L4 and L5 bone marrow with edema, as well as the same findings as described in A and of the same intensity. (C) Sagittal T1WI shows hypointensity of the bone marrow within L4 and L5, and loss of height of the intervertebral space with hypointensity of the disc. The anterior epidural collection is isointense with body bone marrow. (D) Sagittal contrast-enhanced T1WI shows homogeneous enhancement of the bone marrow and the epidural collection, indicating that the anterior epidural space in L5 is also compromised. (E) Axial contrast-enhanced T1WI shows an epidural anterior collection with diffuse and homogenous enhancement (phlegmon) and epidural peripheral abnormal sac enhancement.

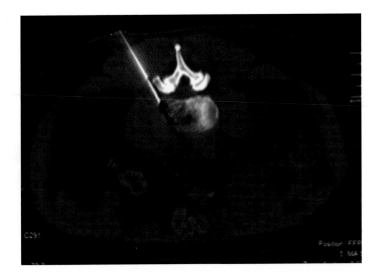

Figure 4.4 Axial CT, bone window image with the patient in the prone position. Needle guidance for a para-vertebral collection biopsy is shown.

• Type IA: disease located in the vertebra, degeneration in one disc, with no collapse, no abscess and no neurological deficits.

• Type IB: abscess formation, degeneration in one or two discs with no neurological deficit.

• Type II: vertebral collapse (pathological fracture), abscess formation, anterior compression deformity correctable with anterior surgery, stable deformity with or without neurological deficit and sagittal index less than 20°.

• Type III: severe vertebral collapse, abscess formation, severe kyphosis, unstable deformity with or without neurological deficit and a sagittal index greater than 20°.

Vertebral involvement The vertebral involvement can be seen in the posterior elements or in the vertebral body, where three patterns of vertebral involvement can be seen: para-discal, anterior and central lesions [19]. Para-discal lesions involve the body adjacent to the endplates. They are the most common pattern of spinal TB and can cause herniation of the disc through the endplate or directly affect the disc [19,22] (Figure 4.5). The anterior lesions are typically noted with the subligamentous spread of the disease through the anterior longitudinal ligament. The abscess strips the anterior periostium and makes the body susceptible to infection [19] (Figure 4.6). Central lesions are seen in the middle of the vertebral body and can cause vertebra plana where the vertebral body collapses.

Imaging is essential in the detection of early spinal TB, ensuring prompt treatment and avoiding further complications. The imaging features of early disease are not easily recognized [13,14], although modern imaging allows a better demonstration of the spinal involvement [23].

CT is a great tool to demonstrate calcifications and bony erosions. Four patterns of bony destruction have been described: fragmentary, osteolytic, subperiostial and well-defined lytic with sclerotic margins [24]. The fragmentary type is the most common presentation, seen in about half of patients. Assessment of the epidural extent of disease is less accurate than with MRI. Abscesses are better seen with this modality if calcification is present [25] (Figure 4.7).

MRI can better evaluate bone marrow disease and the soft tissue components [25]. It can also identify the presence of an epidural abscess and evaluate for cord compression [12]. In the early stages of the disease, the vertebral involvement will be seen as an increase in the bone marrow signal on the T2W fat-saturated sequences and a decreased signal on the T1WIs. Other findings include sparing of the neighboring intervertebral discs and involvement of the posterior elements [26]. As the disease progresses, an anterior fluid collection (cold abscess) is typically identified and involvement of other vertebral bodies can be visualized [25]. The disc is involved later in the disease. The abscess shows thick irregular enhancement with gadolinium DTPA.

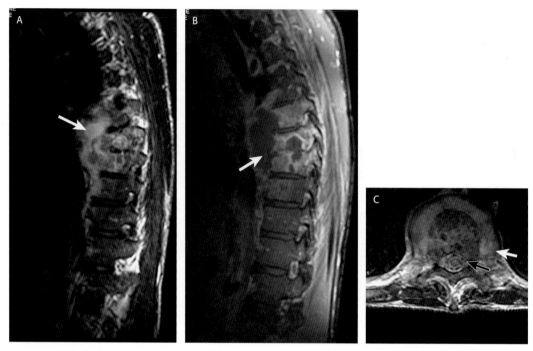

Figure 4.5 Pott's disease. (A) Sagittal short tau inversion recovery (STIR) image shows increased signal of the vertebral bodies along with a fluid collection spanning the anterior longitudinal ligament (arrow). (B) Sagittal and (C) axial fat-saturated T1WIs with gadolinium contrast show enhancement of the affected vertebral bodies and peripheral enhancement of the anterior fluid collection (white arrow) consistent with an abscess formation. The enhancement extends to the epidural space (black arrow).

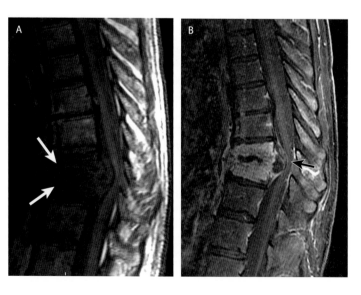

Figure 4.6 Cord compression. Patient with spinal involvement of tuberculosis. (A) Sagittal T1WI without contrast shows diffuse hypointensity of two adjacent mid-thoracic vertebral bodies (arrows). (B) T1WI with gadolinium contrast shows the diffuse enhancement of the vertebrae with a posterior extension of a lesion that shows mild peripheral enhancement, consistent with an epidural abscess. The lesion is severely narrowing and compressing the thoracic cord (arrow).

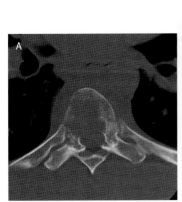
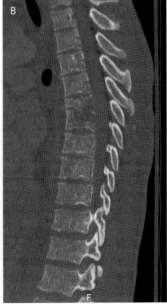
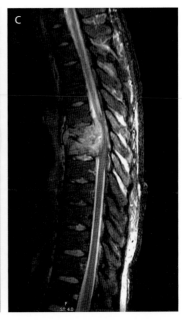

Figure 4.7 Spinal tuberculosis. (A) Axial CT and (B) sagittal reformatted images of the thoracic spine show central erosion of the vertebral body with involvement of two adjacent levels. (C) Sagittal T2WI shows increased signal in the vertebral bodies including the intervertebral disc. A fluid collection fills the epidural space at the same level, compressing the thoracic cord and showing increased signal due to cord edema.

The differential diagnosis of TB spondylitis includes tumors and pyogenic and fungal infections. Young *et al.* described diagnostic clues that allow differentiation of tuberculous spondylitis from pyogenic spondylitis on MRI [27]. Patients with tuberculous spondylitis have an increased incidence of a well-defined para-spinal abnormal signal, a thin and smooth abscess wall, the presence of a para-spinal or intraosseous abscess, subligamentous spread of three or more vertebral bodies, thoracic spine involvement and hyperintense signal on T2WIs. Involvement of the posterior elements and collapse of the vertebral body, such as in Gibbous deformity, makes neoplasms such as lymphoma part of the differential diagnosis.

Spinal canal disease
Spinal canal disease is a rare complication of TB. It is most frequently seen secondary to intracranial disease. The pathology can affect the meninges as tuberculous arachnoiditis, the central nervous system as tuberculous radiculomyelitis, or both (as it typically occurs).

Tuberculous arachnoiditis is rarely seen without spinal involvement, a feature that allows its differ-

entiation from other causes of arachnoiditis. It can occur as a primary process or secondary to vertebral or cerebral involvement. The main feature is a cerebrospinal fluid (CSF) block, frequently present at the level of the conus [28–30]. The imaging changes are seen both in the duramater and in the leptomeninges and include an irregular thecal sac, nodular sac thickening, adhesions and loculations [28,29].

Tuberculous radiculomyelitis presents in patients as subacute paraparesis, bladder disturbance, radicular pain and paralysis [29,31]. There is an extensive and expanding exudate that can have a compressive effect [32]. The imaging findings include linear intradural enhancement or, less typically, an intraspinal nodular enhancing lesion, also referred to as a tuberculoma (Figure 4.8) [28,29].

Brucellosis
Brucella spp. are small Gram-negative encapsulated coccobacilli [26] that are transmitted to humans through ingestion of unpasteurized milk or through exposure of shepherds or farmers to small ruminants [33]. Human-to-human infection is unusual, but has been reported [34,35]. It typically affects

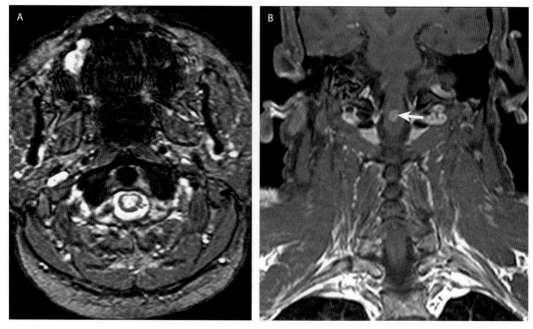

Figure 4.8 Intramedullary tuberculoma. (A) Axial gradient echo (GRE) sequence shows a focus of increased central hyperintensity of the proximal cervical spine. (B) Coronal T1W with gadolinium contrast sequence shows ring enhancement of the lesion (arrow). (Courtesy of Dr Sidhardth Jadhav MD.)

middle-aged adults. Confirmation of the diagnosis should be made by serological testing of the brucellosis [36].

Two forms of vertebral brucellosis have been described: focal and diffuse spondylitis [26]. In the focal form, the anterior aspect of the endplate at the junction with the intervertebral disc is affected (typically L4). In the diffuse form, there is initial involvement of the endplate that extends to two consecutive vertebrae and involves the intervertebral disc. The affected vertebral bodies and discs enhance with gadolinium [36].

The MRI findings are similar to those for pyogenic spine infection, but less severe. Some patients can present with epidural or para-spinal abscesses; however, the vertebral bodies do not show deformities and the endplates are typically intact. Owing to the lack of specific imaging findings, serological testing is recommended if brucellosis is suspected [36].

Subligamentous spread or involvement of the posterior vertebral elements has not been reported with brucellosis.

Fungal osteomyelitis and discitis

Fungal infection of the spine is a rare disease with a high rate of mortality. The occurrence of fungal infections has risen in the last decade with the increasing numbers of immunocompromised patients [6,37]. The two most common pathogens are *Candida* and *Aspergillus* [37–39].

Manifestations in the spine include osteomyelitis, discitis and meningitis. Infection can be by direct implantation or hematogenous spread [6]. Symptoms usually appear late after onset of infection.

MRI is extremely useful in the evaluation of spinal canal infections, although fungal infections share MR characteristics with pyogenic infections (Figure 4.9).

Fungal spondylodiscitis presents as hypointensity of the vertebral bodies on T1WIs and minimal hyperintensity or isointensity of the vertebra on T2WIs, findings that vary depending in the host's immune status [37]. Involvement of posterior elements is more frequent than in pyogenic spondylodiscitis, especially of the pedicles. There can be minimal to moderate para-spinal inflammation. Fungal disease does not show hyperintensity of the discs on T2WIs and the intranuclear cleft is typically preserved in all discs, which can indicate that the intervertebral disc may be spared from fungal invasion and inflammatory changes [37]. Findings can be similar to tuberculous spondylitis in immu-

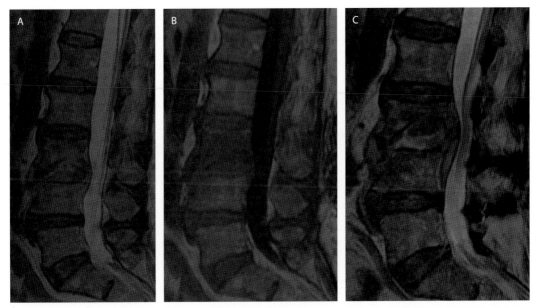

Figure 4.9 *Candida albicans* spondylitis in a 74-year-old female with type 2 diabetes mellitus and previous antibiotic treatment for a urinary infection. (A) Sagittal T2WI shows fracture of the inferior cortical plate of L3 with hyperintensity of the surrounding bone marrow. The disc shows little, poorly defined hyperintensity. (B) Sagittal T1WI shows the same features as in (A), as well as an anterior perivertebral hypointense mass. The patient's pain and infection markers persisted; however, culture of CT-guided biopsy continued to be negative. (C) Sagittal T2WI control showed an epidural hyperintense collection, hyperintensity of the disc and reorganization of the prevertebral collection.

nocompromised patients and this differential diagnosis should always be considered [40,41].

Post-procedural spondylodiscitis

Spinal procedures vary from diagnostic (discography, myelography) to therapeutic (disectomy, percutaneous blockade). Invasive modalities have a risk of post-procedural infection proportional to the magnitude of the intervention [42]. The incidence of post-procedural spondylodiscitis is relatively low and varies depending on the type of surgery and the anatomical site. The incidence of infection of the surgical site after laminectomy, discectomy and fusion is 3% or lower, but with instrumentation may increase to as high as 12% [42,43]. The incidence of post-procedural discitis is approximately 0.2% [44] (Figure 4.10).

The pathogenesis of infection after surgery is multifactorial. The possible sources for microbiological contamination are direct inoculation during surgery, wound infection in the early postoperative phase, or hematogenous spread.

The etiology of many post-procedural infections remains unknown even after needle aspiration or open biopsy. The most common agents are Gram-positive cocci: *S. aureus* being the most common pathogen, followed by *Staphylococcus epidermidis* and β-hemolytic streptococci. Gram-negative pathogens, especially from postoperative wound infection, include *Klebsiella pneumoniae*, *E. coli*, *P. aeruginosa* and *Proteus* spp. [42,44]. Prophylactic antibiotic therapy is used to decrease the infection rate. Clinical factors such as advanced patient age, spinal trauma and diabetes mellitus increase the susceptibility to postsurgical spine infections.

Surgical infections are classified as superficial (without fascial involvement) or deep (occuring below the lumbodorsal fascia or ligamentum nuchae), and can involve the discs, bone and epidural space. Infections can be classified according to time as acute (within 3 weeks of the procedure), chronic, or delayed (after 4 weeks of the procedure).

The most frequent clinical sign is pain; in the initial post-procedural period, the patient usually feels relief from the preoperative symptoms; then pain worsens from 1 to 4 weeks after surgery. Usually the intensity of back pain is not proportional to the physical findings. It is very rare for

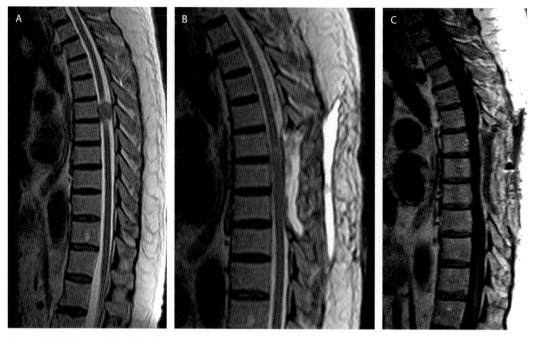

Figure 4.10 A 52-year-old male with lower limb paresthesia. (A) Sagittal T2WI shows an intradural, extramedullary neoplastic lesion of homogenous intermediate signal. (B) After surgery pain persisted and the white blood cell count indicated infection. New images were acquired. Sagittal T2WI shows dorsal laminectomy with superficial and deep fluid collections. The deep collection compresses the dural sac and reduces the subarachnoid space. (C) Sagittal contrast-enhanced T1WI delineates the peripheral rim enhancement, indicating an abscess.

patients to have constitutional symptoms. Superficial infection is usually silent, but there can be wound drainage and erythema [42,44].

The usual laboratory tests for post-procedural infection are blood cell count, ESR, CRP and blood cultures. The CRP, considered to be an acute-phase marker, is the most sensitive indicator of postoperative infection and effectiveness of treatment.

Conventional radiography
Usually there are no changes in the first 3 weeks. In case of discitis, from the fourth to the sixth postoperative weeks, disc space narrowing and endplate changes can be seen. Blurring of contours of paravertebral soft tissues could be a sign of paravertebral abscess. Plain films are also useful in inspecting lysis and alignment of surgical devices.

CT imaging
This imaging tool is useful in visualizing the early bone changes of the vertebral endplates. They appear as erosive and destructive lesions, accompa-

nied by narrowing of the affected disc space height. Soft tissue collections can also be seen. CT is used as a guide for tissue biopsy or needle aspiration for microbiological diagnosis.

MR imaging
MRI is the imaging modality of first choice in post-procedural pain or suspicion of infection, particularly with contrast, with 93% sensitivity and 97% specificity [42,44]. It is helpful earlier than the other two imaging modalities described above, although it is usually not reliable in the first 3 weeks after surgery. Differentiating early postoperative changes from discitis is challenging. If pain persists and there are no MR changes, MRI should be repeated 4 weeks later.

MR findings include decreased signal in the disc space on T1WIs and increased signal on T2WIs. Vertebral endplates show decreased signal intensity on T1WIs and increased signal intensity on T2WIs (called Modic 1 changes in the degenerative disc disease).

MR appears more useful for the exclusion of than the confirmation of post-procedural spondylodiscitis [45]. Boden *et al.* [46] suggested that intervertebral disc space enhancement, annular enhancement and vertebral bony enhancement can lead to the diagnosis of infection. Ross *et al.* [47] stated that this enhancement can be seen in any discectomy, including in asymptomatic patients, and the pattern of enhancement with infection is an amorphous enhancement of the disc. The para-spinal tissues can be seen with contrast enhancement [47, 48]. The epidural abscess is isointense to the cord on T1WIs and hyperintense on T2WIs, with enhancement after contrast administration [6,49] (Figure 4.11).

Imaging differential diagnoses include dialysis-related spondyloarthropathy, pseudoarthrosis, granulomatous spondylitis and neoplasm.

The majority of patients need a nonsurgical treatment approach, including spinal bracing and antibiotics. A minority of patients require operative intervention, usually consisting of debridement and autograft bone reconstruction or posterior instrumented fusion.

Role for therapy follow-up and patient management

MRI is used to monitor response to treatment in patients with spine infection (Figure 4.12). The literature suggests that MR changes may persist or even worsen during treatment despite clinical improvement [2]. Kowalski *et al.* [50] compared baseline MR images with images at 4–8 weeks' follow-up and concluded that para-spinal inflammation and epidural enhancement lessen in

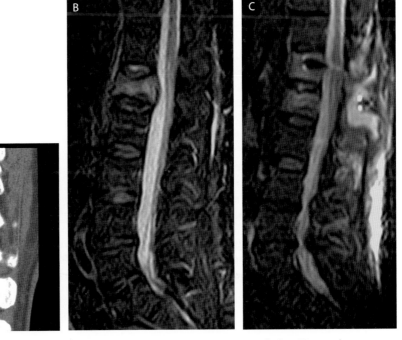

Figure 4.11 A post-traumatic, painful and unstable fracture that required surgery. (A) Multislice CT sagittal reconstruction image shows post-traumatic fracture of L1. (B) Sagittal fat-suppressed T2WI shows fracture of L1 with hyperintensity of the bone marrow, indicating contusion and edema. (C) After surgery, the patient's pain persisted. Sagittal fat-suppressed image shows the surgical hardware placement from T12 to L2, along with laminectomies and usual collection related to it. New bone marrow edema is identified in the L1 and T12 vertebral bodies, the latter not being seen before surgery. A CT-guided biopsy showed *S. aureus* infection.

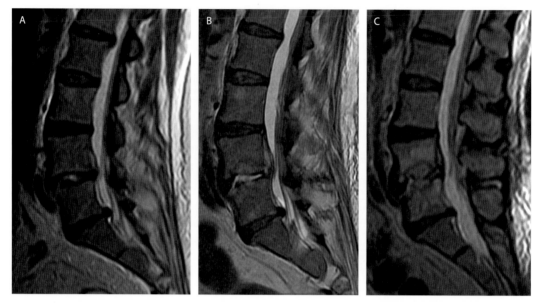

Figure 4.12 Follow-up sagittal T2WIs in a case of *S. aureus* spondylodiscitis. (A) Loss of height of the last two interverterbral spaces is seen, with central hyperintensity of the L4–L5 disc. (B) Two months later, the disc shows diffuse hyperintensity and an anterior epidural collection that compresses the dural sac. (C) Four months later, the disc still shows hyperintensity, there is destruction of the endplates and the epidural collection is diminished.

follow-up studies, while vertebral body enhancement and bone marrow edema were equivocal or even worse compared to the initial studies. However, none of these findings was associated with the patients' clinical status. The efficacy of treatment may be estimated in individual cases from clinical improvement (diminution of pain, resolution of fever), resolution of leukocytosis and decrease in ESR [2,6,50–52].

CT with multiplanar reconstruction and plain radiographs are used to diagnose body height changes, instability, deformities and osseous complications, but are not recommended for follow-up due to the high risk of radiation exposure.

For post-procedural infection, all imaging tools are used for patient follow-up, especially dynamic conventional radiographs and MRI.

References

1. Calderone R, Larsen J. Overview and classification of spinal infections. *Orthop Clin North Am* 1996;27: 1–8.
2. GouliourisT, Aliyu SH, Brown NM. Spondylodiscitis: update on diagnosis and management. *J Antimicrob Chemother* 2010;65 (Suppl 3):iii11–24.
3. Sobottke R, Seifert H, Fätkenheuer G, Schmidt M, Goßmann A, Eysel P. Current diagnosis and treatment of spondylodiscitis. *Dtsch Arztebl Int* 2008;105: 181–187.
4. Bettini N, Girardo M, Dema E, Cervellati S. Evaluation of conservative treatment of non specific spondylodiscitis. *Eur Spine J* 2009;18 (Suppl 1):143–150.
5. Modic MT, Steinberg PM, Ross JS, Masaryk TJ, Carter JR. Degenerative disk disease: assessment of changes in vertebral body marrow with MR imaging. *Radiology* 1988;166:193–199.
6. De Santo J, Ross JS. Spine infection/inflammation. *Radiol Clin North Am* 2011;49:105–127.
7. Ledermann HP, Schweitzer ME, Morrison WB, Carrino JA. MR imaging findings in spinal infections: Rules or myths? *Radiology* 2003;228:506–514.
8. Mylona E, Samarkos M, Kakalou E, Fanourgiakis P, Skoutelis A. Pyogenic vertebral osteomyelitis: a systematic review of clinical characteristics. *Semin Arthritis Rheum* 2009;39:10–17.
9. Modic MT, Feiglin DH, Piraino DW *et al.* Vertebral osteomyelitis: assessment using MR. *Radiology* 1985; 157:157–166.
10. Golimbu C, Firooznia H, Rafii M. CT of osteomyelitis of the spine. *AJR Am J Roentgenol* 1984;142:159–163.
11. Dagirmanjian A, Schils J, McHenry M, Modic MT. MR imaging of vertebral osteomyelitis revisited. *AJR Am J Roentgenol* 1996;167:1539–1543.

12. Gautam MP, Karki P, Rijal S, Singh R. Pott's spine and paraplegia. *JNMA J Nepal Med Assoc* 2005;44: 106–115.

13. McLain RF, Isada C. Spinal tuberculosis deserves a place on the radar screen. *Cleveland Clin J Med* 2004; 71:537–539.

14. Rezai AR, Lee M, Cooper PR, Errico TJ, Koslow M. Modern management of spinal tuberculosis. *Neurosurgery* 1995;36:87–97; discussion 97–98.

15. Lifeso RM, Weaver P, Harder EH. Tuberculous spondylitis in adults. *J Bone Joint Surg Am* 1985; 67:1405–1413.

16. Farinha NJ, Razali KA, Holzel H, Morgan G, Novelli VM. Tuberculosis of the central nervous system in children: a 20-year survey. *J Infect* 2000;41:61–68.

17. Bidstrup C, Andersen PH, Skinhøj P, Andersen AB. Tuberculous meningitis in a country with a low incidence of tuberculosis: still a serious disease and a diagnostic challenge. *Scand J Infect Dis* 2002;34: 811–814.

18. Titone L, Di Carlo P, Romano A *et al.* Tuberculosis of the central nervous system in children: 32 year survey. *Minerva Pediatr* 2004;56:611–617.

19. Moorthy S, Prabhu NK. Spectrum of MR imaging findings in spinal tuberculosis. *AJR Am J Roentgenol* 2002;179:979–983.

20. Ahmadi J, Bajaj A, Destian S, Segall HD, Zee CS. Spinal tuberculosis: atypical observations at MR imaging. *Radiology* 1993;189:489–493.

21. Oguz E, Sehirlioglu A, Altinmakas M *et al.* A new classification and guide for surgical treatment of spinal tuberculosis. *Int Orthop* 2008;32:127–133.

22. Smith A, Weinstein M, Mizushima A *et al.* MR imaging characteristics of tuberculous spondylitis vs vertebral osteomyelitis. *AJR Am J Roentgenol* 1989; 153:399–405.

23. Boachie-Adjei O, Squillante RG. Tuberculosis of the spine. *Orthop Clin North Am* 1996;27:95–103.

24. Jain R, Sawhney S, Berry M. Computed tomography of vertebral tuberculosis: patterns of bone destruction. *Clin Radiol* 1993;47:196–199.

25. Sinan T, Al-Khawari H, Ismail M, Ben-Nakhi A, Sheikh M. Spinal tuberculosis: CT and MRI feature. *Ann Saudi Med* 2004;24:437–441.

26. Sharif H. Role of MR imaging in the management of spinal infections. *AJR Am J Roentgenol* 1992;158: 1333–1345.

27. Jung N, Jee W, Ha K, Park C, Byun J. Discrimination of tuberculous spondylitis from pyogenic spondylitis on MRI. *AJR Am J Roentgenol* 2004;182: 1405–1410.

28. Chang K, Han M, Choi Y, Kim I, Han M, Kim C. Tuberculous arachnoiditis of the spine: findings on myelography, CT, and MR imaging. *AJNR Am J Neuroradiol* 1989;10:1255–1262.

29. Hernández-Albújar S, Arribas JR *et al.* Tuberculous radiculomyelitis complicating tuberculous meningitis: Case report and review. *Clin Infect Dis* 2000;30): 915–921.

30. Vlcek B, Burchiel KJ, Gordon T. Tuberculous meningitis presenting as an obstructive myelopathy. Case report. *J Neurosurg* 1984;60:196–199.

31. Freilich D, Swash M. Diagnosis and management of tuberculous paraplegia with special reference to tuberculous radiculomyelitis. *J Neurol Neurosurg Psychiatry* 1979;42:12–18.

32. Dastur DK, Manghani DK, Udani PM. Pathology and pathogenetic mechanisms in neurotuberculosis. *Radiol Clin North Am* 1995;33:733–752.

33. Tsolia M, Drakonaki S, Messaritaki A *et al.* Clinical features, complications and treatment outcome of childhood brucellosis in central Greece. *J Infect* 2002;44:257–262.

34. Mesner O, Riesenberg K, Biliar N *et al.* The many faces of human-to-human transmission of brucellosis: congenital infection and outbreak of nosocomial disease related to an unrecognized clinical case. *Clin Infect Dis* 2007;45:e135–140.

35. Kato Y, Masuda G, Itoda I, Imamura A, Ajisawa A, Negishi M. Brucellosis in a returned traveler and his wife: probable person-to-person transmission of *Brucella melitensis. J Travel Med* 2007;14:343–345.

36. Pourbagher A, Pourbagher MA, Savas L *et al.* Epidemiologic, clinical, and imaging findings in brucellosis patients with osteoarticular involvement. *AJR Am J Roentgenol* 2006;187:873–880.

37. Williams R, Fukui M, Meltzer C, Swarnkar A, Johnson D, Welch W. Fungal spinal osteomyelitis in the immunocompromised patient: MR findings in three cases. *AJNR Am J Neuroradiol* 1999;20:381–385.

38. Saigal G, Donovan M, Kozic D. Thoracic intradural aspergillus abscess formation following epidural steroid injection. *AJNR Am J Neuroradiol* 2004;25: 642–644.

39. Peman J, Jarque I, Bosch M *et al.* Spondylodiscitis caused by *Candida krusei*: Case report and susceptibility patterns. *J Clin Microbiol* 2006;44: 1912–1914.

40. Son J, Jee W, Jung C, Kim S, Ha K. Aspergillus spondylitis involving the cervico-thoraco-lumbar spine in an immunocompromised patient: a case report. *Korean J Radiol* 2007;8:448–451.

41. Tew C, Han F , Jureen R, Tey BH. Aspergillus vertebral osteomyelitis and epidural abscess. *Singapore Med J* 2009;50:e151.

42. Chaudhary SB, Vives MJ, Basra SK, Reiter MF. Postoperative spinal wound infections and postprocedural diskitis. *J Spinal Cord Med* 2007;30:441–451.

43. Weinstein MA, McCabe JP, Cammisa FP Jr. Postoperative spinal wound infection: a review of 2,391

consecutive index procedures. *J Spinal Disord* 2000; 13:422–426.

44. Silber JS, Anderson DG, Vaccaro AR, Anderson PA, McCormick P; NASS. Management of postprocedural discitis. *Spine J* 2002;2:279–287.

45. Van Goethem JW, Parizel PM, van den Hauwe L, Van de Kelft E, Verlooy J, De Schepper AM. The value of MRI in the diagnosis of postoperative spondylodiscitis. *Neuroradiology* 2000;42:580–585.

46. Boden SD, Davis DO, Dina TS *et al*. Postoperative diskitis: distinguishing early MR imaging findings from normal postoperative disk space changes. *Radiology* 1992;184:765e71

47. Ross JS, Zepp R, Modic MT. The postoperative lumbar spine: enhanced MR evaluation of the intervertebral disk. *AJNR Am J Neuroradiol* 1996;17: 323–331.

48. Babar S, Saifuddin A. MRI of the post-discectomy lumbar spine. *Clin Radiol* 200;57:969–981.

49. Duda JJ Jr, Ross JS. The postoperative lumbar spine: imaging considerations. *Semin Ultrasound CT MR* 1993;14:425–436.

50. Kowalski T, Layton, Berbari E *et al*. Follow-up MR imaging in patients with pyogenic spine infections: Lack of correlation with clinical features. *AJNR Am J Neuroradiol* 2007;28:693–699.

51. Kowalski T, Berbari E, Huddleston P, Steckelberg J, Osmon D. Do follow-up imaging examinations provide useful prognostic information in patients with spine infection? *Clin Infect Dis* 2006;43:172–179.

52. McHenry MC, Easley KA, Locker GA. Vertebral osteomyelitis: Long-term outcome for 253 patients from 7 Cleveland-area hospitals. *Clin Infect Dis* 2002;34: 1342–1350.

Clinical cases

Case 1

S. aureus spondylodiscitis in a 33-year-old male who presented with back pain.

The initial conventional radiograph was considered normal (Figure 4.13), laboratory results showed markers for infection and MR images showed infection at the L4–L5 intervertebral level (Figure 4.14). A CT-guided biopsy was performed to identify the pathogen (Figure 4.15). The patient completed therapy, but after being discharged the pain persisted and corticosteroids were prescribed. The patient returned to hospital with infection recurrence (Figure 4.16). After a second long-term regimen of intravenous antibiotic treatment and 8 months after the onset of symptoms, an MR demonstrated persistence of the changes (Figure 4.17). The spine showed clinical instability and the patient underwent surgery for surgical stabilization (Figure 4.18).

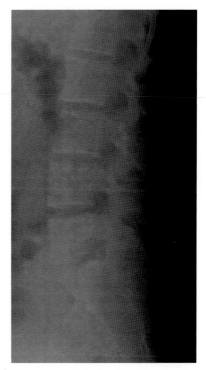

Figure 4.13 Lateral plain film at symptom onset; no bone or intervertebral abnormalities are seen.

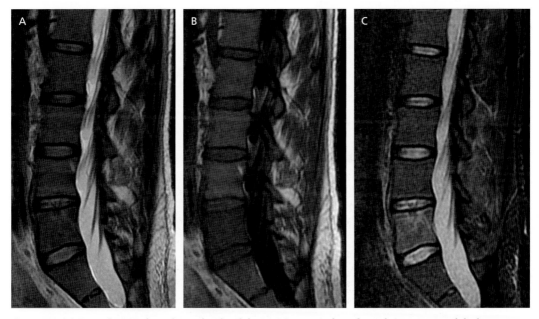

Figure 4.14 (A) Sagittal T2WI shows loss in height of the L4–L5 space with moderate hyperintensity of the bone marrow of L5. (B) Sagittal T1WI shows decreased intensity in the bone marrow of L5. (C) Sagittal fat-suppressed T2WI shows hyperintensity in the bone marrow of L5 with a hyperintense collection in the anterior intervertebral space in L4–L5.

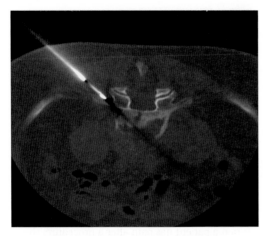

Figure 4.15 Axial CT image of guided biopsy.

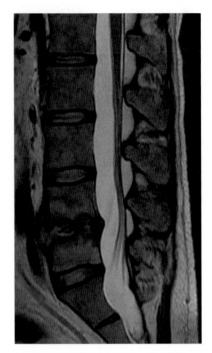

Figure 4.17 Sagittal T2WI 8 months after diagnosis shows more destruction of the vertebral plates, loss of height of L4 and L5, and hyperintensity of the disc with an anterior collection. Plain dynamic films confirmed instability.

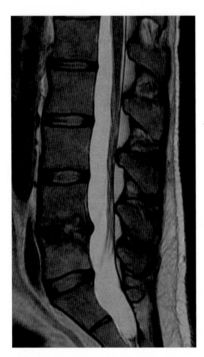

Figure 4.16 After receiving an inadequate course of steroids patient shows clinical and imaging recurrence of infection (4 months after initial therapy) The sagittal T2WI shows cortical destruction of the endplates, loss of height of the intervertebral space, hyperintensity of the central portion of the disc and hyperintensity of the bone marrow adjacent to the endplates.

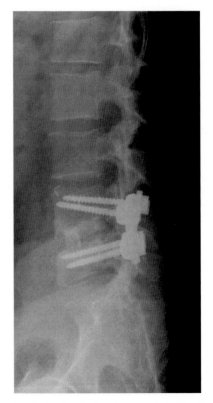

Figure 4.18 Lateral plain film shows posterior fixation and the intradiscal device.

Teaching points
• Initial imaging findings for spine infection can be normal, but if clinical symptoms persist, a contrast-enhanced MR should be repeated at 4 weeks.
• The most reliable MRI findings are evidence of para-spinal or epidural inflammatory tissue, contrast enhancement of the disc, hyperintensity or fluid equivalent signal on T2WIs and erosion or destruction of vertebral endplates on T1WIs.
• MR changes may persist or even worsen after adequate treatment.

Case 2
S. aureus spondylodiscitis in a 52-year-old male with back pain 3 weeks after minimally invasive discectomy.

Laboratory tests and MRI demonstrated infection. MRI showed major signs of infection, including disc hyperintensity on T2WIs, anterior epidural phlegmon (fluid collection with homogenous enhancement) with dural sac compression and endplate disruption along with bone marrow abnormalities indicating edema and infection. The patient required posterior decompression with laminectomies (Figures 4.19 and 4.20).

Teaching points
• When a patient has pain after a procedure, there must be suspicion of infection.
• MRI with contrast enhancement is the imaging modality of choice for evaluation of postsurgical complications.

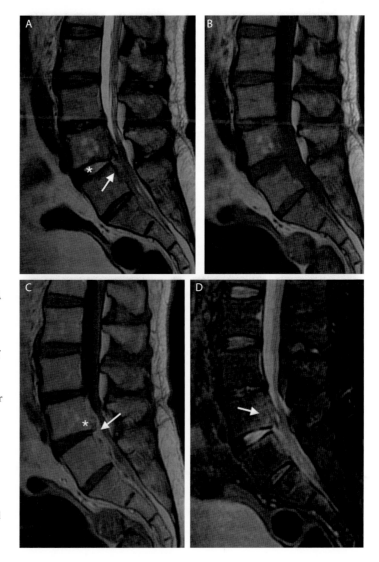

Figure 4.19 (A) Sagittal T2WI shows loss of height in the L4–L5 intervertebral space with hyperintensity of the disc (asterisk). A hyperintense epidural anterior collection (arrow) extends from L4 to S1 and compresses the dural sac. (B) Sagittal T1WI shows hypointensity of the endplate bone marrow; the epidural collection is isointense with the L4–L5 disc. (C) Sagittal T1WI after contrast shows enhancement of the bone marrow (asterisk) and an epidural collection (arrow; phlegmon), confirming dural sac compression. (D) Sagittal fat-suppressed T2WI shows hyperintensity of the endplates and bone marrow adjacent to the disc and a hyperintense epidural collection (arrow).

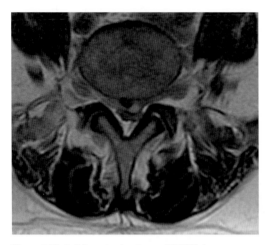

Figure 4.20 Axial contrast-enhanced T1WI shows an anterior epidural collection with diffuse enhancement and a central focal hypointensity corresponding to fluid and abscess within phlegmon and confirming dural sac compression.

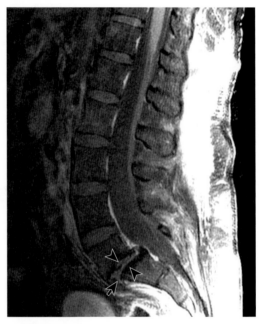

Figure 4.21 Sagittal contrast-enhanced T1WI of the lumbar spine shows increased disc signal at L5–S1 (arrow), listhesis of L5 on S1 and irregular adjacent endplates (arrowheads) with no endplate enhancement.

• If possible, MRI should be performed 3 weeks after surgery in order to differentiate complications from early postsurgical changes.
• Complications include epidural collections, seromas and abscesses.
• Comparison with the presurgical images is essential.
• If there are no MR changes but pain persists, MR should be repeated 4 weeks later.

Case 3

A 29-year-old male with a history of low back pain and chronic cough for the last year. The initial MRI showed anterior listhesis of L5 on S1 with increased disc signal (Figure 4.21). The patient was given pain medication. He consulted a week later for worsening of the back pain and night sweats. Plain radiographs showed anterior listhesis of L5 on S1 and disc space narrowing at L2–L3 with indistinct endplates (Figure 4.22). An MRI with contrast enhancement was repeated and the lesion showed advanced erosion of the inferior endplate of L2 and the supe-

rior endplate of L3 (Figure 4.23) along with a prominent preverterbal soft tissue enhancing lesion consistent with an abscess (Figures 4.23 and 4.24). Antibiotic treatment was initiated empirically to treat bacterial spondylodiscitis. The patient showed no improvement and 2 weeks later a third MRI was performed, showing worsening of the vertebral involvement and the para-spinal abscess, now narrowing the spinal canal (Figure 4.24). A CT-guided biopsy proved the diagnosis of TB.

Teaching points
• The initial stages of bacterial and tuberculous spondylodiscitis can be very difficult to differentiate.
• TB has to be a consideration in spondylodiscitis that does not respond to antimicrobial therapy.
• Isolation of Gram-negative bacilli is not always possible.

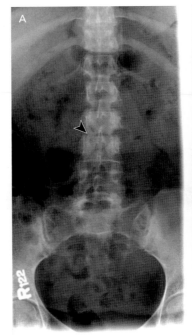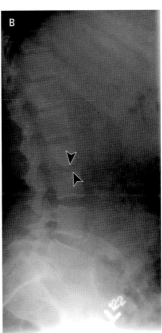

Figure 4.22 (A) Anteroposterior and (B) lateral plain films of the abdomen show decreased intervertebral space at L2–L3 (arrowheads), with irregular endplates. The changes in the lumbosacral junction persist (arrow).

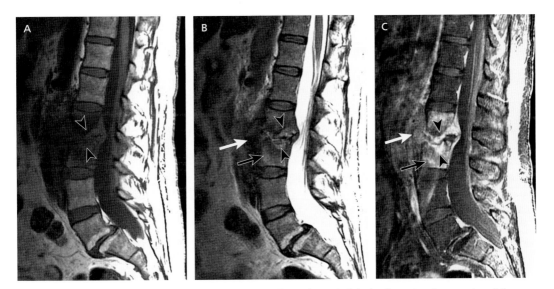

Figure 4.23 (A) Sagittal T1WI, (B) T2WI and (C) contrast-enhanced T1WI of the lumbar spine show erosion of the endplates adjacent to the L2–L3 intervertebral disc (arrowheads). The vertebral bodies show enhancement and increased T2 signal (black arrows). A prevertebral soft tissue mass is seen (white arrows).

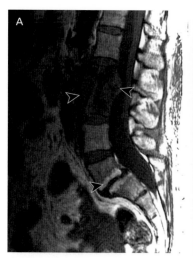

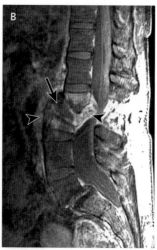

Figure 4.24 (A) Sagittal T1WI and (B) contrast-enhanced T1WI of the spine show collapse of the L2 and L3 vertebral bodies with a large fluid collection in the intervertebral space (arrow) that is contiguous with the enlarging para-spinal enhancing fluid collection (arrowheads). The epidural spread of disease narrows the spinal canal.

CHAPTER 5

Radiological Imaging of Soft Tissue Infections

Carolina Whittle and Giancarlo Schiappacasse

Universidad del Desarrollo, Santiago, Chile

Introduction

Soft tissue infections can occur in any body segment. Skin covers the body and is exposed to different insults. This chapter considers the most prevalent infectious diseases that may affect soft tissue.

Basic knowledge of the clinical problem

Soft tissues are composed of various layers: skin (epidermis, dermis and hypodermis, also known as subcutaneous fat tissue); and deep layers (aponeurotic fascia, tendons and muscles; ending at the periostium). Inflammatory or infectious processes can be found in all of these layers and the presentation is sometimes even pseudotumoral. Most appear clinically as areas of increased volume or palpable mass, with discoloration of the skin surface, hypersensitivity or regional pain.

The clinical questions

The clinician must be aware of the capabilities and limitations of each imaging technique in order to better decide the best modality to use to study these lesions: conventional radiography (X-ray), high-resolution ultrasound (HRUS), computed tomography (CT), magnetic resonance imaging (MRI) and nuclear medicine techniques (the latter are discussed in Chapter 12).

Conventional radiography is of very limited use in soft tissue evaluation. It is used mainly when lesions are suspected to extend to osteoarticular tissues or to rule out or detect foreign materials. Only 15% of wooden foreign bodies are radio-opaque [1] and 40% can be detected on plain films.

HRUS is indicated for superficial or small lesions and for follow-up, and MRI is used for the study of deeper or more extensive lesions, or when it is necessary better to characterize lesions that have been detected on HRUS. CT can be used for deep lesions and when calcifications are suspected. Overall, HRUS and MRI have the highest diagnostic performance.

The referring physician will be concerned as to whether there is an infectious process, as this will influence the therapeutic approach. Some laboratory findings can be of assistance, such as leukocytosis with neutrophilia, high C-reactive protein (CRP) and raised erythrocyte sedimentation rate (ESR). The most specific imaging findings for infection are fluid collections and intralesional gas. If these findings are found, percutaneous needle aspiration guided by US, CT or MRI can be performed to provide a definitive diagnosis [2].

Diagnostic Imaging of Infections and Inflammatory Diseases: A Multidisciplinary Approach, First Edition. Edited by Alberto Signore and Ana María Quintero.

Methodological considerations

Ultrasound

Ultrasound (US) is an accessible and transportable imaging technique that can be easily performed at the patient's bedside. It does not involve ionizing radiation and therefore is the imaging modality of choice in children and pregnant women.

US study of soft tissue should be performed with a broadband multifrequency linear transducers (7–20 MHz) as, depending on the location of the lesion and patient characteristics, different depths will need to explored. Color Doppler examination should also be performed, searching for slow flows in the different soft tissue layers. There should be an appropriate calibration of the sample volume size, smallest possible area of study and use of low pulse repetition frequency and low wall filter. Images must be obtained in at least two planes, transverse and longitudinal. The use of harmonic spatial compounding software and contrast resolution will improve tissue contrast and is useful for further characterization [3].

In the study of lesions of the dermoepidermal and subcutaneous tissue, which are at a depth of less than 2 cm, the use of a gel pad allows better investigation of the focal area and maximum lateral resolution. The high-resolution transducers are ideal for the study of superficial lesions.

US has high sensitivity in detecting fluid collections and can guide diagnostic needle biopsy or collection drainage. Among its limitations are its operator dependency, slow learning curve and non-specific findings.

CT imaging

CT images can provide isotropic reconstructions that better characterize different infectious processes. Reconstructions using soft tissue and bone algorithms should be performed. The first are used for the better assessment of the injury itself and the second to detect the presence of intralesional calcification or ossification. The lung window can be used [4] and may allow better detection of gas in some infectious processes. Intravenous contrast can be used to evaluate the uptake parameters of a soft tissue mass [4]. It is worth mentioning the association of CT with positron emission tomography (PET), a technique that is used primarily with [18F] fluorodeoxyglucose ([18F]FDG) to quantify the metabolism of lesions. In the setting of infections, [18F]FDG uptake is based on the increased glucose metabolism of mononuclear polymorphonuclear cells involved in this process (see Chapter 12).

MR imaging

MRI is an advanced imaging technique that allows an accurate characterization of the infectious processes of soft tissue. It is the preferred modality as it does not involve ionizing radiation and it has high spatial resolution. This technique requires T1- and T2-weighted, short-T1 inversion recovery (STIR) and contrast-enhanced T1 sequences to be obtained. Usually, spin echo (SE) and fast spin echo (FSE) sequences are best suited for the identification and characterization of soft tissue abnormalities; they locate abnormalities, particularly those located deep in the subcutaneous layer or muscle. At least two orthogonal planes are required for better assessment. In some cases, gradient echo (GRE) sequences are necessary for the evaluation of lesions due to its sensitivity in detecting magnetic susceptibility artifacts, such as gas, blood, or metallic products. The visual field is determined by the extent of the lesion [5,6].

Normal findings and artifacts

The different imaging techniques assess soft tissue using different approaches. In conventional radiography and CT, images are dependent on the characteristic soft tissue densities; fat tissue on CT has a specific density range with low Hounsfield units.

On US, the layers of different echogenicity are associated with specific tissues. Normally, the dermoepidermal complex appears on HRUS as a regular band of less than 3 mm. At the surface, a hyperechoic line represents the gel–epidermis interface. The dermal layer has a more echogenic superficial component but at a deeper level it becomes hypoechoic. The subcutaneous tissue is usually hypoechoic, with thin echogenic septa. The fascia has an echogenic fibrillar pattern parallel to the skin surface and lies between the deep subcutaneous layer and muscle. The localized presence of fluid and gas within a focal area allows the diagnosis of fluid collection or infection. It should be noted that the presence of reverberation produced by air may also be the result of trauma or a medical procedure. It is important to consider that the shadowing produced may impede a proper visualization of the deeper layers. Anechogenic lesions with posterior acoustic enhancement may allow confident identification of a fluid interface; however, some fluid lesions have different composition (such as of proteins or debris) and will have a different intensity on acoustic enhancement, making the diagnosis more difficult.

CT artifacts may impair image quality in some cases but in others may aid the diagnosis. Amongst those that impair the image quality are beam hardening artifact, produced when the X-ray beam flows through high-density structures, which filter the low energy photons, generating black lines; partial volume artifact, which may be seen when a component's voxel density differs from the mean voxel density; and movement artifacts.

In MRI, artifacts can impair the image and generally should be avoided. However, some artifacts may be useful and assist in diagnosis. A clear example of this is the chemical shift artifact, which allows the tissues with intracytoplasmic fat to be distinguished, and plays a key role in the identification of lipid-rich lesions. Another is the magnetic susceptibility artifact, which distorts an image when tissues or materials with a very distinct susceptibility are close to each other.

Pathological findings and significance

Soft tissue infectious and inflammatory processes can be divided into superficial lesions (skin layer) or deep lesions (aponeurotic fascia and musculotendinous layers) and in some cases involve more than one layer.

In the skin, including the dermoepidermal complex and the hypodermis or subcutaneous layer, the most common infectious–inflammatory lesions are dermatitis, folliculitis and pyoderma, panniculitis, foreign body granulomas, seroma, abscesses, lymphadenopathy, cat scratch lymphadenitis and bursitis. In the deeper layers, lesions include fasciitis, tendinitis, peritendonitis, tenosynovitis, myositis in its different forms, hydatid disease and abscesses.

The pathological study of skin biopsies can be interpreted according to the patterns of tissue reaction and inflammation. There are four patterns of distribution of inflammatory cells in the skin: superficial perivascular inflammation; superficial and deep dermal inflammation; folliculitis and peri-

folliculitis; and panniculitis. Panniculitis and folliculitis are considered to be the main histological patterns [7].

Dermatitis

Dermatitis is defined as inflammation of the superficial or deep dermis. The predominant cell type is usually the lymphocyte, but there may be a mixture of other cell types. It can be caused by multiple diseases, such as lupus and scleroderma, arthropod bites, parasitic or dermatophytos infection, drugs, urticaria, or secondary to sun exposure, among others [8].

If imaging is considered, HRUS may be useful in focal dermatitis as it can show diffuse thickening of the dermis, which may be hyperemic, and the underlying subcutaneous tissue whose echostructure should be preserved. The findings are nonspecific.

Folliculitis

Folliculitis is the inflammation of the hair follicle, usually owing to bacterial infection. Inflammatory cells are present within the lumen and wall of the hair follicle. When it involves perifollicular connective tissue, which sometimes extends to the adjacent dermis, it is called perifolliculitis. The cause may be infectious (impetigo, fungus, herpes) or noninfectious. It occurs most often in those body segments with thick hair, such as the scalp, neck, chin, underarms, buttocks and limbs [7].

In most cases, clinical evaluation is straight forward and no imaging studies are required. HRUS can show a small (a few millimeters) dermal hypoechoic lesion in the area of the inflamed hair follicle, sometimes associated with thickening and hyperemia of the adjacent dermis (Figure 5.1).

Pyodermia

This is the term for pyogenic infections of the skin, including impetigo and its variants, and folliculitis. *Staphylococcus aureus* is the most common organism in impetigo. In previous decades, β-hemolytic Group A streptococcus was the most prevalent. Typical US findings are folliculitis, dermatitis and cystic lesions (Figures 5.2 and 5.3).

Cellulitis

Cellulitis is acute infection of the skin involving the subcutaneous tissue. It presents as a diffuse

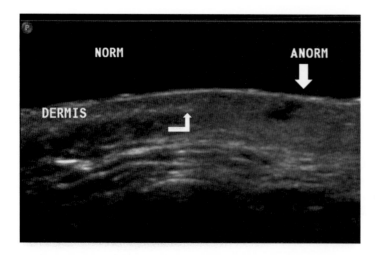

Figure 5.1 Ultrasound shows a 3-mm hypoechoic focus in the superficial dermis (arrow) associated with focal thickening of the dermis (right-angled arrow), consistent with folliculitis and perifolliculitis.

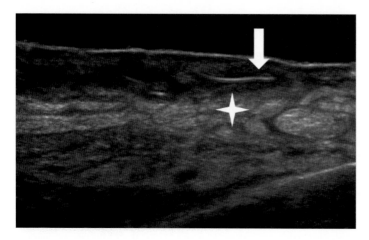

Figure 5.2 Pyodermia. Inflammatory changes of the dermis and subcutaneous tissue of the cheek. These layers are shown to be thickened with edema of the subcutaneous tissue (star) and presence of hairs (arrow).

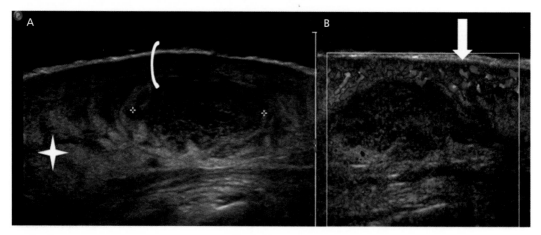

Figure 5.3 Pyodermia. Thickening of the dermis. (A) Subcutaneous edema (star) and abscessed foci (curved arrow) and (B) regional hyperemia (arrow).

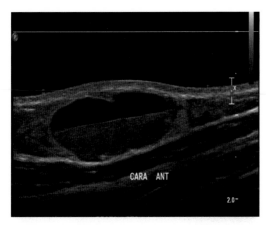

Figure 5.4 Subcutaneous collection with a fluid–fluid level that shows a slight increase in the echogenicity of the surrounding fat tissue.

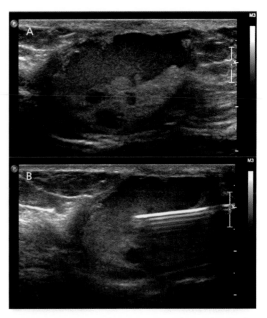

Figure 5.5 (A) Fluid collection in the abdominal wall of irregular contour. It presents with echoes and a fluid–fluid level. (B) Diagnostic percutaneous puncture is performed with fine needle aspiration.

swelling of the connective tissue of the skin or deeper soft tissue, usually from the dermis to subcutaneous tissue. It can be caused by various microorganisms, including *S. aureus* and *Streptococcus pyogenes*. Clinically, it presents as an ill-defined area of erythema, with an orange-peel appearance and painful zone. Microscopically, it is characterized by infiltration of neutrophils. It may progress to necrosis [9,10].

On HRUS, cellulitis shows a diffusely increased echogenicity of subcutaneous tissue of unspecified aspect; sometimes there is a heterogeneous reticular pattern of hypoechoic bands (inflammatory exudative dissection). In some cases, color Doppler shows regional hyperemia (Figures 5.2 and 5.3). HRUS will detect the regional fluid collection or gas bubbles (Figure 5.4).

On CT there is an increase in the fat attenuation coefficient, with loss of well-defined margins between fat and muscle. Thickening and edema of the planes involved can also be seen. Although CT is less sensitive than MRI, it does differentiate superficial cellulitis from a deeper lesion. It is helpful in distinguishing between uncomplicated cellulitis and cellulitis complicated by collections. In advanced cases or virulent infections, cellulitis manifests as necrotizing cellulitis with the presence of gas and abscesses.

On MRI STIR sequences there is an increase in the signal with varying degrees of edema that can be laminar and this is associated with wall thickening. On T1-weighted images (T1WIs) discrete areas of hypointensity in adipose tissue can be seen. If the

process continues, collections or abscesses can be seen, corresponding to fluid areas ringed by a wall that enhances with contrast and surrounded by edema.

Abscesses

Abscesses are localized collections of pus in a space, tissue or organ. They are composed of necrotic tissue, white blood cells and bacteria. Clinically, they present as areas of erythema, pain and in some cases, areas of tenderness fluctuating with palpation.

HRUS visualizes fluid collections, even clinically occult collections, providing an excellent guide for diagnostic aspiration puncture (Figure 5.5) [2]. Biopsy is often indispensable for the differential diagnosis of seroma, hematoma, cystic or necrotic tumor and abscess.

Abscesses may occur as anechoic, hypoechoic, isoechoic or slightly hypoechoic collections and less frequently as hyperechoic collections. The collection may be surrounded by an echogenic wall, with internal septa or echoes. The presence of gas is a characteristic finding of infection and it is hyperechoic with reverberation artifact (Figures 5.6 and

5.7). HRUS can also detect the presence of foreign bodies within the lesion or sinus tract to the surface or deep layers.

On CT, abscesses appear as areas of fluid attenuation. The attenuation coefficient depends on the contents of the abscess. Gas is easily detected with this imaging modality. With the use of intravenous contrast, peripheral enhancement surrounded by edema is usually seen.

Foreign body granuloma

Foreign body granuloma is characterized by the presence of a localized collection of epithelioid cells, often interspersed with multinucleated giant cells, lymphocytes, plasma cells, fibroblasts and macrophages surrounding a foreign body. A foreign body can enter tissues through trauma (thorns, glass, etc.) or inoculation (parasites, silicone, etc.) and is able to move into the deep layers. When a foreign

body reaction occurs, there is a secondary fibrohistiocytic inflammatory reaction.

HRUS shows the foreign body inside the lesion. It is seen as an echoic or hyperechoic image, which may or may not have posterior shadowing artifact. In general, the artifact is not seen for wood or thorns. Acoustic shadow artifact is seen for bone and stone, and reverberation or comet tail artifact for glass, plastic and metal. The foreign body is surrounded by a hypoechoic halo that corresponds to fibrin, granulation tissue and a collagen capsule. The neovasculature may have a hypervascular pattern of a reactive nature (Figure 5.8) [1,11].

Lymphadenitis

Lymphadenitis is a swollen lymph node. It can be found in different locations, but predominantly in the subcutaneous layer, where lymph nodes are the first line of defense against and response to a

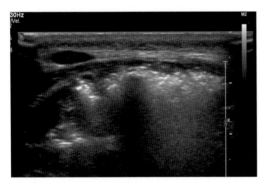

Figure 5.6 Patient with a sharp cervical injury complicated by infection. A cervical collection with air is seen on the left side.

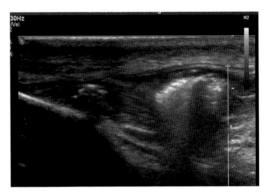

Figure 5.7 Air bubbles in the sternocleidomastoid muscle.

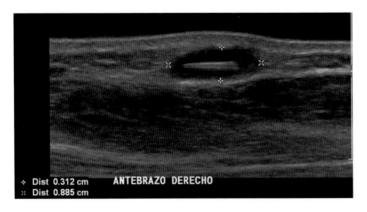

Figure 5.8 Granuloma to a foreign body (a small thorn) in the center of subcutaneous tissue.

number of pathogens, including bacteria, fungi, viruses and parasites. The enlarged lymph nodes also represent the host's response to foreign bodies and can be located in the vicinity of the infection entry port. There are many non-neoplastic systemic diseases that also present as adenitis.

Lymph nodes are seen on US as elongated hypoechoic nodules with a central echogenic hilum that contains lymphatic tissue and blood vessels. When inflamed, as a result of infection or not, lymph nodes may increase in size, remaining oval or becoming round, and appear hypoechogenic with the increase in vascularity. Vascularity of the adjacent soft tissues can also increase and this is generally associated with increased echogenicity of the perilymphatic adipose tissue. Some infections, usually bacterial *Staphylococcus* spp., *Streptococcus* spp. and some mycobacteria, may form abscesses and these are seen as avascular hypoechoic areas with posterior acoustic enhancement.

On CT, normal lymph nodes have a central fatty hilum; in adenitis, the lymph node enlarges, becomes more rounded and may be associated with varying degrees of increased density of the surrounding subcutaneous tissue. Typically, the infectious process results in an increase in the number of lymph nodes, which can be present in groups.

Lymph nodes can be differentiated more effectively on MRI than on CT, as it has greater sensitivity for abscess formation and perinodal compromise of the subcutaneous surrounding tissues. Moreover, deeper compromise can be characterized and complications of the fascia and muscles and development of fistulas can be detected.

Cat scratch lymphadenitis

Cat scratch lymphadenitis is a benign condition secondary to *Bartonella henselae* infection acquired through contact with cats or a cat scratch (90% of cases). It is generally a self-limiting illness and presents as papules or non-pruritic pustules. Regional lymph nodes appear between 3 and 4 weeks after exposure. The most frequently involved zones are the epitrochlear, cervical and inguinal regions. Lymph nodes may be single or multiple and are usually less than 5 cm in length.

On US, lymph nodes are increased in size and tend to be hypoechoic or heterogeneous, single or multiple. There may be discrete perinodal inflammatory changes. Hyperemia of the hilum can be observed with color Doppler; in other cases, lymph nodes are hypovascular.

Bursitis

Bursitis is the focal inflammation of a bursa, or inflammation of the synovial lining structures associated with tendons, muscles and bones. Bursae reduce the friction produced by movements between these structures. As they are covered with synovial tissue, they can be affected by the same processes that affect synovial joints, including inflammatory arthropathy, dialysis-related amyloidosis, crystal arthropathy and infection. They can also be affected by repeated friction or trauma [12]. The most frequently involved bursae are the olecranian and prepatellar.

On US, bursae are seen as hypoechoic–anechoic structures with a small amount of internal fluid and an echogenic rim that corresponds to the synovial membrane. In bursitis, thickening and hyperemia of the synovial membrane can be seen. The production of synovial fluid expands the lumen and there can be a small increase in the echogenicity of the surrounding fat tissue. Features of subacute or chronic bursitis are septa or suspended echoes within the fluid and thin bursa walls. If the content is purulent or hemorrhagic, a fluid–fluid level may be seen (Figure 5.9). HRUS is useful in detecting the collection of fluid and guiding its puncture for aspiration.

CT is unhelpful in the evaluation of bursae.

MRI is the imaging method of choice, especially for deeply located bursae or those in contact with flat bones. Cystic structures can communicate with

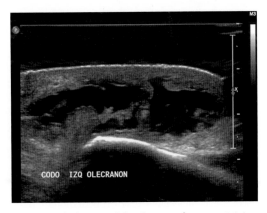

Figure 5.9 Thickening of the olecranon bursa containing fluid and synovial hypertrophy.

a joint or can be located near myotendon structures. They appear as fluid collections with a hypointense wall on T1-weighted (T1WIs) and T2-weighted images (T2WIs), with variable enhancement with contrast; in some cases septa are present. The fluid is usually hyperintense on T2WIs, but if pus or hematic content is present, it can be hypointense on T2WIs and hyperintense on T1WIs. Additionally, MRI delineates adjacent structures such as muscles, tendons and joints, which are sometimes affected by the process.

Proliferative fasciitis

Proliferative fasciitis is a benign non-neoplastic lesion composed of immature spindle-shaped fibroblasts and basophilic giant cells. It usually occurs in patients over the age 40 years, and the forearm and thigh are the most common locations. Patients present with firm and hard subcutaneous nodules, which can be confused with a sarcoma. On imaging it appears as a non-specific solid soft tissue mass that is well-defined or infiltrated (Figures 5.10 and 5.11). The treatment is marginal excision with a free margin.

Nodular fasciitis

This lesion is a non-neoplastic proliferation of fibroblasts and usually occurs in young adults. It is one of the most common lesions of fibrous tissue

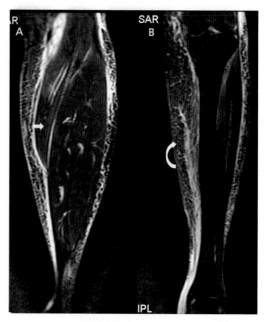

Figure 5.10 Eosinophilic fasciitis. Coronal STIR sequence show (A) mild thickening of the aponeurotic fascia (arrow) and (B) thickening and diffuse edema of the subcutaneous tissue in the left leg (curved arrow). Biopsy revealed an eosinophilic fasciitis.

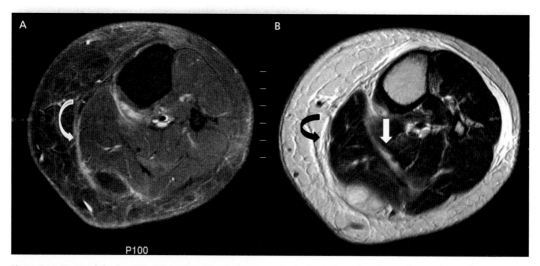

Figure 5.11 Eosinophilic fasciitis. (A) With contrast, the aponeurotic fascia is evident (curved arrow). (B) The T2W sequence shows diffuse edema of the subcutaneous tissue (curved arrow) associated with laminar intermuscular fluid collection (arrow).

origin. It is characterized by rapid growth and its most common location is the upper extremities [13]. Lesions are usually small (1–3 cm) and solitary. There are three types of nodular fasciitis: subcutaneous, intramuscular and fascial. Histologically, the lesion may be mistaken for a sarcoma due to its hypercellularity and mitotic activity. The treatment is excision with free margin and recurrence is uncommon.

On MRI, a well-defined superficial mass or one deeper to the fascia is seen that has middle to low intensity signal on T1WIs and T2WIs because of its high fibrous content. On US, this high fibrous content means that relative to muscle the mass appears as a hypoechoic solid nodule that is usually poorly vascularized.

Necrotizing fasciitis

This is an inflammatory process affecting the fascial planes and is of an infectious nature. The most common infectious agents are *S. aureus* and *S. pyogenes*. It progresses rapidly, forming a collection and gas in the affected soft tissues. Most cases require surgical treatment with extensive debridement of the affected tissue and, sometimes, amputation of a limb.

In the early stages, MRI shows thickened tissue similar to cellulitis, with edema and increased signal on T2WIs. Within hours, the process progresses in extent and depth. The fascia thickens and deep loculated or lamellar small collections accumulate, often with muscle involvement and fibrillar edema and gas.

CT is less sensitive but allows the diagnosis of necrotizing processes by demonstrating a lack of fascia contrast enhancement [14].

On US, thickening of the fascia is a non-specific finding, but if it is associated with increased echogenicity of deep subcutaneous layers it may suggest an inflammatory condition. Gas bubbles are hyperechoic and easily detected on US.

Paratenonitis or peritendinitis

Paratenonitis or peritendinitis is an inflammatory process that affects tendons containing a paratendon, the best example of which is the Achilles' tendon. There is thickening of the tendon (>5 mm in the anteroposterior diameter) and a slight decrease in the echogenicity of the fibers on US, with an increase in the echogenicity of the sur-

rounding adipose tissue. Intrasubstance calcifications may be present and in some cases focal tears.

On MRI, loss of normal morphology (kidney-shaped) is commonly seen, replaced by a rounded or bi-convex shape of greater than 5–6 mm in diameter. In general, the T1 signal is preserved and is slightly increased on STIR. A high signal on T2WIs may indicate focal tears.

Tenosynovitis

Tenosynovitis is an inflammatory entity that affects tendons that are covered by synovium, usually in the extremities. Inflammation can be secondary to repeated mechanical injury, collagen diseases, or foreign bodies, wounds, or bites. The most common infectious agents are *S. aureus* and *S. pyogenes*. If there is a history of a bite, more aggressive bacteria should be considered, including anaerobes.

On HRUS the presence of a peritendineal collection can be detected, sometimes with debris in suspension, nodularity or thickening of the tendon sheath. In some cases the hyperemic tendon sheath can be seen (Figure 5.12).

MRI shows thickening of the involved tendons and increased signal on STIR. Increased fluid in the synovium can enhance with contrast. There may also be varying degrees of thickening, nodularity

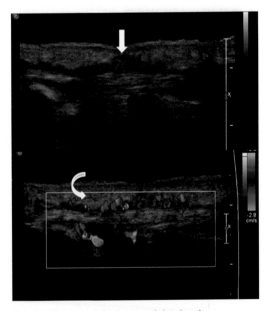

Figure 5.12 Marked thickening of the sheath surrounding the flexor tendon of the finger with a fluid laminar band (arrow) and regional hyperemia (curved arrow) suggesting tenosynovitis.

and irregularity of the synovia, depending on both the chronicity and the etiology.

Proliferative myositis

Proliferative myositis is a rare and self-limiting intramuscular process of inflammatory origin. It presents at an average age of 50 years as a heterogeneous lesion with calcifications. It consists of a rapidly growing mass that diffusely infiltrates the muscle tissue with spindle cells and other giant ganglion-like cells; it can simulate a tumor. No specific treatment is required.

Being a rare entity, there is scarce literature regarding its appearance on MRI. However, in isolated reports it is seen as an ill-defined enlargement in muscle volume of slightly lower signal than normal muscle on T1WIs and slight hyperintensity on STIR, with variable enhancement with contrast. Its infiltrating appearance means it can be confused with muscle tumor lesions such as sarcomas and primary lymphoma.

Infectious myositis (pyomyositis)

This infection, usually bacterial, affects large muscles of the extremities. It occurs mainly in immunosuppressed patients (HIV/AIDS and diabetes) [15]. One study revealed that up to 17% of Americans with pyomyositis were HIV positive and pyomyositis is considered one of the most common complications in this group. Deep wounds, previous surgery and immunocompromise secondary to neoplastic diseases are also risk factors for pyomyositis. It can also result from minor trauma or local hematoma formation, with the hematoma providing a nest for the development of infection [16,17]. Muscles in the extremities are most commonly affected as they are more frequently subjected to trauma and injury; the most common locations are the quadriceps, gluteus tendons and ileopsoas, with the latter commonly infected with *Mycobacterium tuberculosis*. The most common causative organisms are *S. aureus*, *S. pyogenes* and, in developing countries, *M. tuberculosis* and some parasites.

There are three clinical stages: invasive (with pain secondary to muscle edema), suppurative (secondary fever develops due to the presence of an abscess) and late (where, due to the extension of the process, there is life-threatening toxemia).

On CT, the volume of the muscular plane is increased and attenuation decreased by swelling. It is helpful in distinguishing a subcutaneous process from muscle edema. Collections can be seen, but are more easily observed on MRI. Uptake of contrast by the muscle as well as the extent of the process are variable. On MRI, uptake of contrast is also variable. On STIR images, increased signal represents inflammatory edema of the muscle. It is important to mention if there are areas that do not enhance with contrast, a necrotizing component is implied, giving a worse prognosis.

Myositis ossificans

Myositis ossificans is a self-limiting benign condition that occurs as an intramuscular mass predominantly in the extremities. Its name is not appropriate since it is not an inflammatory disease. It is the result of a direct contusion or repeated microtrauma and is a proliferative response in the affected tissue with the development of heterotopic ossifications. There is a focal pattern of maturation with a central area of necrotic muscle tissue, areas of hemorrhage and fibroblasts, a central area of immature bone formation and a peripheral area of mature bone.

On MRI it manifests as a focal alteration of the muscle. Initially, an ill-defined edema is visible that progresses to a tumor or high-signal mass on T2WIs during the first days or weeks after trauma. In this state it may simulate a sarcoma. It takes approximately 4–6 weeks for a metaplastic ossification to develop at the periphery of the lesion; this is difficult to see on MRI, but it is easily distinguished on CT. Later there is progressive ossification toward the center of the lesion, reflecting the degree of maturation of the osteoid tissue, which is greater at the periphery. On MRI, ossification is seen as areas of low signal on T2WIs and middle signal on T1WIs. Myositis ossificans has high signal on STIR and significant contrast capture (Figures 5.13, 5.14, 5.15 and 5.16).

Role for therapy follow-up and patient management

Soft tissue lesion follow-up will depend on its depth and therapy response. If the lesion is well assessed by US, this should be the preferred method. When complications are suspected, or the process involves deeper layers, it should be followed up with MRI or contrast-enhanced CT.

US is considered the diagnostic imaging modality of first choice, since it offers real-time assessment.

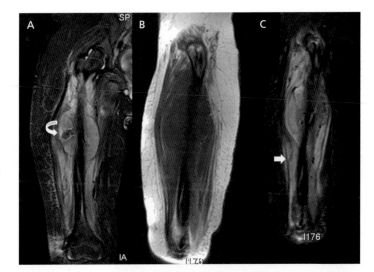

Figure 5.13 Myositis ossificans. (A) T2 STIR, (B) T1W spin echo and (C) T1 fat-saturated, contrast-enhanced sequences. A soft tissue inflammatory process is seen around the fractured shaft of the femur and involves the muscular plane: high signal on T2 STIR (curved arrow, A) and low signal on T1W spin echo (B). It shows significant contrast uptake (arrow, C).

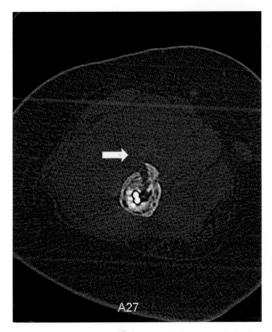

Figure 5.14 CT with axial image in the bone window. Fine foci of ossification are seen within the soft tissue mass (arrow).

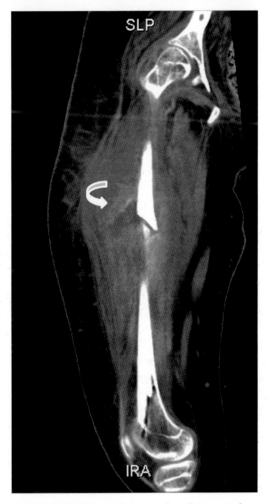

Figure 5.15 CT with sagittal image in the soft tissue window. Fine foci of ossification are seen within the soft tissue mass (curved arrow), characteristic of myositis ossificans.

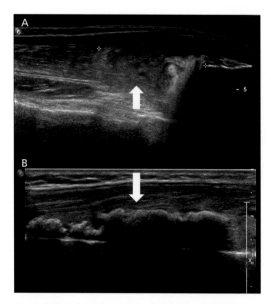

Figure 5.16 Volume increase is observed in the thickness of the triceps muscle with loss of the sharp contours of the fibrillar pattern (top, arrow); 10 days after, US control shows intralesional calcification compatible with myositis ossificans (bottom, arrow).

Biopsies of small lesions can be performed with US guidance, which is less expensive than with CT or MRI [2]. US, CT and MRI can detect fluid collections, even clinically occult collections, and are an excellent guide for diagnostic aspiration puncture (see Figure 5.5) [2]. These techniques are often indispensable for the differential diagnosis of seroma, hematoma, abscess and cystic or necrotic tumor.

Conclusion

Soft tissue infectious–inflammatory symptoms correspond to a varied spectrum of pathologies with different clinical connotations. They are very common in clinical practice. Early diagnosis of septic processes is very important for improvement of the prognosis. Imaging allows their characterization, but the diagnosis is not always accurate. Imaging can detect fluid collections and guide diagnostic puncture. The study of the fluid is important for definitive etiological determination.

References

1. Jacobson A, Powell A, Craig JG, Bouffard JA, Van Holsbeeck MT. Wooden foreign bodies in soft tissue: detection at US. *Radiology* 1998;206:45–48.

2. Douglas BR, Charboneau JW, Reading CC. Ultrasound-guided intervention: expanding horizons. *Radiol Clin North Am* 2001;39:415–428.

3. Winter TC, Teefey SA, Middleton WD. Musculoskeletal ultrasound: an update. *Radiol Clin North Am* 2001;39:465–483.

4. Fayad LM, Carrino JA, Fishman EK. Musculoskeletal infection: role of CT in the emergency department. *RadioGraphics* 2007;27:1723–1736.

5. Beltran J. MR imaging of soft tissue infection. *Magn Reson Imaging Clin North Am* 1995;3:743–751.

6. Struk DW, Munk PL, Lee MJ, Ho SG, Worsley DF. Imaging of soft tissue infections. *Radiol Clin North Am* 2001;39:277–303.

7. Weedon D. Acercamiento a la interpretación de las biopsias cutáneas. In: *Pielpatología*, vol 1. Harcourt Health Science Edition en español Marban Libros, SL, 2002, pp. 3–14.

8. Weedon D. Infecciones e infestaciones cutáneas: patrones histológicos e infecciones bacterianas y por rickettsias. In: *Pielpatología*, vol 2. Harcourt Health Science Edition en español Marban Libros, SL, 2002, pp. 519–548.

9. Loyer E, DuBrow R, David C *et al.* Imaging of superficial soft-tissue infections: sonographic findings in cases of cellulitis and abscess. *AJR Am J Roentgenol* 1996;166:149–152.

10. Bureau NJ, Chhem RK, Cardinal E. Musculoskeletal infections: US manisfestations. *RadioGraphics* 1999; 19:1585–1592.

11. Whittle C, González P, Horvath E *et al.* Detección y caracterización por ultrasonido de cuerpos extraños de partes blandas. *Rev Méd Chile* 2000;128: 419–424.

12. Kransdorf M, Murphy M. Masses that may mimic soft tissue tumors.In: *Imaging of Soft Tissue Tumors*, 2nd edn. Philadelphia: Lippincott Williams & Wilkins, 2006; pp. 511–572.

13. Kransdorf M, Murphy M. Benign fibrous and fibrohistiocytic tumors. In: *Imaging of Soft Tissue Tumors*, 2nd edn. Philadelphia: Lippincott Williams & Wilkins, 2006; pp. 189–256.

14. Beauchamp NJ Jr, Scott WW Jr, Gottlieb LM, Fishman EK. CT evaluation of soft tissue and muscle infection and inflammation: a systematic compartmental approach. *Skeletal Radiol* 1995;24:317–324.

15. Restrepo CS, Lemos DF, Gordillo H *et al.* Imaging findings in musculoskeletal complications of AIDS. *RadioGraphics* 2004;24:1029–1049.

16. Yuh WT, Schreiber AE, Montgomery WJ, Ehara S. Magnetic resonance imaging of pyomyositis. *Skeletal Radiol* 1988;17:190–193.

17. Gordon BA, Martinez S, Collins AJ. Pyomyositis: characteristics at CT and MR imaging. *Radiology* 1995; 197:279–286.

Clinical cases

Case 1

A 21-year-old male patient with no morbid history. He had previously traveled to Ecuador and presented with two skin lesions in the left lower extremity, one on the leg and the other in the suprapatellar region, characterized by increased focal volume, reddening and pain. Soft tissue ultrasound suggested two foreign bodies each of 15 mm in diameter and surrounded by a hypoechogenic halo (Figure 5.17). They were located in the subcutaneous layers and there was increased echogenicity of the fat surrounding them. Minimum intralesional movement was observed and a diagnosis of myiasis was considered.

Surgery was performed and two larvae were extracted, one from each lesion. The patient progressed well with postoperative antibiotic therapy and remained in good health.

Teaching points
• If the patient has traveled to endemic jungle areas, myiasis must be considered in the differential diagnosis of inflammatory skin lesions of the exposed extremities.
• In the presence of echogeneic foreign bodies with minimum intralesional movement, larvae should be suspected.

Case 2

A 55-year-old male with a history of abdominal pain mainly located in the right upper quadrant and a palpable mass in the left inguinal cord. Laboratory tests showed only a small elevation in alkaline phosphatase. A CT was performed.

A cystic multilobulated mass was found in the inguinal region. It was localized to the fat tissue, adjacent to the femoral vessels. The cyst was a well-defined lesion with several septations and a thick wall. No inflammatory changes were seen (Figure 5.18). The cystic mass extended into the pelvic and abdominal cavities, including into the liver (Figures 5.19 and 5.20).

The inguinal mass was resected and histopathological biopsy diagnosed a hydatid cyst. Following surgery the patient received medical treatment.

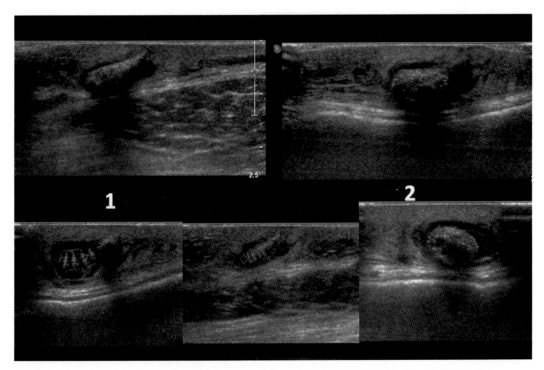

Figure 5.17 US suggested two subcutaneous foreign bodies of 15 mm each surrounded by a hypoechogenic halo. Minimum intralesional movement is observed.

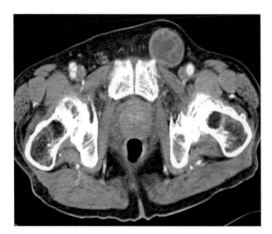

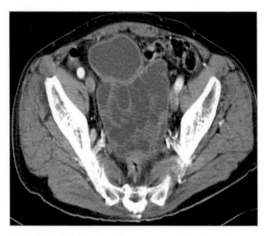

Figure 5.18 CT of the inguinal cord. A cystic well-defined multilobulated mass is identified in the subcutaneous tissue, adjacent to the femoral vessels. The lesion shows several septations and a thick wall. No inflammatory changes are seen.

Figure 5.19 CT showing the mass extending into the pelvic space.

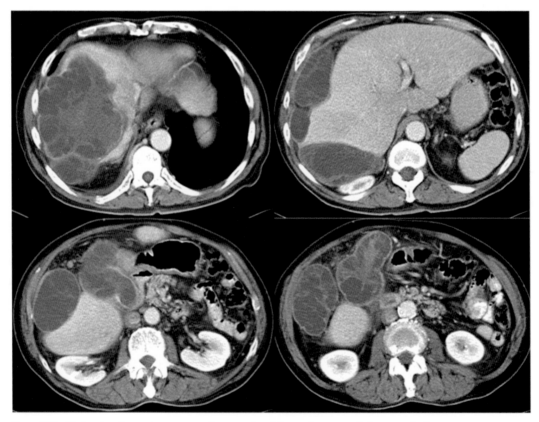

Figure 5.20 CT showing the cystic mass extending into the abdominal cavity, including into the liver.

Teaching points

• Hydatid disease is an endemic zoonotic disease in developing countries and is particularly common in southern Chile.

• If on diagnostic imaging a mass is identified, proper follow-up ensuring resolution should be performed. Otherwise this disease could be missed.

• In areas where hydatid disease has a high prevalence, unusual extrahepatic abdominal locations may be seen, such as the spleen, pancreas and peritoneum.

• With these unusual locations there is often a history of liver hydatid cyst surgery, with secondary peritoneal seeding, or they may be secondary to re-infection.

• The presence of liver cysts is characteristic. On US, cystic membranes, septa or hydatid sand can be seen. CT can better demonstrate wall calcification and cyst infection.

Case 3

A 32-year-old male, single, agronomist with no morbid background. He presented with 48 hours of gradually increasing malaise and fever. Acute pain and compromised function of the left wrist and mild pain in the right carpus, left shoulder and left leg began 24 hours ago. There was no diarrhea or urethritis.

On physical examination, temperature was 37.6°C. There was local pain in his left wrist, with a little swelling and redness, mild pain in the left shoulder and right carpus and a sore left Achilles area with mild redness and pain on dorsiflexion of the foot. The urethral meatus was irritated and red but without any secretion. A clinical diagnosis of asymmetric acute oligoarthritis of the large joint was made.

Laboratory results were white blood cell count 14 000 µL, with 80% neutrophils with no left shift; ESR of 18 mm/h; and CRP of 7. The hepatic profile showed a slight increase in pyruvic and glutamic transaminases. Urethral culture for *Chlamydia trachomatis* was negative.

Left wrist and carpal X-ray and US detected left tenosynovial enlargement and wrist fluid. It was decided to perform fluid puncture under US (Figures 5.21, 5.22, 5.23 and 5.24) and, with difficulty, a drop of left tenosynovial fluid was extracted and sent for Gram blood and bacterial culture, which were negative but there was a slight predominance of PMN leukocytes.

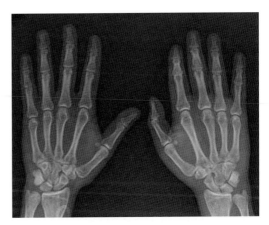

Figure 5.21 Normal left wrist and carpal X-ray.

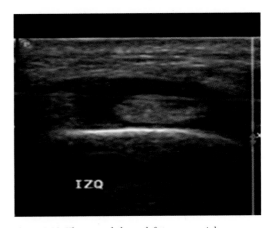

Figure 5.22 Ultrasound shows left tenosynovial enlargement.

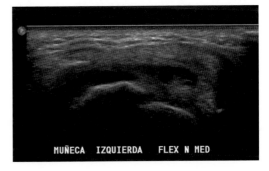

Figure 5.23 Ultrasound show fluid in the wrist.

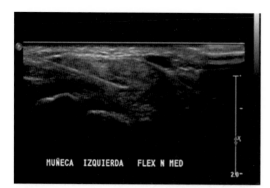

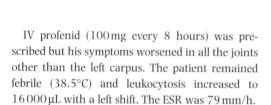

Figure 5.24 Diagnostic fluid puncture under US guidance.

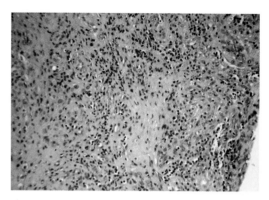

Figure 5.25 Biopsy showed synovial tissue with moderate inflammatory infiltrate.

IV profenid (100 mg every 8 hours) was prescribed but his symptoms worsened in all the joints other than the left carpus. The patient remained febrile (38.5°C) and leukocytosis increased to 16 000 μL with a left shift. The ESR was 79 mm/h.

After 48 hours a positive culture for *Neisseria gonorrhoeae* was obtained and gonococcal arthritis and tenosynovitis was diagnosed. The patient was treated with ciprofloxacin and surgical drainage. Drainage 72 hours after starting antibiotics showed abundant pus and marked acute synovitis.

Biopsy of synovial tissue showed a moderate inflammatory infiltrate consisting of lymphocytes, plasma cells, histiocytes and numerous neutrophil granulocytes, with newly formed vessels with prominent endothelium, increased stromal cellularity, edema, hyperemia and synoviocytes with reparative changes (Figure 5.25). Gram staining showed no infection. A final diagnosis of leukocyte synovitis in granulation was made.

Teaching points
• Synovial and peritendon infection by *N. gonorrhoeae* is a common cause of synovitis in the USA, occurring in sexually-active young people.
• Synovitis could be a manifestation of disseminated gonococcal disease with bacteremia and localization in the skin, synovium, tendons, etc.
• Symptoms are malaise, fever and oligoarthralgias that may be migratory and most often involve the knee, elbow, wrist, metacarpal bones and ankle.
• Tenosynovitis is observed in two-thirds of patients, mainly in the hands and fingers.
• Imaging shows findings consistent with synovitis of the affected joint or thickening of the affected tendon sheath.
• Preliminary diagnosis is made by culture and Gram stain of joint or peritendinous fluid.
• The differential diagnosis includes reactive arthritis, hepatitis B, rheumatic fever, Still's disease, infective endocarditis, meningococcemia, etc.

CHAPTER 6

Radiological Imaging of Abdominal Infections and Inflammatory Disease

Carolina Whittle[1], Giancarlo Schiappacasse[1] and Francesca Maccioni[2]

[1] Universidad del Desarrollo, Santiago, Chile
[2] "Sapienza" University, Rome, Italy

Introduction

This chapter focuses on infectious intra-abdominal processes, which have an acute presentation with abdominal pain or fever syndrome and are among the most frequent reasons for presentation to the emergency room.

Basic knowledge of the clinical problem

There are numerous causes for abdominal pain or sepsis. The most frequent intestinal pathologies are appendicitis, enteritis, ileitis, colitis, and diverticulitis; urinary pathologies are pyelonephritis and perinephric abscess; biliary-pancreatic pathologies are hepatitis, cholecystitis, cholangitis and liver abscess); and other pathologies are peritonitis, appendangitis, perihepatitis and panniculitis.

Patients consult for acute, diffuse or focal abdominal pain, fever and chills, vomiting, altered bowel transit and general malaise, among other symptoms. Laboratory tests are requested by physicians in search of infectious etiologies. These include hemogram with white blood count, erythrocyte sedimentation rate (ESR) and C-reactive protein (CRP). Conventional radiography, ultrasound (US), computed tomography (CT) and magnetic resonance imaging (MRI) are helpful diagnostic imaging modalities which may be aided by nuclear medicine techniques in some cases (see Chapter 13).

The clinical questions

Patient information regarding age, sex, ethnic group and pain characteristics, such as localization and intensity, should be collected. All findings at physical examination and laboratory results are important in obtaining a proper differential diagnosis and therefore in determining the appropriate imaging required. The radiologist's role is to determine the diagnostic approach that will answer questions posed by the referring physician, e.g. Is an infectious disease involved? Is emergency surgery needed?

Most imaging modalities are useful in these settings, including US, CT and MRI, and are usually available in any department of radiology of a large

Diagnostic Imaging of Infections and Inflammatory Diseases: A Multidisciplinary Approach, First Edition. Edited by Alberto Signore and Ana María Quintero.
© 2014 John Wiley & Sons, Inc. Published 2014 by John Wiley & Sons, Inc.

hospital or clinic. In general, for acute abdominal pain, an abdominal US study is the first-line examination and, according to the findings, the diagnostic algorithm can stop here or continue with CT or MRI. The choice of imaging (i.e. US) is especially important in the pediatric and pregnant female populations, given the need to avoid radiation exposure. In the female population, where differential diagnosis will include gynecological diseases, proper technique which depicts these entities should be used [1].

Methodological considerations

US techniques
Ultrasonographic study should be performed with medical sonographic instruments and using low-frequency broadband and multifrequency convex transducers (1–5 MHz) and high multifrequency linear transducers (7–12 MHz), according to the lesion location and patient characteristics. High-resolution ultrasound (HRUS) examination performed with linear transducers at 7 MHz or higher frequencies is mandatory to evaluate the bowel wall. The images must be obtained in at least two planes, transverse and longitudinal. Imaging with harmonics, spatial compounding software and contrast resolution improves the tissue contrast, reduces the artifacts from intestinal gas and improves the evidence for fluid collections.

It is useful to integrate the US examination with a color Doppler analysis to detect either normal vascularization or absence of flow or hyperemia at the level of a given inflammatory tissue. A slow but adequate flow filter is recommended for assessing bowel wall vascularity.

Generally, the patient with an acute infection is an emergency patient. Therefore, the initial conventional abdominal US study may be performed without previous fasting. The area of interest and site of pain should be located if possible, followed by progressive focal compression in flanks in the right or left lower quadrant. The colon, cecal appendix, ileum and ileocecal valve should be recognized using HRUS. Furthermore, size and content, parietal alteration or peri-intestinal inflammatory changes should be assessed.

US has technical and operator limitations. Technical limitations are: adipose tissue thickness, mobility, cooperation, bloating, intense pain, which affect adequate scan compression. Operator limitations are particularly related to the operator's experience and knowledge of the pathological findings in the various entities.

CT imaging
In the evaluation of a patient with an acute abdomen, multislice CT technology is recommended due to its speed, which avoids or at least drastically reduces patient motion artifact; and its ability to acquire the study with submillimeter thickness collimators, thus providing high-definition images with multiplanar reconstructions. It is completely independent of patient constitution, allows a rapid examination and diagnosis is independent of the operator.

Generally, preliminary patient preparation involves the oral administration of a neutral contrast (water) or positive contrast medium (iodinated contrast), which allows adequate distension and subsequent evaluation of the gastrointestinal tract. Occasionally, in specific inflammatory processes of the small intestine and colon [i.e. inflammatory bowel disease (IBD)], preparation with enteroclysis is required. Intravenous iodinated contrast agents allow better detection, characterization and diagnosis of any inflammatory disease. It should be mentioned that it is particularly helpful in the analysis of acquired images to use an appropriate workstation in order to obtain high-quality reformatted images.

MRI imaging
MRI has gained increasing importance in the evaluation of some abdominal inflammatory conditions, given the development of ultrafast high-resolution sequences that have improved the image quality and speed of sequences. Its high spatial resolution capability is especially useful in the evaluation of structures such as the bile duct, gallbladder, small intestine and colon walls. T2- and T1-weighted fat-saturated sequences with the use of intravenous contrast (gadolinium-chelate) are highly recommended. Sequences can also be obtained in ciné mode, thus allowing better assessment of intestinal peristalsis.

MRI has acquired increased importance in the study of IBD, pregnant women and children (due the absence of ionizing radiation), and in the evaluation of patients allergic to iodine contrast as it uses a different contrast medium (paramagnetic).

Recently, diffusion-weighted MRI (DWI) sequences have been increasingly used in the evaluation of abdominal diseases [2]. DWI allows visualization and measurement of the random Brownian extra- and intra-cellular motion of water molecules, which can be altered in several pathological benign or malignant processes. This technique can differentiate between a benign and a malignant lesion, and between fluid collections and an abscess, due to the different behavior of water molecules in these pathological conditions. Whole-body DWI can highlight both oncological and non-oncological lesions, particularly infectious and inflammatory diseases, throughout the entire body, similarly to single-photon emission computed tomography (SPECT)/CT and positron emission tomography (PET)/CT, although on a different biochemical basis.

Normal findings and artifacts

Different imaging modalities allow assessment of the structures of abdominal organs. Some findings, such as free abdominal fluid and pneumoperitoneum, are always associated with pathological entities.

Intraluminal abdominal gas is always present, due to both ingested air and gas produced by normal intestinal bacterial flora. However, any gas within solid viscera such as the liver and intestinal wall or free in the peritoneum is abnormal and may be associated with a poor prognosis. Fluid within the intestine is a non-pathological finding, although any fluid collection or free fluid in the abdominal cavity should be considered abnormal and precise diagnosis should be pursued.

Most abdominal structures are surrounded by adipose tissue and one of the most sensitive findings for infectious or inflammatory disease is a focal increase in the surrounding fat density or echogenicity. When assessing the intestinal walls, increased thickness or vascularization is also a finding suspicious for a developing disease.

Every imaging modality has its individual artifacts, some of which are useful in the identification of normal or pathological tissues. Examples include US acoustic shadowing (allows determination of calcifications), reverberation (presence of gas) and posterior acoustic enhancement (confident diagnosis of the presence of fluid).

MRI motion artifacts related to bowel peristalsis and respiratory movements can severely degrade the image quality. Most of them can be avoided by using fast acquisition sequences or respiratory triggering. Some artifacts, however, may assist diagnosis. Chemical shift artifact allows tissues with intracytoplasmic fat to be distinguished and plays a key role in the identification of lipid-rich lesions, such as adrenal adenomas. Another useful artifact is magnetic susceptibility artifact, which distorts image when tissues or materials with very distinct susceptibility are close to each other.

Some CT artifacts may degrade image quality, while others aid diagnosis. The former include beam hardening artifact, produced by the X-ray beam flowing through high-density structures, which filter the low energy photons and generate black lines; and partial volume artifact that arises when a voxel contains many different types of tissues – automatic computer averaging may produce bands and streaks in the image.

Pathological findings and significance

Appendicitis

Embryologically, the cecal or vermicular appendix develops along the cecum, to which it is connected. It is a tubular structure with an average length of 8–10 cm. The mesoappendix surrounds it. Its central lumen is narrow, usually measuring between 1 and 3 mm. Lumen obstruction leads to acute appendicitis, a disease first described in 1886 by Reginald Heber Fitz.

Acute appendicitis is a highly prevalent disease and is one of the most common causes of acute abdominal pain in the young. If untreated it generally evolves progressively to peritonitis and spontaneous resolution is rare. Since the length and location of the appendix is variable, the clinical presentation of appendicitis is heterogeneous. This is the reason why images have played a key role in its diagnosis.

The differential diagnosis includes cecal diverticulitis, epiploic appendagitis and omentum infarction, infectious ileitis and colitis, among others.

For its diagnosis, CT and HRUS are valuable examinations, while the role of MRI is still under investigation. Moreover, since a large percentage of patients with acute appendicitis are children, US is the examination of first choice.

Several studies have demonstrated the high sensitivity and specificity of both CT and HRUS in the diagnosis of acute appendicitis. The meta-analysis by Doria *et al.* reported pooled sensitivity and specificity of US studies for diagnosis of appendicitis in children of 88% and 94%, and 94% and 95% for CT studies, and for diagnosis in adults of 83% and 93% for US studies and 94% and 94% for CT studies [3]. CT has a significantly higher sensitivity than US for the diagnosis of appendicitis; however, as the US sensitivity is reasonably high, it is the recommended study in children, in whom reduction of radiation

is of special concern [3]. Depending on the US findings, the clinician can decide on surgery, clinical follow-up or further imaging with CT [4].

The most sensitive findings for both CT and US modalities are appendiceal dilatation of greater than 5 mm and an increase in thickness of its wall. Alteration of the density or echogenicity of pericolonic fat and the presence of a coprolite obstructing the lumen at the level of the appendiceal origin are diagnostic findings (Figure 6.1). CT is also specific if there is no opacity of the lumen when oral contrast has been given. A non-compressible lumen of the appendix is another sensitive US finding. Secondary findings include engorgement of the periappendicular vessels, reactive thickening in the distal ileum and free fluid adjacent to the appendix (Figure 6.2). Appendicitis can be complicated by necrosis of

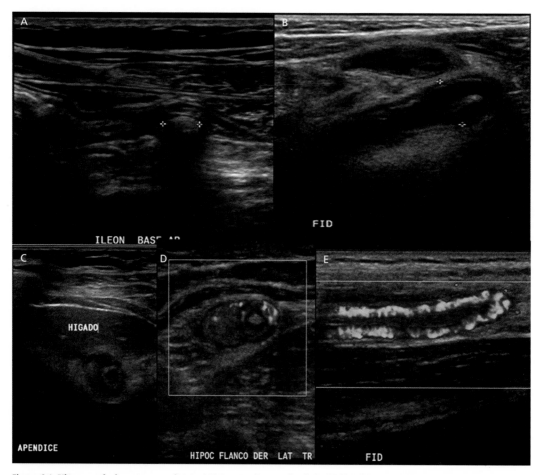

Figure 6.1 Ultrasound of acute appendicitis. (A) Proximal appendicolith, (B) distal lumen distension with mild wall thickening and increased echogenicity of the periappendicular fat, (C) subhepatic location and (D,E) parietal hyperemia.

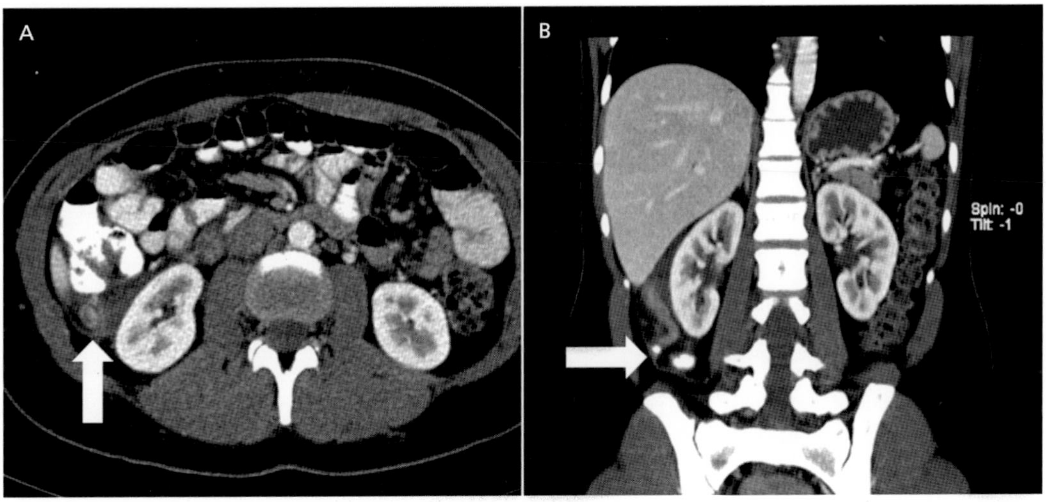

Figure 6.2 (A) Axial CT and (B) coronal reconstruction of ascending retrocecal acute appendicitis (arrows).

the wall, leading to perforation. In these cases, extraluminal gas and collections can be observed. CT has a greater sensitivity and specificity than US for the detection of these complications.

MRI is used only in specific cases since it is less sensitive and specific than CT, e.g. in patients allergic to iodinated contrast or pregnant women in whom US imaging has not been conclusive. An appendix diameter larger than 6 mm with a thickened wall and increased T2W signal can be easily visualized. Periappendicular adipose tissue and regional collections can also show increased signal. Recently, the use of DWI has proved to be particularly sensitive for the detection of acute appendicitis [5].

Diverticulitis

Diverticula are focal protrusions of the mucosa that have herniated through the muscular layers at weak spots in the wall. As they do not involve all the layers of the wall, they are actually pseudo-diverticula. On barium enema, diverticula are observed as small round protrusions of the colonic profile.

Diverticulosis (presence of diverticula) is common in the colon of the adult western population by the age of 50 years (33–50%).

Diverticulitis is an inflammatory process that is usually self-limiting and responds to medical treatment. Only 15–30% of patients with colonic diverticulosis develop symptomatic diverticulitis. Age at presentation is variable. The most common loca-

tions are the descending and sigmoid colon [6]. Clinical presentation is with diffuse or focal abdominal pain, fever and, sometimes, a palpable abdominal mass. Leukocytosis is a common finding. Differential diagnoses include acute appendicitis, colitis and ileitis.

Suspicion of diverticulitis should prompt study with CT or US and HRUS. Depending on the operator's experience, inflamed diverticula and regional inflammatory changes may be visible on HRUS. US and CT findings in diverticulitis include wall thickening of the colon; increased echogenicity or density of pericolonic fat; presence of diverticula; thickening of the fascia; presence of inflamed diverticulum; and free fluid or pericolonic abscess [7]. On HRUS, concentric thickening of the wall by hypertrophy of the hypoechoic muscle can be observed. The edematous diverticulum is rounded and hypoechoic, and the pericolonic fat shows increased echogenicity (Figure 6.3). The presence of fluid or a regional collection can also be detected. It is sometimes difficult to identify extraluminal gas as it can be confused with intraluminal gas in adjacent loops.

CT is one of the best methods for diagnosis. A thick-walled diverticulum is frequently observed, which may enhance with intestinal contrast and its lumen may be seen to be filled with fluid or feces. Increased density of pericolonic fat and thickening and hyperemia of the mesentery of the affected colonic segment are usually observed (Figure 6.4).

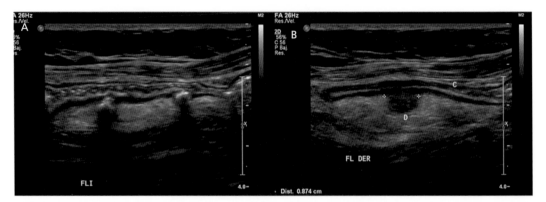

Figure 6.3 Ultrasound of diverticula. (A) Hyperechoic permeable diverticulum and (B) colon wall (C) with a hypoechoic swollen diverticulum (between calipers) and increased echogenicity of the pericolonic fat.

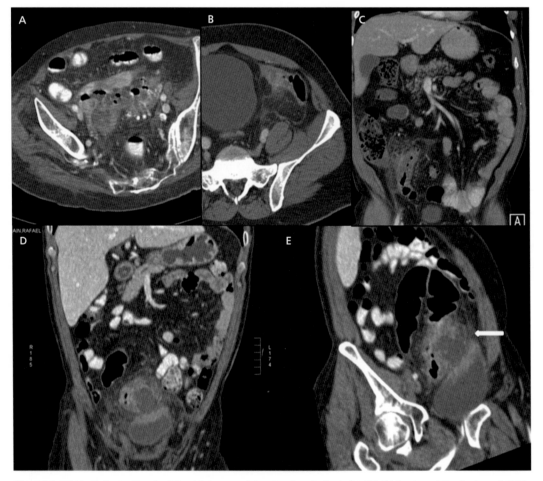

Figure 6.4 CT. (A–C) Acute diverticulitis with increased density of pericolonic fat, (B) thickening of the fascia and (D,E) pericolonic fluid collection.

The sensitivity and specificity of CT for diagnosis are both over 95% and certainly higher than for US. Use of multislice CT with the possibility of multiplanar reconstruction has significantly improved the diagnostic accuracy of this method. Complications such as intestinal perforation, abscesses, fistulas, diffuse or focal peritonitis are best demonstrated by CT. Perforation is detected by the presence of extraluminal gas and the eventual development of a pericolonic abscess. Coloenteric, colovesical, colouterine and coloparietal fistulas and also postinflammatory stenosis may develop.

Percutaneous drainage of abscesses can be performed under US or CT guidance (Figure 6.6).

MRI is rarely used in the diagnosis of diverticulitis, other than in pregnant patients. A thickened wall with increased signal from the pericolonic fat tissue may be easily detected on MRI as on CT. The presence of fluid or local collections can be observed, particularly on fat-suppressed T2-weighted images (T2WIs). However, the overall sensitivity of MRI for the detection of complications is lower than for CT as its visualization of extraluminal gas is poor.

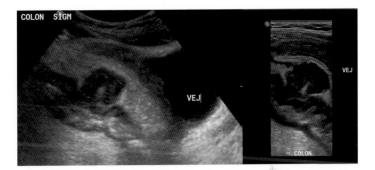

Figure 6.5 Complicated diverticulitis. Presence of abscess between the sigmoid colon and bladder (vej).

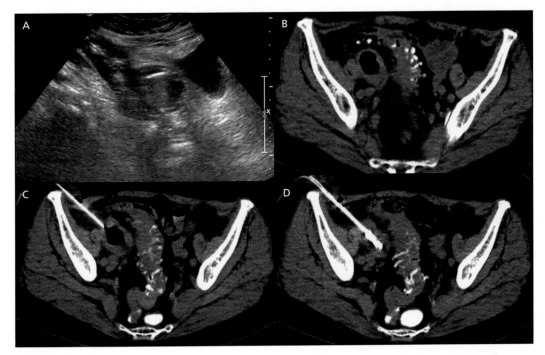

Figure 6.6 (A–D) Pericolonic abscess with visible air bubbles in CT and US. Percutaneous drainage with CT guidance.

Right diverticulitis is a less common localization (Figure 6.7). This condition is usually caused by obstruction and inflammation of a solitary and congenital diverticulum. It is seen in younger patients, more frequently female and the Asian population.

Ileitis, colitis and infectious enteritis

Ileitis, colitis and enteritis are intestinal inflammatory conditions and may involve one or more bowel segments. The causes are multiple, the most common etiologies being infectious and ischemic. Infections include bacteria (*Yersinia* spp., Salmonella spp., *Campylobacter* spp., tuberculosis); parasites (amoebas); and fungi (histoplasmosis). IBD

often affects the colon and is discussed later in this chapter. Special consideration should be given to pseudo-membranous colitis which is associated with the use of broad-spectrum antibiotics and caused by toxins produced by *Clostridium difficile* [8–10].

Imaging can detect dilated loops, whether of the small or large intestine; thickening of the wall of the jejunum, ileum, colon and ileocecal valve; increased peristalsis; and in some cases, increased echogenicity or density of the peri-intestinal fat or presence of enlarged regional lymph nodes.

On CT and HRUS, colitis is seen as a diffuse or segmental thickening of the colon wall. In some cases CT can also differentiate between different

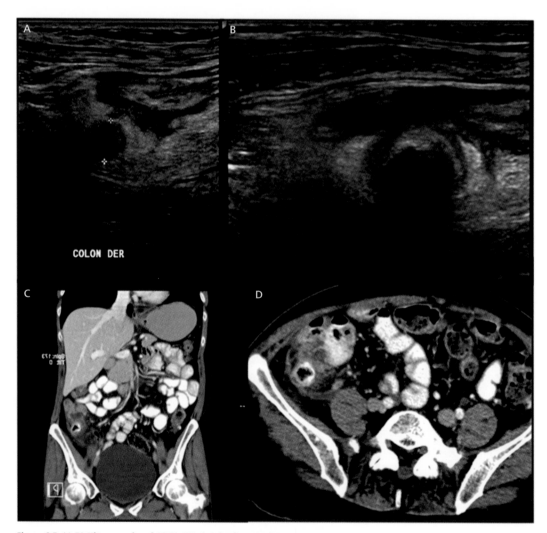

Figure 6.7 (A,B) Ultrasound and (C,D) CT of right diverticulitis.

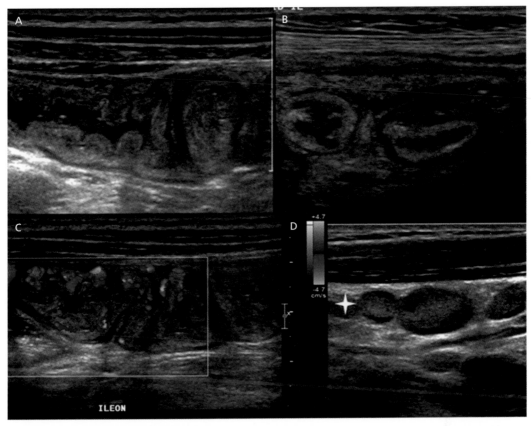

Figure 6.8 (A–D) Ultrasound of ileitis showing concentric thickening of the ileus wall, especially the submucosal layer, hyperemia and enlargement of local lymph nodes.

etiologies. Among the important features to highlight are the degree of wall thickening, extent and anatomical distribution, and complications such as abscesses, fistulas and parietal necrosis (Figure 6.8).

Pseudo-membranous colitis shows marked thickening of the wall and interhaustral folds with obliteration of the lumen, affecting the entire colon or right colon segmentally. There may be alteration of the pericolonic fat and the presence of ascites [10].

Colitis caused by bacteria such as *Shigella* spp., *Salmonella* spp. and *Campylobacter* spp. usually involves the right colon, sometimes associated with ileitis. Mild thickening and edema of the wall associated with local lymphadenopathy is observed. It is rarely complicated by perforation or abscess. Colitis caused by cytomegalovirus is usually found in immunocompromised patients; primary involvement of the right colon is observed with moderate

wall thickening and pericolonic edema that may mimic pseudo-membranous colitis. In infection with *Shistosoma japonicum* it is common to observe disorder of the left colon: obliteration of the normal haustral pattern, discrete wall thickening and presence of curvilinear calcifications in the wall. Other forms of colitis are secondary to viral infections, producing diffuse wall thickening and neutropenia, and causing mainly typhlitis with or without extramural gas with peri-colonic fluid. Tuberculosis disorder presents with a significant thickening of the cecal wall associated with regional adenopathies.

Enteritis may be diffuse, but it mainly affects the ileum and may be associated with colitis, usually of the right colon. Most cases are infectious and secondary to bacterial or viral infection (*Shigella* spp., *Campylobacter* spp., *Yersinia* spp. and tuberculosis). In general, it is common to observe mild thickening and uptake of contrast by the wall of the affected segment with varying degrees of edema of the submucosa and hyperemia of the mesentery. There may be perforation and development of abscesses, although the latter are unlikely to be observed. There may also be regional adenopathy, which in the case of tuberculosis has a hypodense center of caseous necrosis.

Yersinia enterocolitica is the cause of acute terminal ileitis in 50–80% of cases and it can present as pseudoappendicitis. It may be associated with secondary manifestations such as erythema nodosum and monoarticular arthritis.

MRI is not the usual modality for the diagnosis of infectious enteritis and colitis, although it can be a very specific method for assessing the extent of the process throughout the gastrointestinal tract and the characterization of the affected gut wall. It is also used for the evaluation and detection of complications. MRI findings of enteritis and colitis include a thickened wall (>3 mm), increased uptake of gadolinium and, if there is edema of the submucosa, a target sign with wall stratification [9]. Sinus tracts and abscesses can be characterized accurately by this imaging method.

Crohn's disease

Crohn's disease is a chronic disease characterized by transmural and discontinuous inflammation of the digestive tract wall from the mouth to the anus. The term inflammatory bowel disease (IBD) refers either to Crohn's disease or ulcerative colitis, both sharing an unknown etiology and a chronic relapsing–remitting course lasting for the patient's lifetime. To date, the pathogenesis of IBD remains unknown, although recent studies have shown an important role for environmental enteric, immune and genetic factors.

Crohn's disease is frequently diagnosed in young or pediatric patients. The small intestine is affected in nearly 80–90% of cases, particularly in adults. In pediatric patient the colon, particularly the descending colon and rectum, is more frequently involved than the distal ileum [11]. The colon is affected in approximately 50% of patients, frequently in association with the small bowel. The most common region of involvement is the terminal ileum, which represents the hallmark of the disease.

The inflammatory process starts in the submucosa, consisting of lymphoid hyperplasia and lymphedema. At this stage, barium studies may show aphthoid ulcers. With progression of the inflammatory process, it extends to the serosa, mesenteric adipose tissue and wall thickening. Lumen stenosis, abscesses and fistulas can be observed, more accurately using a cross-sectional rather than an endoluminal imaging modality. Cross-sectional imaging, including high-resolution US (HRUS), multislice CT (MSCT) and MRI allow the characterization of the typical transmural and extramural lesions of Crohn's disease [12,13]. The main finding of this disease is a concentric and usually marked wall thickening of intestinal or colonic segment, ranging from 4 to 20 mm in more severe disease, that can be easily visualized on US, CT and MRI. On MRI and CT, wall thickening is frequently associated with marked wall enhancement after intravenous injection of a contrast agent. Other findings, assessable with cross-sectional imaging and particularly with CT and MRI, include fibrofatty proliferation of the mesenteric fat adjacent to the affected bowel loop, increased number and size of local mesenteric lymph nodes and possible complications, such as phlegmons, abscesses and enteroenteric.fistulas. The disease activity can be established with all these imaging modalities, but most accurately with MRI.

US examination is the first-line examination, due to its wide availability and accessibility, as well as repeatability and safety [13,14]. When performed with high-resolution probes (7.5–12 MHz), HRUS may show in great detail the typical wall thickening of the distal ileum and colon. In the early stages, the US appearance of Crohn's disease looks like ileitis or colitis, while in the chronic phases the US pattern shows typical stratification and other findings that are characteristic of the disease: a multilayered pattern with increased thickening (>4 mm) and echogenicity of the submucosal layer (Figure 6.9A). Moreover, Crohn's disease should be strongly suspected whenever the thickened and stratified wall is also rigid and characterized by reduced or absent peristalsis, with increased echogenicity of the fat surrounding it, and the presence of adenopathies or signs of fistula and para-intestinal abscess. Color Doppler analysis allows detection of the typical mural and mesenteric hypervascularity (Figures 6.9B). Recently, contrast-enhanced US (CEUS) examination, performed after intravenous injection of specific intravascular contrast agents based on

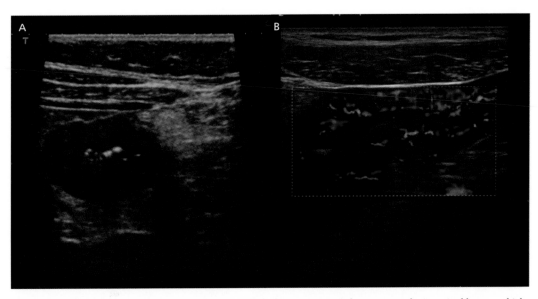

Figure 6.9 (A) HRUS showing the typical concentric wall thickening (>4 mm) that narrows the intestinal lumen, which is associated with fibrofatty proliferation. (B) Implementation of the color Doppler module shows the increased wall vascularization, which is a well-established sign of inflammatory activity.

stabilized gas microbubbles, has been successfully used to assess the increased vascularity of the bowel wall in Crohn's disease [15]. Both color Doppler US and CEUS have shown a good correlation with disease activity.

MSCT is an accurate diagnostic tool in the overall evaluation of Crohn's disease that is able to detect inflammatory lesions at the level of both the small and large bowel [8,13,14]. CT accuracy is improved by administration of an oral contrast agent, with enteroclysis or enema (CT enterography, CT enteroclysis, CT colonography). When the intestinal lumen is properly distended using contrast agent, either an iodinated contrast or an isomolar water solution (positive and negative contrast agents, respectively), the characteristics of the edematous wall and the presence of strictures or fistulas can be evaluated with high accuracy [13,14] (Figure 6.10). Contrast-enhanced MSCT can also detect most of the main complications associated with Crohn's disease, particularly wall thickening and fibrofatty proliferation, as well as its inflammatory activity. It is considered the gold standard for the detection of complications of Crohn's disease, such as fistulas and abscesses or perforations. However, because it requires radiation exposure, use of CT should be limited to occasional rather than periodic evaluation of Crohn's disease patients.

MRI is considered to be the most valuable alternative to CT in the evaluation of Crohn's disease. Since it allows a good characterization of the main features of Crohn's disease without irradiating the patient and has high contrast resolution, MRI is the method of choice for the overall evaluation of Crohn's disease, particularly if performed with the use of specific intestinal contrast agents (MR enterography and MR enteroclysis). Intestinal contrast agents for oral administration include negative superparamagnetic agents, consisting of iron oxides particles and producing a black lumen effect on T1- and T2-weighted imaging, and biphasic agents, usually isomolar water solutions, that induce a bright lumen effect on T2WIs and a dark lumen effect on T1WIs [16]. It allows an excellent description of the length, activity and location of the disease in both the small and large bowel, similar to MSCT (Figure 6.11) [13,14,16–18]. Moreover, it provides a more accurate detection and staging of perianal disease.

MRI is currently considered the most sensitive diagnostic modality for the assessment of Crohn's disease inflammatory activity [16,19]. This

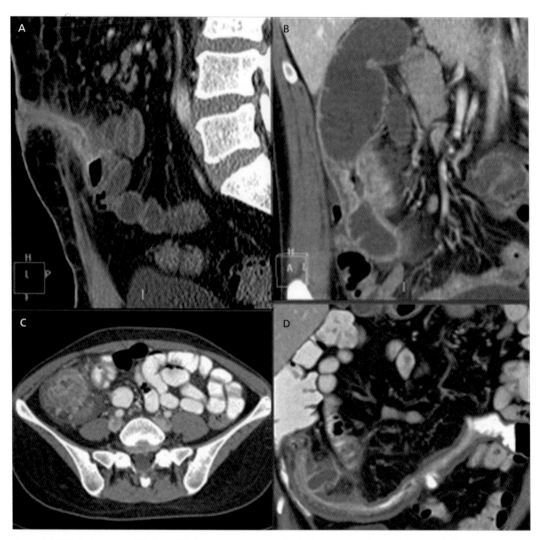

Figure 6.10 Crohn's disease. (A) Axial CT shows a sinus tract with inflammatory changes of the wall that connects a loop of intestine (ileum) to the anterior abdominal wall (Crohn's disease with enterocutaneous fistula). (B) Coronal CT scan shows localized small bowel thickening of 4 cm in length with a significant stenotic lumen and proximal dilatation (Crohn's disease: inflammatory, stenosing). (C) Axial CT shows marked inflammatory thickening of the right colon with increasing density of the pericolonic adipose tissue and the presence of some regional lymph nodes. (D) Oblique CT reconstruction of inflammatory Crohn's disease with segmental distal ileum associated with a small parietal collection (abscess) in the mesenteric border. Note the engorgement of the vasa recta.

evaluation is crucial in therapeutic planning, particularly in monitoring drug effects, and has been based on a combination of clinical symptoms, physical findings, laboratory parameters, endoscopy, nuclear medicine and several imaging modalities, particularly US and color Doppler US. MRI has shown great accuracy both in characterizing

disease lesions, between predominantly inflammatory and predominantly fibrous lesions, and in evaluating the degree of inflammation by using different imaging parameters, both at the level of the affected wall and of the perivisceral fat tissue. Inflammatory parameters include increased wall gadolinium enhancement on T1WIs, and wall

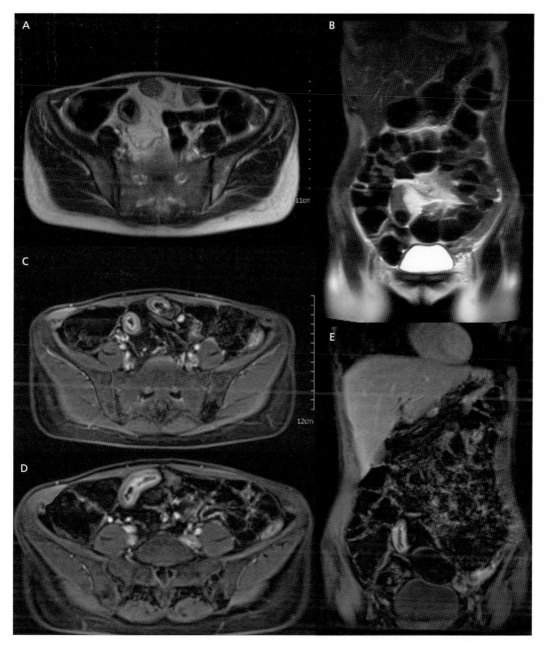

Figure 6.11 Female patient affected by long-standing Crohn's disease with a typical localization in the terminal ileum. (A,B) Axial and coronal T2WIs showing marked wall thickening of the terminal ileum, associated with fibrofatty proliferation. The lumen is dark due to the oral administration of a negative super-paramagnetic contrast agent (MR-enterography) [17,18]. (C–E) Axial and coronal T1W gadolinium-enhanced images showing marked thickening and enhancement of the wall of the terminal ileum, with the characteristic layered pattern frequently observed in long-standing Crohn's disease.

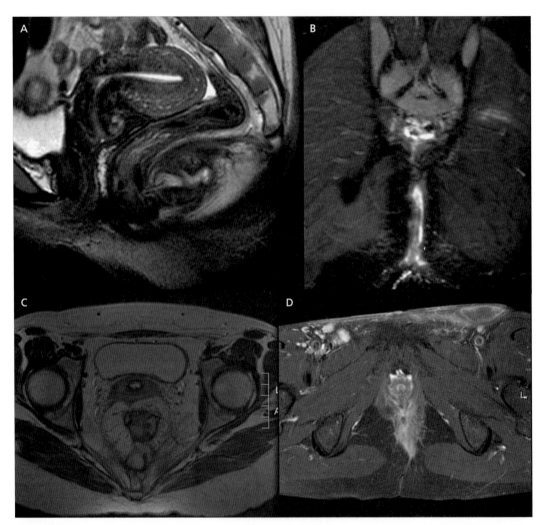

Figure 6.12 (A) Sagittal T2 MRI sequence shows ischiorectal space collection. (B) Coronal T1W fat-saturated sequence with gadolinium shows an intersphincteric fistula presenting a downward path that drains into the gluteal fold. (C) Axial T1WI shows wall thickening of the rectoanal region with two fistulas at 10 and 3 o'clock. Note the fibrofatty proliferation of perirectal fat tissue. (D) Axial T1W fat-saturated sequence with gadolinium shows a perianal fistula at 6 o'clock with inflammatory changes in local fat tissue that takes up contrast.

edema and mesenteric edema on T2WIs, particularly after selective suppression of the fat signal (Figure 6.12). These are typical findings of an active Crohn's disease and direct expressions of its typical transmural inflammation, which involves all wall layers, the serosa and the fat immediately outside the intestinal wall. A direct correlation between these findings and active Crohn's disease was reported in several studies [13,14,16–19]. Recently, MRI has been defined as a valuable alternative to endoscopy in the assessment of ileocolonic Crohn's disease [19]. Some have found an excellent correlation between several MRI parameters of active inflammation (wall thickness, wall enhancement, presence of edema and ulcers) and the endoscopic signs of inflammation, thus proposing an MRI index of inflammation that correlates well with the CD Endoscopic Index of Severity (CDEIS). DWI has been recently investigated in the evaluation of disease activity, with satisfactory preliminary results [20].

Ulcerative colitis

Ulcerative colitis is an inflammatory disease of unknown etiology that affects the colon and mostly presents in young individuals between 15 and 40 years old. The inflammatory reaction is mostly confined to the colonic wall and involvement of the small intestine is rare. The different clinical behavior of ulcerative colitis and Crohn's disease should be recognized. Crohn's disease may involve any portion of the gastrointestinal tract, usually the small and/or the large bowel, typically in a discontinuous and unpredictable way, although most frequently affecting the terminal ileum. Conversely, ulcerative colitis is characterized by a predictable course and localization, extending continuously from the rectum to the colon, involving first the left and then the transverse and right colon, very rarely the distal ileum (so-called "backwash ileitis"). The different patterns of ulcerative colitis are commonly called "ulcerative proctitis", "ulcerative sigmoiditis", "left-sided colitis" or "pancolitis". At endoscopy, a rectosigmoid localization is present in up to 95% of patients with ulcerative colitis, whereas it is rarely observed in Crohn's disease. On the other hand, the mucosal inflammation of the terminal ileum, a hallmark of Crohn's disease, it is rarely observed in ulcerative colitis, developing only in the presence of a pancolitis, the so-called "backwash ileitis"; in those cases, it is very difficult to differentiate ulcerative colitis from Crohn's disease.

On cross-sectional imaging, particularly CT and MRI, it is common to observe a regular continuous thickening of the colonic wall, frequently associated with signs of hyperemia in the submucosa of the long colonic segments [9,17]. The thickening of the colonic wall is usually lower in ulcerative colitis than in Crohn's disease, with a mean value of 7 mm versus 13 mm; it can be easily visualized on T1- and T2-weighted sequences and preferably on axial images [21]. On HRUS, the main findings are concentric regular wall thickening of the colon associated with increased echogenicity of the regional fat, usually not exceeding 6–8 mm. Fistulas or abscesses are extremely rarer in ulcerative colitis than in Crohn's disease, since the inflammatory process is confined within the wall rather than having a transmural extent.

Other findings of ulcerative colitis, particularly on coronal CT and MRI images, include the loss of haustration of the involved colonic segments, widening of the presacral mesorectal space and, occasionally, several severe complications, such as massive bleeding, toxic megacolon, tight bowel strictures or perforation, and later, colorectal cancer.

MRI plays an increasing role in this disease because it is able both to detect the typical disease abnormalities and to assess disease activity without being invasive [17].

A few publications have reported on the utility of MR diffusion sequences as a predictor of parietal inflammation in IBD [20–22]. The typical wall stratification of ulcerative colitis, already described on CT [23], is detectable on MRI as well, and well observed on T2-weighted plain images as a bright wide line within the two dark stripes of the mucosal and muscularis propria [21].

Thanks to its panoramic and multiplanar capability, MRI is usually able to distinguish between a proctitis, a left-sided colitis or a pancolitis, according to the findings observed on axial or coronal planes. Coronal planes are very useful to exclude involvement of the terminal ileum, thus helping in differentiating ulcerative colitis from Crohn's disease. To assess rectal disease, it is important to use a sagittal plane too, since it better displays the typical widening of the rectosacral space [21]. Wall gadolinium enhancement on T1-weighted fat-suppressed images is another relevant finding of IBD, usually observed both in active Crohn's disease and in ulcerative colitis [21].

A recent study comparing diffusion with contrast-enhanced T1W fat-saturated sequences showed that diffusion is more sensitive in detecting intestinal segments with active inflammation and differentiating them from those that are normal [22].

To conclude, although ulcerative colitis activity and extent are routinely assessed by endoscopy, MRI can play an important role in the overall management of the disease, similar to its role in Crohn's disease. MRI can assess the extent and severity of the disease when endoscopy is incomplete or contraindicated, particularly in hyperacute phases. In severe patients, MRI can detect a toxic megacolon and determine the severity and activity of mucosal lesions without any risk to the patient. Moreover, MRI can assess disease activity at any time, including in quiescent phases, by distinguishing submucosal edema from fat. In addition, MRI can help to distinguish Crohn's disease from ulcerative colitis in uncertain cases by assessing the sparing of the distal ileum and the continuity of the colonic involvement [21].

Hepatitis

Hepatitis is an inflammation of the hepatic parenchyma. It has various etiologies, the main ones being infection by hepatotropic viral agents, drugs and alcohol. In the acute phase (>3 weeks), imaging findings are non-specific so clinical and hepatic laboratory studies showing elevated transaminases and positive serology are required for early diagnosis. The key role of imaging is to rule out other etiologies that produce similar clinical and laboratory abnormalities, such as extrahepatic cholestasis, hepatic metastatic disease and cirrhosis [24].

On US, most cases of hepatitis will not show any abnormalities. However, in some cases, the hepatic parenchyma appear less diffusely echogenic with prominence and increased echogenicity of the portal walls (periportal cuffing). There may be hepatomegaly and gallbladder wall thickening from the edema of the gallbladder wall without distension of its lumen. The presence of enlarged lymph nodes in the hepatic hilum is not a common finding.

Mild hepatomegaly and diffuse periportal edema can be found on CT and MR. CT reveals heterogeneous parenchymal enhancement, which may include low-density areas that are relatively well-defined and reflect periportal edema. On MRI, edema appears as areas of high signal on T2WIs and low signal on T1WIs. It is usually located in the periportal regions. Extrahepatically it is common to find thickening from edema of the gallbladder submucosa and less common to find ascites.

Hepatic abscesses

Abscesses can be pyogenic or less frequently amebic. Pyogenic abscesses may be secondary to hematogenous spread via the portal vein (gastrointestinal infections) or via the artery (sepsis disseminated), ascending cholangitis, or necrosis infection of pre-existing hepatic lesions. Some abscesses, especially if they are isolated, can be of cryptogenic origin.

The US presentation of liver abscesses is varied. Most have a cystic appearance with fluid content that can be anechogenic and of varied echogenicity. In some cases, they are observed as hypoechoic lesions that resemble a solid lesion, or as solid lesions with a necrotic component and irregular contour or with air bubbles from gas-producing bacteria. There may be a fluid–fluid level, air–fluid level, or presence of septa of variable thickness.

CT can diagnose more than 90% of pyogenic abscesses, which can be divided into micro- (<2 cm) or macro-abscesses (>2 cm). They can be single or multiple; the latter may adopt a clustered pattern as they coalesce with each other. Sometimes microabscesses coalesce focally in the center of the lesion. Microabscesses may progress over time to form large abscesses. On CT they appear as multiple small hypodense images with a peripheral ring corresponding to the wall that captures the contrast; sometimes they are seen adjacent to each other when they adopt a clustered pattern. There may be perilesional edema, a finding that differentiates them from cysts or other cystic lesions that are not inflammatory. Large abscesses are usually hypodense and homogeneous, with a well-defined thick wall that takes up contrast. There may be intralesional septa. The presence of gas is not common.

Abscesses have variable signal on T1W and T2W MRI sequences, depending on their protein content. In general, they are of intermediate-to-high signal on T2WIs with a low signal wall that captures the contrast. It is common to observe perilesional edema.

On MRI, an amebic abscess usually appears as a single rounded lesion near the hepatic capsule, with a low density (similar to fluid), a thick wall (>3 mm) and a peripheral area of edema. The central area may have septa or detritus–fluid levels and rarely areas of hemorrhage or gas. They have homogeneous low signal on T1WIs and high signal on T2WIs, and perilesional edema is observed in approximately 50% of cases. MRI may be extremely helpful in distinguishing simple fluid collections from abscesses, both in the liver parenchyma and at any level of the abdomen and peritoneal cavity. Pus is characterized by restricted diffusion of water molecules and thus is enhanced by DWI; the signal from the abscess increases progressively with increasing b-values (increased diffusion weighting), while from a simple fluid collection it decreases progressively. Therefore, DWI may allow detection and characterization of inflammatory fluid collections at any level of the abdominal cavity. Although to date DWI has been predominantly used in neuroimaging, routine use in the detection of infectious collections in the liver and at any level of the abdomen is likely in the near future [2].

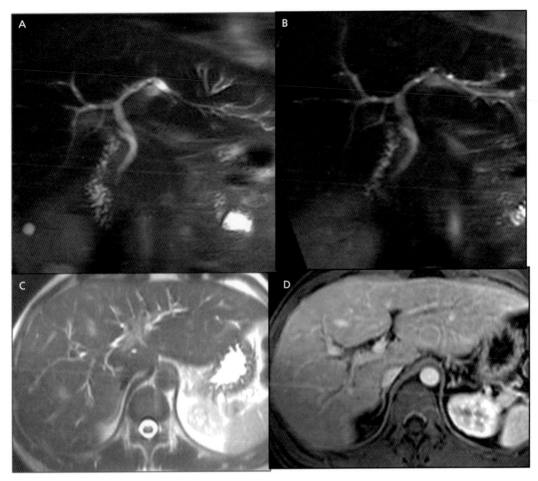

Figure 6.13 Cholangitis. (A,B) Cholangiographic T2W MRI sequence shows discrete parietal irregularities of the intrahepatic bile ducts. (C) HASTE T2W axial MRI sequence shows mild dilatation of the intrahepatic bile ducts. (D) Axial T1W fat-saturated MRI sequence with contrast shows minimal enhancement of the intrahepatic bile duct wall.

Acute bacterial cholangitis

Cholangitis is the suppurative infection of the bile duct, in most cases secondary to obstruction of the bile duct. Its most frequent cause is choledocho-lithiasis, the presence of bile duct stones, and this may be primary (gallstones formed in the common bile duct) or secondary (gallstones that migrate from the gallbladder). Choledocho-lithiasis may be complicated by obstruction and jaundice, cholangitis and pancreatitis [25]. The clinical triad of fever, pain in the right upper quadrant and jaundice is seen in 50–75% of patients with cholangitis.

Imaging is necessary in most cases to assess the condition of the bile duct and changes in the hepatic parenchyma, and to exclude of complications. Concentric wall thickening of the bile duct can be seen. It is unusual to see dilatation of the extrahepatic

segment, but this depends on the level and etiology of the obstruction, i.e. whether the bile duct dilatation is intra- or extra-hepatic. If the etiology is choledocho-lithiasis, dilatation at the start of the bile duct is more commonly observed [26,27].

US can detect the presence of intraductal echogenic content which corresponds to sediment. Visualization of ductal stones is better the more dilated the common hepatic duct is and the more proximally the stone is located, but it is highly dependent on observer experience.

MRI (Figure 6.13) and US can both detect dilatation of the bile duct. US with a sensitivity and specificity of greater than 95% for the detection of a dilated bile duct is the first examination. Visualization of gallstones on US is highly specific but less sensitive (40–70% according to different series and highly dependent on operator experience). The sensitivity of MRI for detecting gallstones is 93%. Diagnostic endoscopic US has shown high sensitivity and specificity for detecting stones, even small stones. Wall reinforcement of the bile duct is visualized on MRI in up to 92% of cases if gadolinium contrast is used [28].

Acute cholecystitis

Acute cholecystitis is an inflammation of the gallbladder, usually secondary to cystic duct obstruction by a gallstone (approximately 90–95% of cases). Approximately one-third of patients with gallstones present with symptoms of acute cholecystitis. The sequelae are the obstruction of bile disposal, intraluminal hypertension and development of parietal ischemia, which in turn can become necrotic and lead to perforation.

Direct signs of gallbladder inflammation include pain or sonographic Murphy's sign on compression with the transducer, presence of gallstones and visualization of an impacted and obstructing gallstone in the cystic duct, which does not move with gravitational maneuvers.

On abdominal plain films only 67% of the black-pigmented gallstones are visible and less than 20% of the cholesterol gallstones are visible. For this reason, conventional radiography is not a sensitive imaging technique for the diagnosis of lithiasis or its complication.

US is the imaging method of choice if there is suspicion of acute cholecystitis. It is highly sensitive and specific in detecting gallstones in the gallbladder (>95% sensitivity and specificity in different series). Gallstones are visualized as hyperechoic images with acoustic shadow, since they absorb and reflect ultrasound. The stones move in the movement with gravity-dependent maneuvers [29]. Gallbladder wall thickening greater than 4 mm, a distended gallbladder, biliary sludge and fluid or a perivesicular collection can be observed. Three layers of wall thickening are seen: a central hypoechoic band between two hyperechoic lines of edema (Figure 6.14). The positive predictive value of the presence of gallstones and sonographic Murphy's sign or wall thickening is 92% and 95%, respectively. Visualization of the impacted gallstone in the cystic duct has a positive predictive value of 92%.

If gallbladder wall thickening is observed in a collapsed gallbladder, it should be ascertained if

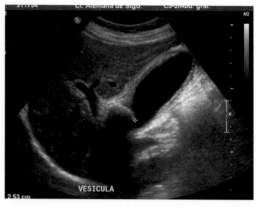

Figure 6.14 Diffuse gallbladder wall thickening is seen as three layers: a central hypoechoic band between two hyperechoic lines of edema and impacted gallstone.

the patient has recently ingested food or if there is a non-obstructive inflammation associated with another symptom (hepatitis, ascites, etc.). Focal perivesicular fluid is observed as a fluid collection, usually anechogenic or hypoechoic, and is a sign of acute cholecystitis, probably complicated (perforated), but it may also be observed in pancreatitis or complicated ulcer. Another complication is emphysematous cholecystitis, which is more common in diabetics. It is associated with gas-producing bacteria so air bubbles can be seen in the wall or inside the lumen, which appears as a hyperechogenic focus with posterior artifact the in comet tail artifact.

The remaining 5–10% of cases of acute cholecystitis are acalculous cholecystitis. This condition is more difficult to diagnose and sometimes requires successive US examinations.

CT detects 75% of gallstones. Major criteria for the diagnosis of acute cholecystitis are the presence of gallstones, gallbladder wall thickening, perivesicular fluid and subserosal edema, and minor criteria are vesicular distension and biliary sludge [30]. CT has a sensitivity of 91.7%, specificity of 94% and accuracy of 94% for the detection of one major and two minor criteria, whereas MRI has a sensitivity of 91%, specificity of 79%, positive predictive value of 87% and negative predictive value of 85%. On MRI it is easier to identify the presence or absence of gallstones in the gallbladder lumen or cystic duct. The wall is thickened by the increased signal from the submucosal edema and capture of the mucosa and serosa. Perivesicular inflammatory changes and complications such as wall perforation or perivesicular abscesses may be visualized [31].

Perihepatitis

Perihepatitis is inflammation of the peritoneal capsule of the liver. Classically it has been linked to the pelvic inflammatory disease called Fitz–Hugh–Curtis syndrome. It is considered to be the result of the intraperitoneal spread of infection from the peritoneal cavity [32]. It is associated with infection with *Neisseria gonorrhoeae* and *Chlamydia trachomatis*. It may also be associated with systemic lupus erythematosus, perforated cholecystitis, perforated hepatic abscess and tuberculous peritonitis secondary to radiation [33]. The most common clinical presentation is acute right upper quadrant abdominal pain; thus, it is frequently confused with acute cholecystitis or pleuritis.

On CT and MRI it manifests as a significant strengthening of the surface of the liver. Capsular strengthening can be seen in arterial phase images that reflect hyperemia of the inflamed liver capsule, while strengthening of the late stage reflects an initial liver fibrosis.

Pancreatitis

Pancreatitis is a multifactorial inflammatory disease of the pancreas. It can have an acute or chronic course. The diagnosis is based on the clinical presentation and laboratory tests. The severity of the presentation is extremely variable and can be classified according to the Ramson and Balthazar criteria [34].

When complications of pancreatitis are suspected, specifically if there is early fluid collection, fluid collection with air bubbles, a developing pseudocyst, or a pseudocyst with bubbles, it is important to rule out the existence of an infection.

US is a useful diagnostic tool for detecting biliary stones as the cause of pancreatitis, as well as for evaluating for the presence of peripancreatic fluid, ascites or pleural effusions. It is also helpful in the follow-up of complications and in supporting interventional procedures.

CT has proven to be important in predicting the evolution of the inflammation in an acute pancreatitis, detecting necrosis and fluid collection (Balthazar criteria) and in guiding percutaneous procedures [34].

MRI is the imaging modality of choice in the evaluation of gallbladder and biliary duct stones. It can detect pancreatic duct variants, such as pancreatic divisum, which is a risk factor for recurrent pancreatitis. MRI is a valuable tool for evaluating pancreatic parenchyma, particularly when chronic or autoimmune pancreatitis is suspected. It is also helpful for studying the pancreatic duct and for detection of stenosis, wall irregularities and stones in the Wirsung duct. The value of DWI MRI is questionable in the study of pancreatitis. It is possible to detect affected pancreatic areas with inflammation, but these finding are not definitive for the diagnosis.

Imaging is crucial in supporting interventional procedures, either diagnostic or therapeutic. CT is necessary for planning the procedure, which will depend on the location of the fluid collection and the presence of a wall, septum or necrosis. When drainage requires a gastric approach, endosonographic US guidance may be necessary. For retroperitoneal percutaneous procedures, US or CT guidance can be used. A recent report described the use of broad drainage with a self-expandable stent installation, which allows extraction of necrotic tissue [35].

Pyelonephritis and perirenal abscess

Acute pyelonephritis is the interstitial tubule inflammation of the kidney. Infections (of which *Escherichia coli* and *Staphylococcus aureus* are the most common) can reach the kidney by ascending infection (85% of cases) or through hematogenous spread. This condition is more common in young women.

Imaging is necessary to support the diagnosis and rule out complications.

On US the kidney may appear normal or show a slight increase in size, with alteration in structure and hypoechoic or hyperechoic foci in the parenchyma, usually hypovascular on color Doppler. There may be dilatation of the renal pelvis and thickening by edema of the mucosa. Pain on renal compression by the transducer is common.

CT is the imaging modality of choice for evaluating acute bacterial pyelonephritis because it provides anatomical and functional information on intra- and extra-renal pathological conditions. Non-contrasted CT visualizes gas, stones, hemorrhagic areas, enlarged kidneys, inflammatory masses and obstruction. However, in many cases, non-contrasted CT can be normal. After intravenous administration of contrast, areas of hypoperfusion, which are wedge-like or have a stretch mark pattern, in the cortical parenchyma can be observed. There may be a persistent and late enhancement after contrast administration [36].

Secondary signs of pyelonephritis can be observed in some patients: overall increase in kidney size, perirenal edema and complications. If pyelonephritis is not treated, renal abscesses can form. There is greater risk of this in patients with diabetes, urinary tract obstruction, infected kidney stone, immunocompromise, drug abuse or chronic illnesses.

Renal abscesses are usually solitary. They look like a hypoechoic complex mass, sometimes with posterior enhancement artifact. There may be a septum, debris and variable wall thickness. In its evolution it may spontaneously drain the collecting system or perirenal space, creating a perirenal abscess.

Abscesses are seen as round or oval collections, sometimes with a septum and wall enhancement.

MRI is an excellent imaging modality for the diagnosis of pyelonephritis. It is particularly useful in patients with allergy to iodinated contrast media or those in whom the avoidance of radiation is desirable. Edema, hemorrhage, congestion of the parenchyma, abscesses and perirenal collections can be observed. Inflammatory lesions and collections are hypointense on T1WIs and hyperintense on T2WIs. Wedge-like hypovascular lesions with a focal or diffuse stretch-mark pattern can also be observed. Gadolinium helps to better visualize the lesions.

Emphysematous pyelonephritis is an infection caused by gas-producing bacteria. It is more common in diabetic women and between the ages of 50 and 60 years. It is usually unilateral, but may be bilateral in 5–10% of cases. Gas may be seen in the collecting system, at foci of destruction of the parenchyma, or as bubbles in the renal or perirenal collections [37].

Appendangitis

Vesalius mentioned the epiploic appendices in 1543. There are approximately 100–150 in the large intestine, which measure between 0.5 and 5 cm. They are composed of fat tissue and vascular structures. If vascular thrombosis or secondary ischemia causes one of these appendices to twist, the clinical manifestation is epiploic appendangitis. The clinical characteristic is acute abdominal pain, generally focused at a specific point. There may be a history of previous physical exercise. On physical examination there may be focal Blumberg or mild muscle endurance. Over 90% of cases show normal results on laboratory tests.

It can be diagnosed by US or CT imaging. On US it appears as an oval hyperechoic, non-compressible and avascular mass. It is attached to the colon wall or to the abdominal wall. A peripheral hypoechoic halo is present in up to 60% of cases (Figure 6.15). There may be a regional fluid laminar band and increased echogenicity of the surrounding fat (94% of cases) [38].

On CT there is a pedunculated mass with fat density surrounded by a dense ring. It attaches to the colon serosa and abdominal wall (Figure 6.16). There is increased density of regional fat. Central dense fine lines, which correspond to the thrombosed vessels, can be seen in 43% of cases. CT can rule out an underlying colonic lesion (diverticulitis or hidden perforation) [39].

Mesenteric panniculitis

This is the non-specific chronic inflammation of the mesenteric fat tissue. It is a benign, uncommon entity that is difficult to diagnose. Biopsy can reveal fatty necrosis, chronic inflammation and fibrosis. There are several names for this disease, but in general it is designated as mesenteric panniculitis when fat inflammation with lipodystrophy predominates and sclerosing mesenteritis when fibrosis predominates. Over 90% of cases involve the mesentery of the small intestine, primarily the root, but it can affect the mesocolon, peripancreatic region, greater omentum, retroperitoneum and pelvis. It occurs most frequently in men (ratio 2:1) in the sixth to seventh decades. Approximately 43% of cases are asymptomatic and only identified on imaging studies or laparotomy. There may be abdominal pain, anorexia, fever, nausea, diarrhea and weight loss, and it is associated with history of trauma or abdominal surgery, vasculitis, neoplasm and peritoneal infections

The diagnostic imaging methods are US, CT and MRI. On US, increased echogenicity of mesenteric fat in a defined area with small oval hypoechoic nodules can be observed, corresponding to lymph

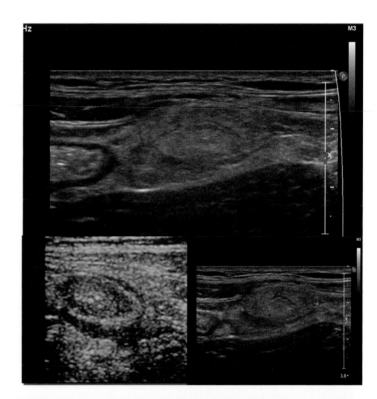

Figure 6.15 Appendangitis. On US a hyperechoic mass adjacent to the descending colon and a hypoechoic peripheral halo are seen.

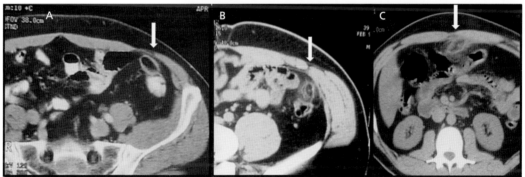

Figure 6.16 Appendangitis. CT shows (A) a fat hypodense nodule surrounded by a dense ring (arrow) and (B) a small dense linear vessel inside (arrow) that (C) is in contact with the abdominal wall (arrow).

nodes, and regional vessels can be seen crossing the area. When fibrosis predominates, a hypoechoic mass of solid appearance and somewhat irregular contour can be visualized [40].

On CT, the most common finding is an increase in adipose tissue attenuation of the mesenteric root that tends to surround the vessels (Figure 6.17). A pseudo-capsule surrounding the lesion has been described in 50% of cases. It can also occur as an infiltrating soft tissue mass when there is fibrosis. Less common findings are calcification or a cystic component [41].

Role for therapy follow-up and patient management

Broadly, pathologies such as diverticulitis, abscesses, perihepatitis, renal abscess or appendangitis can be followed up by US. If complications are suspected, CT is the modality of choice, particularly if extraluminal gas is present, given its higher sensitivity and specificity for the visualization of this imaging feature.

When abdominal collections are present, both CT and US are useful for percutaneous diagnostic guidance and drainage.

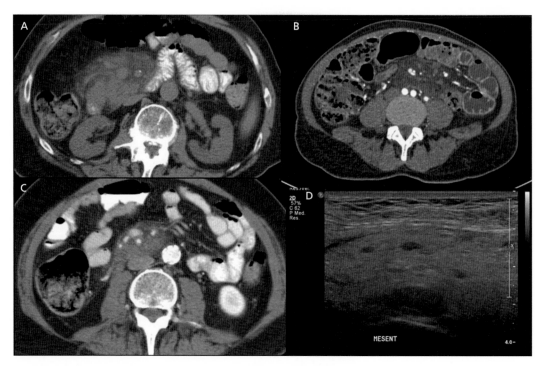

Figure 6.17 Mesenteric paniculitis. (A–C) The increased density of adipose tissue in the root of mesentery is associated with small lymph nodes at that level. (D) US showing similar findings.

Conclusion

Abdominal infectious and inflammatory conditions are common and are considered to be the principal reason for emergency room consultation in a high percentage of cases. As these conditions have different origin and severity, a multidisciplinary team approach is important to assist in their diagnosis and treatment. Knowledge of imaging diagnostic methods, together with their advantages and limitations, is important to optimize time to diagnosis and health resources.

References

1. Solomkin J, Mazuski J, Bradley J *et al.* Diagnosis and management of complicated intra-abdominal infection in adults and children: Guidelines by the Surgical Infection Society and the Infectious Diseases Society of America. *Clin Infect Dis* 2010;50:133–164.

2. Kwee TC, Takahara T, Ochiai R. Whole-body diffusion-weighted magnetic resonance imaging. *Eur J Radiol* 2009;70:409–417.

3. Doria AS, Moineddin R, Kellenberger CJ *et al.* US or CT for diagnosis of appendicitis in children and adults? A meta-analysis. *Radiology* 2006;241:83–94.

4. Krishnamoorthi R, Ramarajan N, Wang N *et al.* Effectiveness of a staged US and CT protocol for the diagnosis of pediatric appendicitis: Reducing radiation exposure in the age of ALARA. *Radiology* 2011;259:231–239.

5. Inci E, Kilickesmez O, Hocaoglu E *et al.* Utility of diffusion-weighted imaging in the diagnosis of acute appendicitis. *Eur Radiol* 2011;21:768–775.

6. Zaidi E, Daly B. CT and clinical features of acute diverticulitis in an urban U.S. population: Rising frequency in young, obese adults. *Am J Radiol* 2006;187:689–694.

7. Laméris W, Van Randen A, Bipat SH *et al.* Graded compression ultrasonography and computed tomography in acute colonic diverticulitis: Meta-analysis of test accuracy. *Eur Radiol* 2008;18:2498–2511.

8. Horton K, Corl F, Fishman E. CT evaluation of the colon: Inflammatory disease. *RadioGraphics* 2000;20:399–418.

9. Maccioni F. MRI of colitis. In: Chapman AH (ed). *Radiology and Imaging of the Colon.* New York: Springer Verlag, 2004, pp. 201–214.

10. Patriarchi F, Rolla M, Maccioni F *et al. Clostridium difficile*-related pancolitis in lung-transplanted patients with cystic fibrosis. *Clin Transplant* 2011;25:E46–51.

11. Maccioni F, Viola F, Carrozzo F *et al.* Differences in the location and activity of intestinal Crohn's disease

lesions between adult and paediatric patients detected with MRI. *Eur Radiol* 2012;22:2465–2477.

12. Tolan D, Greenhalgh R, Zealley I *et al*. MR enterographic manifestations of small bowel Crohn disease. *RadioGraphics* 2010;30:367–384.

13. Panés J, Bouzas R, Chaparro M *et al*. Systematic review: the use of ultrasonography, computed tomography and magnetic resonance imaging for the diagnosis, assessment of activity and abdominal complications of Crohn's disease. *Aliment Pharmacol Ther* 2011;34:125–145.

14. Horsthuis K, Bipat S, Bennink RJ, Stoker J. Inflammatory bowel disease diagnosed with US, MR, scintigraphy, and CT: meta-analysis of prospective studies. *Radiology* 2008;247:64–79.

15. Ripollés T, Martínez-Pérez JM, Blanc E *et al*. Contrast-enhanced ultrasound (CEUS) in Crohn's disease: technique, image interpretation and clinical applications. *Insights Imaging* 2011;2:639–652.

16. Maccioni F. Double-contrast magnetic resonance imaging of the small and large bowel: effectiveness in the evaluation of inflammatory bowel disease. *Abdom Imaging* 2010;35:31–40.

17. Maccioni F, Bruni A, Viscido A *et al*. MR imaging in patients with Crohn disease: value of T2- versus T1-weighted gadolinium-enhanced MR sequences with use of an oral superparamagnetic contrast agent. *Radiology* 2006;238:517–530.

18. Panés J, Ricart E, Rimola J. New MRI modalities for assessment of inflammatory bowel disease. *Gut* 2010;59:1308–1309.

19. Rimola J, Rodriguez S, García-Bosch O *et al*. Magnetic resonance for assessment of disease activity and severity in ileocolonic Crohn's disease. *Gut* 2009;58:1113–1120.

20. Oto A, Kayhan A, Williams JT *et al*. Active Crohn's disease in the small bowel: Evaluation by diffusion weighted imaging and quantitative dynamic contrast enhanced MR imaging. *J Magn Reson Imaging* 2011;33:615–624.

21. Maccioni F, Colaiacomo MC, Parlanti S. Ulcerative colitis: value of MR imaging. *Abdom Imaging* 2005;30:584–592.

22. Oussalah A, Laurent V, Bruot O *et al*. Diffusion-weighted magnetic resonance without bowel preparation for detecting colonic inflammation in inflammatory bowel disease. *Gut* 2010;59:1056–1065.

23. Gore RM, Balthazar EJ, Ghahremani GG, Miller FH. CT features of ulcerative colitis and Crohn's disease. *AJR Am J Roentgenol* 1996;167:3–15.

24. Mortelé KJ, Segatto E, Ros PR. The infected liver: radiologic-pathologic correlation. *RadioGraphics* 2004;24:937–955.

25. Catalano OA, Sahani DV, Forcione DG *et al*. Biliary infections: spectrum of imaging findings and management. *RadioGraphics* 2009;29:2059–2080.

26. Soto J, Alvarez O, Múnera F *et al*. Diagnosing bile duct stones. Comparison of unenhanced helical CT, oral contrast-enhanced CT cholangiography, and MR cholangiography. *AJR Am J Radiol* 2000;175:1127–1134.

27. Lee NK, Kim S, Lee JW *et al*. Discrimination of suppurative cholangitis from non suppurative cholangitis with computed tomography (CT). *Eur J Radiol* 2009;69:528–535.

28. Bader TR, Braga L, Beavers KL, Semelka RC. MR imaging findings of infectious cholangitis. *Magn Reson Imaging* 2001;19:781–788.

29. Ralls PW, Colletti PM, Lapin SA *et al*. Real-time sonography in suspected acute cholecystitis. Prospective evaluation of primary and secondary signs. *Radiology* 1985;155:767–771.

30. Bennett GL. CT findings in acute gangrenous colecititis. *Am J Radiol* 2002;178:275–281.

31. Kalimi R. Diagnosis of acute colecistitis. *J Am Coll Surg* 2001;193:609–613.

32. Dalaker K, Gjonnaess H, Kvile G *et al*. *Chlamydia trachomatis* as a cause of acute perihepatitis associated with pelvic inflammatory disease. *Br J Vener Dis* 1981;57:41–43.

33. Kim S, Kim TU, Lee JW *et al*. The perihepatic space: comprehensive anatomy and CT features of pathologic conditions. *RadioGraphics* 2007;27:129–143.

34. Balthazar EJ, Robinson DL, Megibow AJ, Ranson JH. Acute pancreatitis: value of CT in establishing prognosis. *Radiology* 1990;174:331–336.

35. Navarrete C, Castillo C, Caracci M, Vargas P, Gobelet J, Robles I. Wide percutaneous access to pancreatic necrosis with self-expandable stent: new application (with video). *Gastrointest Endosc* 2011;73:609–610.

36. Stunell H, Buckley O, Feeney J *et al*. Imaging of acute pyelonephritis in the adult. *Eur Radiol* 2007;17:1820–1828.

37. Craig WD, Wagner BJ, Travis MD. Pyelonephritis: radiologic-pathologic review. *RadioGraphics* 2008;28:255–277.

38. Horvath E, Majlis S, Seguel S *et al*. Apendicitis epiploica primaria: diagnostico clínico y radiológico. Primary epiploic appendangitis. Clinical and radiological diagnosis. *Rev Med Chile* 2000;128:601–607.

39. Singh A, Gervais D, Hahn P *et al*. Acute epiploic appendagitis and its mimics. *Radiographics* 2005;25:1521–1534.

40. Heredia C, Saenz R, Soffia P, Schultz M. Paniculitis mesentérica: infrecuente entidad clinic patologica. *Gastroenterol Latinam* 2008;19:221–226.

41. Horton K, Lawler L, Fishman E. CT findings in sclerosing mesenteritis (panniculitis): spectrum of disease. *RadioGraphics* 2003;23:1561–1567.

42. Lee WK, Mossop PJ, Little AF *et al*. Infected (mycotic) aneurysms: spectrum of imaging appearances and management. *RadioGraphics* 2008;28:1853–1868.

Clinical cases

Case 1

A 69-year-old diabetic female with renal failure was admitted to hospital with sepsis, abdominal pain and fever. Laboratory tests showed elevation of C-reactive protein (CRP) and leukocytosis. An abdominal CT scan was requested. Following CT and with a diagnosis of abdominal sepsis, she went to surgery.

Her postoperative outcome was poor and fever and abdominal pain persisted. With clinical suspicion of pancreatitis, a new CT scan was performed and with the images she was immediately taken to surgery (Figures 6.18 and 6.19); an axillary femoral bypass was performed and the aorta was clamped. There was a massive intraoperative bleed and consumption coagulopathy and hemostatic control was not achieved. The patient died in the early postoperative period. The surgeon described the aortic wall as "like butter" [42] (Figures 6.18, 6.19 and 6.20).

Teaching points

• Mycotic aneurysms have the following imaging appearance:

  ○ Rapid onset (days or weeks) of irregularities in the wall and dilatation of an artery.
  ○ Thickening and inflammatory changes of the periarterial fatty tissue.
• There can be multiple aneurysms at different levels in the same artery or in different vessels.
• Aneurysms are associated with debilitating disease, sepsis or decompensated diabetes mellitus.

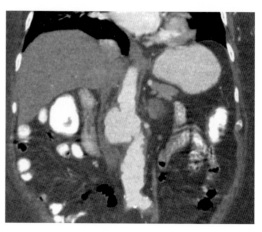

Figure 6.19 CT orthogonal coronal reconstruction of the aorta showing irregularities in the aneurysm wall.

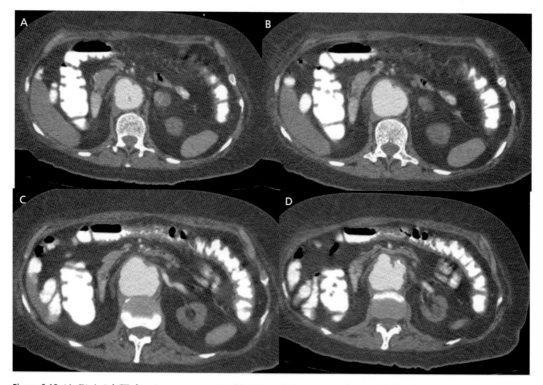

Figure 6.18 (A–D) Axial CT showing aneurysmatic dilatation of the aorta with irregular border.

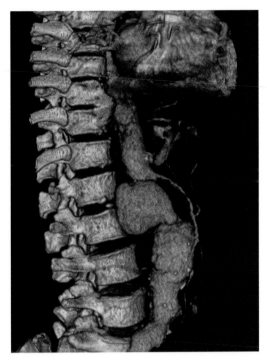

Figure 6.20 Three-dimensional CT reconstruction of an aortic aneurysm.

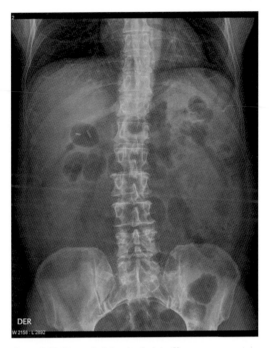

Figure 6.21 Normal abdominal plain film.

• The differential diagnoses to be considered include atherosclerotic aneurysm, perianeurysmal fibrosis (formerly called an inflammatory aneurysm), vasculitis (polyarteritis nodosa, giant cell arteritis, Takayasu's disease), fibromuscular dysplasia and infectious process in the vicinity of the vessel not affecting its wall (i.e. cellulitis, phlegmons or spondylodiscitis).

Case 2

A 69-year-old male with a history of IBD that had been managed for years. The patient related abdominal distension and mild right flank pain for 1 month and abdominal pain and fever 48 hours prior to hospital admittance. Physical examination found right lower quadrant tenderness and discrete muscular resistance of the abdominal wall. Laboratory tests showed leukocytosis with left shift, a CRP of 17 mg/dL and a raised erythrocyte sedimentation rate (ESR) of 50 mm/h. There was cholestatic alteration in liver tests.

Plain abdominal radiography and US were requested (Figures 6.21 and 6.22). Later an abdominal CT was performed and this demonstrated an inflammatory mass in the right lower quadrant

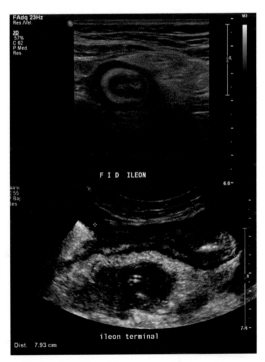

Figure 6.22 Bowel US. Focal wall enlargement in a rigid small bowel loop with mild inflammatory changes in the adjacent fat tissue.

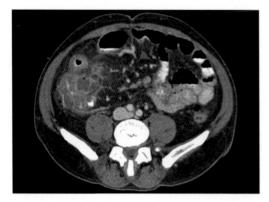

Figure 6.23 Axial CT image of the cecum and terminal ileum with diffuse wall enlargement.

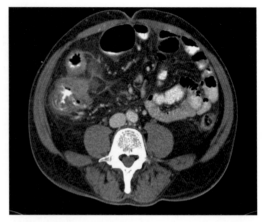

Figure 6.24 Axial CT image of the cecum and terminal ileum with diffuse wall enlargement.

with an abscess in the cecum wall (Figures 6.23 and 6.24).The patient began to vomit and intestinal obstruction was confirmed. Treatment with antibiotics and steroids was established. After 3 months of therapy, images showed stenosis of the distal ileum that required an ileocecal resection. Histological study confirmed Crohn's disease.

Teaching points

• IBD is divided into Crohn's disease, ulcerative colitis and undetermined colitis.

• Crohn's disease is characterized by thickening of the digestive tract wall. It can occur from the mouth to the anus, but the majority occurs in the distal ileum and ileocolic segment. The rectal–anal region is also commonly affected.

• For definitive diagnosis, clinical, radiological and histological criteria should be considered.

• The following imaging findings should always be considered: segmentary thickening of the digestive tract, with a target pattern on the wall, vasa recta hyperemia (comb sign), enlargement of the pericolic fatty tissue or mesenteric tissue near the compromised intestinal segment, presence of a focal area of stenosis, fistula or wall abscess, and discontinuous bowel edematous segments alternating with normal segments.

• The differential diagnoses to be considered are ulcerative, infectious (bacterial, viral, neutropenic, cytomegalovirus), ischemic or pseudomembranous colitis and neoplasms such as lymphoma.

Case 3

A 28-year-old female who related diarrhea during ciprofloxacin treatment. Two days later she presented with abdominal right flank pain exacerbated by postural changes. Physical examination demonstrated tenderness in the lower right quadrant (++), peritoneal reaction and rebound positive signs.

US detected pneumatosis of the right colon (Figure 6.25). PCR was less than 0.5 mg/dL and white blood cell count 6400. A diagnosis of atypical enterocolitis was considered. A CT scan confirmed the US findings (Figure 6.26).

She was admitted for IV antibiotic treatment with metronidazole and ceftriaxone. After 3 days she was released in good health. Cultures remained negative.

Teaching points

• Colitis is a group of inflammatory conditions that affect the large bowel in a diffuse, segmentary, acute or chronic way.

• For diagnosis, clinical, radiological and endoscopic factors should be considered.

• Imaging findings include concentric wall thickening, inflammatory changes within the pericolic fatty tissue, vasa recta hyperemia and, in some case, pneumatosis intestinalis.

• The differential diagnoses to be considered include IBD, ischemic colitis, colonic neoplasm and bowel venous ectasia caused by deep venous thrombosis.

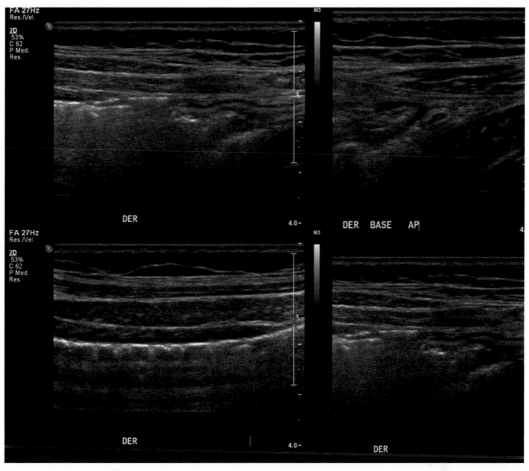

Figure 6.25 US of the abdominal right lower quadrant. The presence of extraluminal and bowel wall gas is depicted.

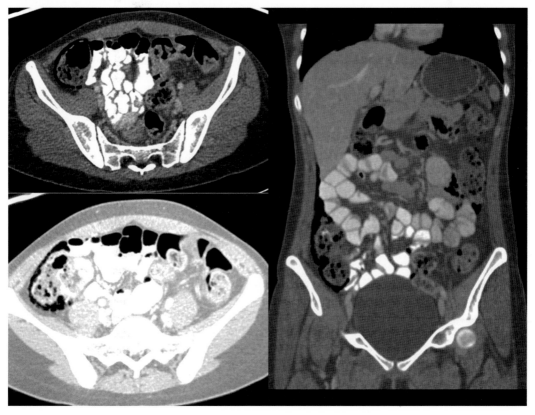

Figure 6.26 CT images that confirm pneumatosis intestinalis and pneumoperitoneum.

CHAPTER 7

Radiological Imaging of Vascular Graft Infection

Alejandro Romero[1], Tobias Zander[2], Jorge Lopera[3], Sergi Quiroga[1] and Manuel Maynar[2]

[1]*Hospital Universitario Valle Hebrón, Barcelona, Spain*
[2]*Las Palmas de Gran Canaria University, Canary Islands, Spain*
[3]*The University of Texas Health Science Center, San Antonio, TX, USA*

Introduction

Prosthetic vascular graft infection is an uncommon complication that was first described more than 30 years ago [1,2]. It is considered the most serious and devastating complication of vascular surgery, and is associated with significant morbidity and mortality rates. For extracavitary vascular grafts, the incidence of infection following vascular reconstructions has been reported to be between 0.5% and 5% [3–5]; 15–30% of patients with this type of prosthetic vascular graft infection suffer limb loss and 20–40% die within 1 year after diagnosis [1,6]. For aortic prosthetic grafts, the incidence of infection is reported to be between 0.5% and 2%, and this is also associated with considerable morbidity and mortality [7,8]. Successful treatment depends on early diagnosis, the extent of the infection, other organ compromise and identification and potential virulence of the infectious pathogens [9]. Because a delay in diagnosis may have a considerable impact on mortality, efficacious imaging is an important contribution to patient care.

This chapter reviews the imaging work-up for prosthetic vascular graft infection with conventional plain films, ultrasound (US), computed tomography (CT) and magnetic resonance imaging (MRI). Nuclear medicine imaging techniques are reviewed in Chapter 14.

Basic knowledge of the clinical problem

Vascular graft infection can develop from days to years after prosthesis placement and can be related to the surgical episode or not; thus, clinical manifestations may vary according to the length of time that has elapsed since the surgical procedure. Diagnosis is suspected from the clinical findings and supported by imaging and microbiological complementary studies. The specific manifestations associated with infection depend on the location of the infected portion(s) of the graft. Signs and symptoms are multiple and depend on the severity of the infection. Fever is present in most cases.

The clinical presentation may not be a challenge in cases of superficial grafts in which swelling, erythema, pain, a pulsatile mass and, occasionally, a draining sinus may be noted. This is particularly common in the femoral region. However, the mani-

Diagnostic Imaging of Infections and Inflammatory Diseases: A Multidisciplinary Approach, First Edition. Edited by Alberto Signore and Ana María Quintero.

festations of a graft infection may be non-specific and, as already described, remote in time with respect surgery. Malaise, back pain, fever, gastrointestinal bleeding, elevated sedimentation rate, hydronephrosis or ischemia from a clotted graft should all be considered potential clinical findings of a graft infection and warrant further diagnostic evaluation.

Aortoenteric fistulas (AEFs) should be considered a subset of aortic graft infection, as also can be the rare finding of an aortoureteral fistula. The radiological signs of an AEF and graft infection overlap, although there is a greater likelihood that perigraft or intraluminal air will be seen with an AEF [10].

Embolic events as a complication of vascular graft infections have been reported and involve either the pulmonary or systemic vasculature, according to the location of the infected device. Occlusion of a graft may lead to distal manifestations of ischemia or necrosis [11]. Pseudoaneurysms can develop at vascular graft anastomosis and are evident from the presenting pulsatile masses. For infection involving percutaneous drivelines and subcutaneously implanted devices, inflammatory signs and purulent drainage at the percutaneous exit site and/or abscess formation are sometimes associated with bacteremia. Sepsis with shock and multiorgan dysfunction is present in some acute cases caused by virulent pathogens such as *Staphylococcus aureus* and *Pseudomonas aeruginosa*. Subacute and chronic presentations can be seen in infections caused by less aggressive microorganisms. These infections might present as bacteremia with fever without any other clinical findings. Immune-mediated events are occasionally seen with chronic infections and include immune complex-mediated nephritis and vasculitis.

In 1972 Szilagyi *et al.* [1] divided extracavitary vascular graft infections into three groups according to the local compromise. The first group includes infections affecting the dermis, the second infections involving the subcutaneous tissue and the third infections affecting the vascular prosthesis. This classification was modified in 1988 by Samson *et al.* [12], who divided graft infections into five groups:
• Group I: infections extending no deeper than the dermis
• Group II: infections involving the subcutaneous tissue but not completely in direct contact with the graft

• Group III: infections involving the body of the graft but none of its anastomosis
• Group IV: infections surrounding an exposed anastomosis but without bacteremia or anastomotic bleeding
• Group V: infections involving a graft-to-artery anastomosis and associated with septicemia and/or anastomotic bleeding at the time of presentation.

The clinical questions

To confirm a graft infection, the radiologist must consider the patient's clinical history and status, particularly in cases of low-grade infections when findings may be subtle. The radiologist should be familiar with the complete information on the patient *before* graft implantation, including the vascular problem that led to the repair and any associated pathological conditions (trauma, local or systemic infection processes, etc.). Essential intraprocedural information, including whether it was an endovascular procedure or open surgical repair, the prosthesis that was used [its type and number, especially in endovascular aneurysm repair (EVAR)], anatomical location and extension of the graft, type of anastomoses, anatomical changes inherent to the repair and postsurgical evolution.

Before undertaking the imaging studies the radiologists should be aware of the patient's current clinical status, including signs, symptoms, clinical examination, laboratory tests, microbiological profile and complementary studies. The radiologist may be able to use this information to indicate the most appropriate imaging modality, optimize acquisition protocols and, if necessary, suggest complementary techniques.

Methodological considerations

Imaging for diagnosis of vascular graft infection can be performed by plain film, US, CT, MRI and digital subtraction angiography (DSA). Vascular grafts can be intracavitary (thoracic or abdominal) or extracavitary (infrainguinal, upper limb, hemodialysis, etc.). Which imaging method is selected depends upon the type of vascular graft and the suspected grade of infection. In high-grade infections, signs of a vascular graft infection may be diagnosed with a high positive predictive value [3]. However, in low-grade infections it may be difficult to confirm the diagnosis and radiological signs may be subtle. A white blood cell (WBC)-labeled radionuclide scan can be helpful to confirm diagnosis. However, false-positive results from other inflammatory causes have been reported [7]. Once infection is confirmed, medical treatment and/or patient reoperation is planned in most cases after performing DSA or CT angiography (CTA). Percutaneous aspiration and drainage placement can be helpful for culture, antibiotic selection and as a first-line treatment, which when combined with antibiotic therapy can be definitive.

Conventional radiography

Plain film does not play a major role in the diagnosis of a local graft infection. It may be helpful in evaluating the integrity of devices based on a metal structure (such as endovascular stents or stent-grafts). Non-metal devices are not visible on plain films.

Other indications for using plain films in the setting of a vascular graft infection include the detection of free air and the evaluation of adjacent radio-opaque anatomical structures to identify pathologies. Therefore, a plain film can be used for follow-up after endovascular stent-graft repair or if osteomyelitis is suspected. Aortic graft infections occasionally manifest as vertebral osteomyelitis. Rarely, lower-extremity heterotrophic osteoarthropathy is associated with aortic graft infection. If there is suspicion of a graft infection adjacent to a bony structure, a plain film can clarify if the bone is involved and this will have an impact on treatment. Periosteal elevation, disruption and interruption of the cortical surface and/or osteolytic lesions can be seen. Conversely, infection with bone involvement, like a sternal osteomyelitis after aortic surgery, can indicate a prosthetic infection as this can spread to an aortic graft [13].

Ultrasound

US is an important imaging modality for basic diagnosis because it is widely available, of low cost and quick to use. It can be applied in the evaluation of groin masses as well as fast bedside follow-up examination after a surgical intervention to check for, for example, changes in size of a previously demonstrated perigraft fluid collection or a pseudoaneurysm [14,15].

It should be pointed out that extreme care must be taken during the examination, since the use of excessive probe pressure on an infected pseudoaneurysm could induce its rupture, with possibly fatal consequences. The quality of the US image evaluation is operator dependent; therefore, US findings are difficult to compare, especially in adverse conditions.

Reviews indicate that as a primary imaging modality US is only useful in the evaluation of superficial grafts if complex or anechoic collections or possibly "gas" are demonstrated around the graft in an appropriate time frame, which is described as 3 months for fluid and beyond 7 weeks for gas. In cases of aortic grafts, its usefulness is usually limited by overlying bowel gas, as well as in patients with a large body habitus. In addition, in most institutions, surgeons would not base a decision to operate on US findings alone; usually they rely on other imaging modalities, such as CT, MRI or angiography, which likely provide a more detailed roadmap.

For arteries and veins that are located superficially, such as carotid arteries, Doppler US is the imaging modality of choice [16]. Superficial structures can be examined using a 7-MHz linear array US transducer. The lower penetration depth is compensated by a higher image resolution. The morphology of a graft as well as its anastomoses and the adjacent native vessel can be studied with Doppler US and at the same time flow disturbances can be evaluated.

It allows a good evaluation of the surrounding tissues and has a high sensitivity for fluid collections, distinguishing serous fluid from hematoma [17]. Factors compromising the evaluation are obesity, edema, surgical wound/air and overlying hematoma.

The assessment of abdominal vascular grafts is more difficult. A 3.5-MHz ultrasound transducer is used for evaluation of intra-abdominal organs and detection of pathologies that could be related to a graft infection, such as cholecystitis, pancreatitis or intra-abdominal abscess. Doppler US has the capacity to assess intra-abdominal and retroperitoneal vessels and has been proposed for the follow-up of EVAR procedures [15].

US does not play a major role in the diagnosis of graft infections in the intrathoracic cavity. The intrathoracic vessels cannot be evaluated in their entirety by US. Even if parts of the thoracic aorta are accessible to transesophageal US, this procedure is invasive and there are better alternatives for visualization of the whole intrathoracic vascular structure, such as CT and MRI.

An invasive method for evaluating the vascular system is intravascular US (IVUS). Its usefulness has been reported in the diagnosis of suspected atypical aortic graft infection as it can improve prosthesis wall evaluation [18]. Finally, US is indicated in the guidance of diagnostic punctures to confirm graft infection [19].

CT imaging

CT is the diagnostic imaging modality of choice for vascular graft infections. It is available in most hospitals and a diagnosis can be obtained in a short time. Every anatomical region of the body is amenable for CT evaluation and a vascular prosthesis can be clearly and entirely visualized. CT has a sensitivity of 94% and a specificity of 85% when the criteria of perigraft fluid, perigraft soft tissue attenuation, ectopic gas, pseudo-aneurysm, or focal bowel wall thickening are used [10]. However, in low-grade infection, sensitivity decreases because the morphological changes are difficult to distinguish from post-surgical changes [20].

Today, multidetector CT angiography (MDCTA) allows a fast evaluation due to its high spatial resolution. It offers images of different contrast phases, such as non-enhanced images, and images in the arterial, venous and late phase. The non-enhanced images provide information about vascular and perivascular masses, ectopic gas and/or fluid collection, and play a major role in the detection of hyperdense blood collections and in helping to distinguish calcium from injected contrast leaks in post-EVAR studies. The arterial phase permits an evaluation of the native adjacent arteries and arterial graft and its lumen, while the venous phase permits an evaluation of the venous system. In the late phase or late venous phase it is also possible to detect other pathologies that could have led to graft infection. Oral contrast administration can help to detect AEFs or may distinguish between enteric loops and abscesses; however, its use is not mandatory and its advantages must be weighed against the disadvantage of more time consuming and laborious maximum intensity projections (MIPs) and volume rendering reconstructions. In the late phase, bleeding after graft infection can be evidenced and also better definition of fluid collections can be obtained.

In recent years, better reconstruction algorithms, such as three-dimensional (3D) reconstructions, maximum intensity projections (MIP) and multiplanar and curved reconstruction images have contributed to clarifying the anatomical relation between the vascular graft, pathological images and other anatomical structures.

CT can also be used to guide diagnostic aspiration of a fluid collection. It has also been used to guide percutaneous drainage placement in patients who are considered at high risk for surgical management or to improve a patient's condition before surgery is contemplated [21].

MR imaging

Magnetic resonance imaging (MRI) has also proven its accuracy in the diagnosis of prosthetic aortic graft infection [22]. It is the alternative imaging modality to CT in cases in whom there is a contraindication to the use of an iodinated contrast medium. The positive predictive value of MRI in intracavitary vascular graft infection has been reported to be as high as 95%, while the negative predictive value in this condition is 80% [3]. Nevertheless, there are disadvantages compared with CT, such as its higher costs, lower availability and time-consuming examination. In some instances, MRI is superior to CT, such as in cases in whom perivascular inflammatory changes and/or small amounts of periprosthetic fluid are suspected, and in these cases MRI evaluation should be the initial technique [23].

MRI images with different protocols can differentiate between tissues. Changes in signal intensity on T1-weighted images (T1WIs) and T2-weighted images (T2WIs) provide useful information if there is a perigraft fibrosis, fluid collection or hematoma [24]. However, it cannot differentiate between sterile or infected fluids, particularly in the postoperative period [22]. In addition, it does not allow differentiation of the signal void produced by calcification from that seen with air.

MR images can be obtained before and after the administration of paramagnetic contrast medium. The addition of contrast medium can provide information about the patency of the vascular graft and can detect an inflammatory process in the vascular wall or surrounding tissue. Additional MR sequences can provide further information, e.g. a short TI inversion recovery (STIR) sequence may better define the extent of infection with a greater fat–fluid contrast [25].

Digital subtraction angiography

In the diagnosis of vascular graft infection, DSA plays only a limited role and is not the primary tool for imaging evaluation. As a diagnostic tool, only intraluminal contrast-enhanced structures can be visualized; therefore, the surrounding structures cannot be evaluated. Furthermore, angiography is unable to show the most important criteria of graft infection: perigraft gas and perigraft fluid [26].

Nevertheless, angiography can be used for diagnosing complications of graft infections, such as pseudo-aneurysm, rupture or thrombosis of a graft. A diagnostic DSA should always be performed in emergency cases before a therapeutic endovascular procedure. Hemorrhage after graft infection is a potentially life-threatening condition that can be diagnosed by DSA and then treated with endovascular embolization or stent-graft deployment to achieve hemostasis [27]. Carbon dioxide (CO_2)-enhanced angiography has also been used in the diagnosis of bleeding. CO_2, a negative contrast, can detect bleeding spots that are not visible on a standard angiogram [28]. Finally, an angiography should be performed before a surgical intervention because it can provide additional information, like proximal and distal vessel status and flow dynamics.

As a therapeutic tool, angiography and stent-graft placement should be considered as a first-line treatment in emergency cases and in high-risk surgical patients [29]. A hybrid approach consisting of emergency stent-graft placement and staged surgical repair has also been reported in cases of rupture of infected anastomotic pseudo-aneurysms [30].

Normal findings and artifacts

Conventional radiography

Plain films are not generally used today. However, plain films are indicated to detect associated osteomyelitis in suspected cases of vascular graft infection. If a graft infection adjacent to a bony structure is suspected, a plain film should be able to clarify if the bone is involved in the infectious process; this has an important impact on treatment.

Ultrasound

The main disadvantage of US evaluation is its operator dependency. On US, endovascular and vascular grafts can be monitored but this depends on their localization. A vascular graft appears as a well-defined anechoic vascular channel with echogenic walls. Superficially located vascular grafts are easily detectable when patent as echo-free channels. For deeper grafts, like abdominal prosthesis, overlying bowel gas and obesity can decrease the quality of the examination [10]. Intra-abdominally located structures can transmit echoes to the inner lumen of grafts and this limits the accuracy of diagnosis. Doppler US adds further information to the evaluation of a graft. In contrast to B-mode US, Doppler US can detect blood flow inside the vessel. With color Doppler US, the flow signal should be seen for the entire graft without any filling defect.

The diameter of the prosthesis and the adjacent vessels should be measured. The US probe should be positioned perpendicular to the vessel as diagonal measurements overestimate graft and arterial diameter. If possible, the whole graft should be visualized to rule out graft infection. The anastomoses are evaluated regarding dilatation or stenosis. Proximal and distal native vessels can be visualized as tubular structures that may show atherosclerotic changes. These atherosclerotic plaques, especially when calcified, have increased echogenicity, although it might be difficult to distinguish atherosclerotic plaques from bacterial vegetations. In addition, severe calcifications cause an intense echo pattern with a distal acoustic shadow, limiting an appropriate evaluation of the vascular lumen.

Other factors that decrease the accuracy of a US graft evaluation are hematomas surrounding the graft and surgical incisions. Ectopic air following a recent open surgical intervention also produces artifacts in the operating field and therefore decreases accuracy.

CT imaging

Vascular grafts can be studied in their entirety on CT scans. The visibility of a vascular graft depends on whether the graft is synthetic, biological, or an endovascular prosthesis with a metallic structure. Synthetic graft materials such as Dacron or polytetrafluoroethylene (PTFE) can often be visualized due to their well-defined tubular shape. Also, PTFE grafts are clearly seen due to their high fluor content. Often, postoperative changes are found on CT, such as infiltration of the perigraft fat tissue, perigraft fluid collection and ectopic air (the latter is only a normal finding in the recent postoperative period).

An endovascular prosthesis is usually based on a metal framework. Its manufacture from radio-opaque materials facilitate its visualization and it can be identified as a metal-density tubular device surrounded by the diseased vessel [31]. However, the impermeable membrane that covers the metal frame cannot be visualized directly on CT.

Non-contrast-enhanced and enhanced CT scans provide valuable information in the follow-up evaluation of a vascular graft. The size of the prosthesis, adjacent vessel diameters and patency can be evaluated with CT. During follow-up, changes should be documented, such as perigraft air/fluid reduction, contours of the prosthesis, excluded aortic lumen after EVAR, morphological changes and metallic mesh integrity. Intramural thrombus and intimal hyperplasia are two other features that can be visualized with contrast-enhanced CT images [31].

However, there are some limitations to CT. Besides motion and flow artifacts, metallic artifacts after surgery affect the quality of images [32]. Surgical clips as well as metallic prosthesis produce streak artifacts. The radiological markers on an endoprosthesis are strategically important during prosthesis placement. However, in the neighborhood of these markers, small amounts of fluid or periprosthetic air and intraluminal thrombosis may be difficult to visualize.

Severe calcification of arteries causes artifacts that overestimate the degree of stenosis of the affected arteries. In small-caliber arteries it may be difficult to distinguish mural thrombi from a patent vascular lumen or to detect small amounts of perivascular fluid in the neighborhood of calcification. In addition, CT does not distinguish between small quantities of perivascular fluid and recent hematoma.

Artifacts on raw data can mimic or miss pathologies; therefore, special care should be taken when evaluating reconstructed images.

MR imaging

Depending on the sequences used during MRI, the acquisition time can be long and motion artifacts from pulsating great vessels may decrease its accuracy in graft evaluation. Nevertheless, MRI can be used to measure the diameters of the vessel and to evaluate the vascular lumen after gadolinium-enhanced gradient echo sequence.

A vascular prosthesis presents as a thin line of low signal on T1WIs and T2WIs. In contrast, an endovascular prosthesis with a metal structure produces susceptibility artifacts due to its paramagnetic properties. A cobalt alloy- or platinum-based stent produces a strong void signal; Nitinol-based stent structures are of less importance. The severity of artifacts depends on the thickness of the metallic meshwork and the lumen of the stent-grafts may not be evaluated accurately in some cases [33]. The operator should therefore be familiar with the paramagnetic properties of the prosthesis in question. The same susceptibility artifacts are frequently seen after open vascular surgery in the vicinity of metal clips, particularly when adjacent to vessels.

MRI has excellent diagnostic accuracy in differentiating the periprosthetic tissue. Perigraft fluid collections usually appear with high signal intensity in T2WIs and with a low signal on T1WIs. For fat-containing tissues, the signal intensity of T1WIs and T2WIs is reversed. Low signal intensity in T1W and T2W sequences is typical for periprosthetic fibrosis [24]. Perigraft hematoma may be visualized as variations in the magnetic characteristics, depending on the time of evolution.

Another limitation of MRI is the poor differentiation between air and calcification.

Digital subtraction angiography

On DSA a graft can be visualized as a patent tube without internal filling defects. The entirety of the anastomotic region should be explored and neither aneurysms nor stenosis should be found.

As already mentioned, angiography has the disadvantage that only the endoluminal structures can be visualized. Therefore, pathological changes in the surrounding tissue cannot be evaluated and the complete extent of pseudo-aneurysms cannot be seen when thrombus is present.

Pathological findings and significance

Vascular graft infection should be suspected if clinical signs and symptoms are present. Abscess formation is the most common presentation followed by false aneurysms and graft thrombosis [34,35]. However, the most significant radiological signs for an infected vascular graft are soft tissue attenuation, periprosthetic air and perigraft fluid, which can be visualized before any clinical presentation is evident [26,36]. In case of low-grade infection, radiological signs may be subtle or undetectable.

The imaging appearance of a graft infection can be broad and to increase the likelihood of detecting graft infection, several different signs may need to be considered. In graft infection with AEF, the most frequent presentation is soft tissue attenuation, ectopic gas and focal bowel wall thickening [36]. Less frequent observations include osteomyelitis and hydronephrosis [37].

Ectopic air

Ectopic air in relation to a vascular graft infection refers to the presence of air in anatomical structures where gas should not be found, such as the vicinity of a vascular graft (periprosthetic air), in the surrounding tissues (subcutaneous emphysema, abscess formations, etc.) and inside an excluded aneurysm or vascular prosthesis (Figure 7.1).

After an open surgical or endovascular graft placement, periprosthetic air is a normal finding. Even in the presence of fever and leukocytosis, free

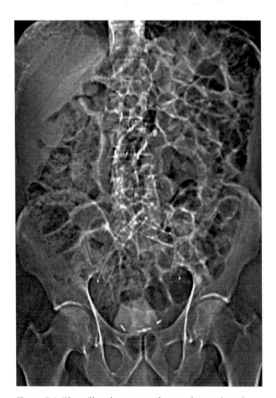

Figure 7.1 Plain film showing endovascular graft with perigraft gas.

air is not necessarily a sign of vascular graft infection [38]. After open surgery, air can be found in the surrounding tissues and the surgical wound due to manipulation of the perivascular tissue. Perigraft air can also be present if the graft is not yet incorporated into the tissue. Ectopic gas might be detected within 1 week after surgery but has been identified up to 7 weeks [10]. After open aortic aneurysm repair, periprosthetic air is a frequent sign, but it is more likely to be found after surgery for aneurysms larger than 6.0 cm. [39]. Ectopic air is also a normal finding after endovascular prosthesis placement. Here, air can invade the space between the vascular wall and the endoprosthesis or can be captured inside an excluded aneurysm due to an insufficiently flushed endoprosthesis.

CT is the leading tool for detecting ectopic air. In case of contrast allergy, air can be detected on a non-enhanced CT.

Even though perigraft air is one of the leading radiological signs for graft infection, air either within or around an open surgical graft was reported in only 25–50% of confirmed graft infections [26,36]. If an increasing volume of air is detected on sequential images, whether inside an excluded aneurysm or perigraft, an infection in combination with a fistula may be the cause. It has been reported that although ectopic air has been noted as a sign of perigraft infection, air in and around an aortic graft is more likely due to a fistulous communication rather than to a gas-producing organism [36].

Imaging modalities other than the CT are of less importance in the diagnosis of ectopic air. US can be useful for guiding the puncture of a superficially located air-containing structure to confirm diagnosis, but if visibility is insufficient, a CT-guided puncture can be an alternative.

Perigraft fluid

Fluid collections surrounding a graft can have different origins, such as inflammatory exudates, purulent fluid, hematomas and lymphocele after iatrogenic disruption of lymphatic vessels. Transudation of fluid through the prosthetic surfaces has also been reported [40].

Perigraft fluid is a normal finding after surgery and is more frequently found in open than in endovascular surgery. It can be detected in 90% of patients 1 week after surgery and should disappear within 24 weeks [24]. If perigraft fluid persists after an open surgery, a low-grade infection might be suspected [41]. After endovascular repair, fluid and pleural effusion can be the consequence of an inflammatory reaction to the foreign body.

Perigraft fluid is not always present when a surgical graft is infected but may be detected in non-infected grafts. Perigraft fluid collections were found in 48% of infected grafts with AEFs, but in only 33–42% of those without AEFs [36]. False-positive results have been reported for perigraft hematoma [42]. Therefore, perigraft fluid alone cannot be used to definitively diagnose a graft infection and must be combined with other signs before a diagnosis is made.

Fluid collections can be diagnosed by CT (Figure 7.2), MRI or, if large or superficially located, US. However, if fluid is found in the vicinity of a graft, CT and US may not differentiate the fluid collection from a soft tissue mass. The most accurate tool for diagnosing perigraft fluid is MRI, as it can detect even small amounts of fluid collections. Moreover it has the capacity to distinguish between hematoma, protein-containing fluid or purely serous fluids. Because MRI cannot distinguish between sterile and infected fluid, CT or US can be used for guiding a diagnostic puncture. Angiography does not play a major role in this setting as it fails to demonstrate perigraft fluid collections. The only diagnostic use for DSA may be in the visualization of a bleeding perigraft hematoma.

Perigraft soft tissue attenuation

Perigraft soft tissue attenuation refers to the radiological finding of a perigraft tissue mass which enhances on contrast-enhanced images. It is a normal finding after open surgery and is interpreted as an inflammatory response to the perigraft tissue in the postoperative period. Even after endovascular repair, a transient periprosthetic thickening of the artery and the surrounding tissues has been described 2 months after stent-graft implantation as a foreign body reaction [43]. After the postoperative period, the tissue surrounding the graft should have the same attenuation as normal fat. However, if soft tissue attenuation is found 1 year after a surgical treatment, an infection must be suspected, especially when associated with periprosthetic fluid [10]. One dilemma with this radiological finding is that non-infected grafts are reported to present peri-

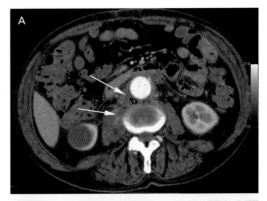

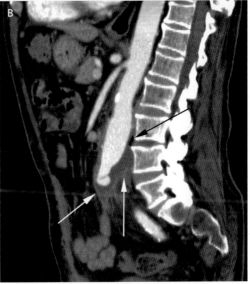

Figure 7.2 (A) Axial CT image shows a fluid collection with gas inside, adjacent to the graft. The collection extends to the right psoas muscle (arrows). (B) Sagittal reconstruction shows a periaortic collection that extends along the right branch of the graft (white arrows) and has gas inside (black arrow), anterior to L3.

graft soft tissue attenuation too [36] and a sterile graft can be misdiagnosed as infected. Also, other clinical entities can mimic soft tissue attenuation, such as pancreatitis, retroperitoneal fibrosis and retroperitoneal lymphoma [44]. However, if a graft is infected, perigraft soft tissue attenuation is almost always present on contrast-enhanced images [26,36].

The best modalities for diagnosing perigraft soft tissue attenuation are contrast-enhanced CT (Figure 7.3) and MRI. In contrast to CT, MRI may be superior in demonstrating the extent of focal

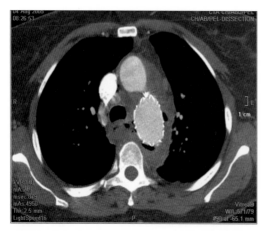

Figure 7.3 Thoracic CT shows mediastinitis signs: perigraft fluid and gas inside the collection. Esophagus planes cannot be seen.

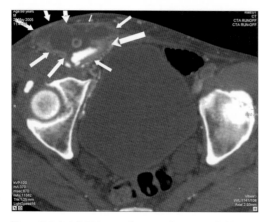

Figure 7.4 Axial CT image shows graft surrounded by fluid and contrast extravasation (arrows).

inflammation as adjacent tissues have an increased signal intensity on T2WIs [22]. If results are inconclusive, other methods such as single-photon emission CT (SPECT), a labeled white blood cell scan or positron emission tomography (PET) can be used to confirm infection (see Chapter 14).

Pseudo-aneurysm

A false aneurysm forms when blood leaks out of a graft or an anastomosis into the adjacent tissue and forms a hematoma with a patent lumen (Figures 7.4 and 7.5). In contrast to a true aneurysm it has no arterial layers around it. Various mechanisms have been identified in the development of a pseudo-aneurysm after open vascular surgery: infection,

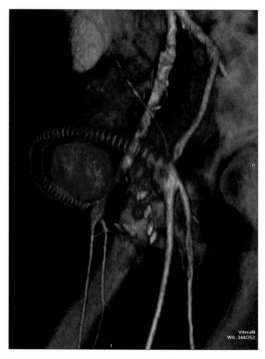

Figure 7.5 Volume-rendering of CT image shown in Figure 7.4.

failure of the suture, hypertension, trauma/necrosis of the native vessel or the biological graft at the site of anastomosis, thrombosis, mismatch of native vessel and graft diameter, and degenerative processes involving the anastomosis site such as atherosclerotic changes [45]. Complications of pseudo-aneurysms include graft thrombosis, distal embolization, aortoenteric/bronchial fistulas, compression of adjacent organs and rupture [46].

After open vascular surgery, the incidence of pseudo-aneurysms has been reported to be between 1% and 4%. The incidence of pseudo-aneurysms may be underestimated, as the time gap between initial surgery and the appearance of this complication can be long; therefore, its true long-term incidence may be up to 25% [47].

One major problem with the radiological finding of a "pseudo-aneurysm" is knowing whether or not there is an infection. Most of these are non-infected but it is difficult to diagnose those patients with infected pseudo-aneurysms. Time of occurrence may be helpful in differentiating infected from non-infected pseudo-aneurysms as diagnosis of a sterile pseudo-aneurysm in the first years after an open aortic surgery is rare [46], and if a pseudo-aneurysm does occur then, an infection has to be suspected. Nevertheless, major perioperative complications, technical errors, recurrent aneurysm, and α-1-antitrypsin deficiency have been associated with the early appearance of pseudo-aneurysms [48–50]. Radiological signs of infected pseudo-aneurysms include a lobulated vascular mass, an irregular arterial wall, perianeurysmal edema, soft tissue attenuation and calcification [51].

US should be the first-line diagnostic tool when a palpable pulsatile mass is detected [14]. US has a sensitivity of 94% and a specificity of 97% for superficially localized pseudo-aneurysms [52]. When Doppler US is used, the "ying–yang sign" can be found (an alternating pulse waveform) and can be visualized as changes from red to blue in color Doppler US. Care should be taken not to apply too much pressure with the transducer as infected pseudo-aneurysms are prone to rupture.

For deeper located pseudo-aneurysms, the preferred method is MDCTA. For detection of pseudo-aneurysms, CT has a reported sensitivity of 95% with a specificity of 99% [32,53]. It can distinguish between true aneurysms and pseudo-aneurysms, and provide information about the neck, surrounding thrombus and feeding artery, and is therefore essential for treatment planning.

MRI can also be useful in patients with iodine contrast allergy and it is reported to be as accurate as CT in detecting pseudo-aneurysms [54]. Angiography can be used in the detection of pseudo-aneurysm; however, its value is limited, as it does not depict the thrombus but only the inner lumen. Because it is an invasive procedure and is inferior to CT and MRI, today angiography should only be used in emergency situations when a therapeutic approach is required [32,53].

Aortoenteric fistula

An AEF is defined as a communication between the aorta and the gastrointestinal (GI) tract and is a life-threatening condition with a high mortality rate [55]. AEF may be primary or secondary. Primary AEF is rare and almost always associated with pre-existing aortic aneurysms. Secondary AEF develops after an aortic reconstructive surgery or endovascular stent-graft placement. Infection, pseudo-aneurysms and erosion have been identified as risk factors for the development of a secondary AEF [56]. Secondary fistulas that result from peri-

graft infection may occur between 2 weeks and 10 years after surgery, but are more frequent after open than after endovascular surgery [57].

The correct diagnosis of an AEF is difficult. If GI bleeding is present in combination with a history of aortic surgery, an AEF has to be suspected. CTA has become the first-line modality for imaging evaluation. Endoscopy and MRI improve the likelihood for detecting an AEF, but clinical suspicion is still most important [56]. Gastroduodenoscopy can be performed when bleeding is present; nevertheless, CTA is potentially more accurate than endoscopy [58]. For detecting ectopic air, CT evaluation is superior to MRI, with a sensitivity of 40–90% and specificity of 33–100% [57]. CT findings that correlate strongly with the presence of AEF have been reported, such as the appearance of prosthesis inside the bowel lumen and active extravasation. Indirect signs of AEF can also be present in graft infection without fistula, such as effacement of the periaortic or perigraft fat plane and the fat plane between the aorta and bowel, perigraft soft tissue, bowel wall thickening adjacent to the graft, perigraft fluid, perigraft hematoma, pseudo-aneurysm and dystrophic vascular graft calcification [58]. Before acquisition of CT images, oral contrast administration may help to confirm the presence of enteral perforation.

The vascular prosthesis that leads to AEF is considered to be infected but can present with or without clinical symptoms of an infection. Because of the high mortality and morbidity associated with secondary AEF, surgical treatment is always recommended [56]. In case of active hemorrhage, open surgery is associated with a high mortality; therefore, the placement of an endovascular endoprosthesis has been suggested to control the bleeding [59]. After endoprosthesis placement, recurrent infections have been reported with an almost three-fold increased risk of persistent/recurrent infection for secondary compared to primary AEF [60]. Elective conversion might reduce mortality in these cases.

Aortobronchial fistula

An aortobronchial fistula (ABF) is a communication between the aorta and the bronchial tree. It is a rare but highly lethal condition if untreated [61]. These types of lesions are commonly seen in patients with thoracic aortic aneurysms following thoracic trauma, but they may occur as postoperative complications after cardiac surgery or stent-graft placement [62]. The reported time from operation to presentation ranges from 4 months to 17 years [63]. ABF develops in the presence of a vascular graft or suture material adjacent to an aneurysm and in the presence of infection. ABF often present with recurrent or massive hemoptysis [64]. This non-specific sign can be found in other pathologies as well. Therefore, an ABF should be suspected if an aneurysmatic disease is known or if the patient has a history of previous aortic intervention.

ABF typically extends from the descending aorta to the left bronchial tree [63]. In these patients, CT is the principal imaging modality in the diagnostic work-up [65]. Chest radiography cannot visualize an ABF; however, it may delineate pulmonary abnormalities in the vicinity of a vascular structure. A CT scan with 3D reconstructions can visualize the relation between the vascular prosthesis and the bronchial tree, and has the potential to detect ectopic air inside an excluded aneurysm. If hemoptysis is the leading symptom, a CTA may identify a leak. If CT is inconclusive, MRI is indicated to detect a fistula [66]. Angiography can detect an ABF, usually in cases with important bleeding. Bronchoscopy is useful for identifying the site of bleeding and it permits direct visualization. Care should be taken in removing blood clots as this can cause catastrophic bleedings [67].

Endoluminal stent grafting is considered to be the preferred treatment alternative to surgery in cases of ABF, but could be a definitive method of treatment [68]. However, even if surgical conversion after endograft infection is not mandatory, close surveillance is necessary to detect recurrence of ABF after an endovascular treatment [69].

Role for therapy follow-up and patient management

Once the infection is diagnosed and the treatment carried out, CT is the preferred imaging modality for follow-up. Post-treatment changes should be documented, like the presence and reduction of perigraft air/fluid, anastomoses, endoprosthesis or graft appearance and morphological changes. The entire prosthesis should be evaluated as well as the adjacent vascular anatomy. Intramural thrombus and intimal hyperplasia are two other features that can be visualized with contrast-enhanced CT scans [31].

References

1. Szilagi DE, Smith RF, Elliot JP, Vrandecic MP. Infection in arterial reconstruction with synthetic grafts. *Ann Surg* 1972;176:321–333.
2. Johnson KK, Russ PD, Bair JH, Friefeld GD. Diagnosis of synthetic vascular graft infection: Comparison of CT and gallium scans. *AJR Am J Roentgenol* 1990; 154:405–409.
3. Shahidi S, Eskil A, Lundof E, Klaerke A, Jensen BS. Detection of abdominal aortic graft infection: comparison of magnetic resonance imaging and indium-labeled white blood cell scanning. *Ann Vasc Surg* 2007;21:586–592.
4. Homer-Vanniasinkam S. Surgical site and vascular infections: treatment and prophylaxis. *Int J Infect Dis* 2007;11 (Suppl 1):S17–22.
5. Treska V, Houdek K, Vachtova M, Smid D, Kormuda S. Management of the prosthetic vascular graft infections – the influence of predictive factors on treatment results. *Bratisi Lek Listy* 2008;109:544–550.
6. Amstrong PA, Back MR, Bandyk DF, Jonhson BL, Shames ML. Selective application of sartorious flaps and aggressive staged surgical debridement can influence long-term outcomes of complex prosthetic graft infections. *J Vasc Surg* 2007;46:71–78.
7. Seeger JM. Management of patients with prosthetic vascular graft infection. *Am Surg* 2000;66:166–167.
8. FitzGerald SF, Kelly C, Humphreys H. Diagnosis and treatment of prosthetic aortic graft infections: confusion and inconsistency in the absence of evidence or consensus. *J Antimicrob Chemother* 2005;56: 996–999.
9. Zetrenne E, McIntosh BC, McRae MH, Gusberg R, Evans GR Narayan D. Prosthetic vascular graft infection: A multi-center review of surgical management. *Yale J Biol Med* 2007;80:113–121.
10. Orton DF, LeVeen RF, Saigh JA *et al.* Aortic prosthetic graft infections. Radiologic manifestations and implications for management. *RadioGraphics* 2000;20: 977–993.
11. Baddour LM, Bettmann MA, Bolger AF *et al.* Nonvalvular cardiovascular device-related infections. *Circulation* 2003;108:2015–2031.
12. Samson RH, Veith FJ, Janko GS, Gupta SK, Scher LA. A modified classification and approach to the management of infections involving peripheral arterial prosthetic grafts. *J Vasc Surg* 1988;8:147–153.
13. Katayama Y, Minato N, Kawasaki H, Sakaguchi M. Surgical strategy for impending rupture of an infected anastomotic pseudoaneurysm of the aorta 9 years after a Bentall procedure: radical surgery involving en bloc resection of the infected sternum, pseudoaneurysm, and artificial vascular graft. *Gen Thorac Cardiovasc Surg* 2008;56:584–588.

14. Polak JF, Donaldson MC, Whittemore AD, Mannick JA, O'Leary DH. Pulsatile masses surrounding vascular prostheses: real-time US color flow imaging. *Radiology* 1989;170:363–366.

15. Chaer RA, Gushchin A, Rhee R *et al*. Duplex ultrasound as the sole long-term surveillance method post-endovascular aneurysm repair: a safe alternative for stable aneurysms. *J Vasc Surg* 2009;49:845–849; discussion 849–850.

16. Knight BC, Tait WF. Dacron patch infection following carotid endarterectomy: a systematic review of the literature. *Eur J Vasc Endovasc Surg* 2009;37:140–148.

17. Paes E, Paulat K, Hamann H *et al*. Early detection and differentiation of periprostheticfluid accumulation after vascular reconstructive surgery. *Surg Endosc* 1988;2:256–260.

18. Duda SH, Schott U, Raygrotzki S. Intravascular ultrasound diagnosis of aortic graft infection. *J Cardiovasc Surg (Torino)* 1998;39:303–305.

19. Mantoni M, Neergaard K, Christoffersen JK, Lambine TL, Baekgaard N. Long-term computed tomography follow-up after open surgical repair of abdominal aortic aneurysms. *Acta Radiol* 2006;47:549–553.

20. Fukuchi K, Ishida Y, Higashi M *et al*. Detection of aortic graft infection by fluorodeoxyglucose positron emission tomography: comparison with computed tomographic findings. *J Vasc Surg* 2005;42:919–925.

21. Rossi P, Arata FM, Salvatori FM *et al*. Prosthetic graft infection: diagnostic and therapeutic role of interventional radiology. *J Vasc Interv Radiol* 1997;8:271–277.

22. Olofsson PA, Auffermann W, Higgins CB, Rabahie GN, Tavares N, Stoney RJ. Diagnosis of prosthetic aortic graft infection by magnetic resonance imaging. *J Vasc Surg* 1988;8:99–105.

23. Modrall JG, Clagett GP. The role of imaging techniques in evaluating possible graft infections. *Semin Vasc Surg* 1999;12:339–347.

24. Spartera C, Morettini G, Petrassi C *et al*. Role of magnetic resonance imaging in the evaluation of aortic graft healing, peri-graft fluid collection, and graft infection. *Eur J Vasc Surg* 1990;4:69–73.

25. Hansen ME, Yucel EK, Waltman AC. STIR imaging of synthetic vascular graft infection. *Cardiovasc Interv Radiol* 1993;16:30–36.

26. Vogelzang RL, Limpert JD, Yao JS. Detection of prosthetic vascular complications: comparison of CT and angiography. *AJR Am J Roentgenol* 1987;148:819–823.

27. Kotsis T, Lioupis C, Tzanis A *et al*. Endovascular repair of a bleeding secondary aorto-enteric fistula with acute leg ischemia: a case report and review of the literature. *J Vasc Interv Radiol* 2006;17:563–567.

28. Sandhu C, Buckenham TM, Belli AM. Using CO_2-enhanced arteriography to investigate acute gastrointestinal hemorrhage. *AJR Am J Roentgenol* 1999;173:1399–1401.

29. Ascoli Marchetti A, Gandini R, Ippoliti A *et al*. The endovascular management of open aortic surgery complications with emergency stent-graft repair in high-risk patients. *J Cardiovasc Surg (Torino)* 2007;48:315–321.

30. Klonaris C, Katsargyris A, Vasileiou I, Markatis F, Liapis CD, Bastounis E. Hybrid repair of ruptured infected anastomotic femoral pseudoaneurysms: Emergent stent-graft implantation and secondary surgical debridement. *J Vasc Surg* 2009;49:938–945.

31. Hoang JK, Martinez S, Hurwitz SR. MDCT angiography of thoracic aorta endovascular stent-grafts: pearls and pitfalls. *AJR Am J Roentgenol* 2009;192:515–524.

32. Miller-Thomas MM, West OC, Cohen AM. Diagnosing traumatic arterial injury in the extremities with CT angiography: pearls and pitfalls. *RadioGraphics* 2005;25 (Suppl 1):S133–142.

33. Hansmann HJ, Dobert N, Kücherer H, Richter GM. [Various spiral CT protocols and their significance in the diagnosis of aortic dissections: results of a prospective study]. *Rofo* 2000;172:879–887.

34. Jones L, Braithwaite BD, Davies B, Heather BP, Earnshaw JJ. Mechanism of late prosthetic vascular graft infection. *Cardiovasc Surg* 1997;5:486–489.

35. Bunt TJ. Vascular graft infections: a personal experience. *Cardiovasc Surg* 1993;1:489–493.

36. Low RN, Wall SD, Jeffrey RB, Jr, Sollitto RA, Reilly LM, Tierney LM, Jr. Aortoenteric fistula and perigraft infection: evaluation with CT. *Radiology* 1990;175:157–162.

37. Perera GB, Fujitani RM, Kubaska SM. Aortic graft infection: update on management and treatment options. *Vasc Endovasc Surg* 2006;40:1–10.

38. Carpenter JP, Baum RA, Barker CF *et al*. Durability of benefits of endovascular versus conventional abdominal aortic aneurysm repair. *J Vasc Surg* 2002;35:222–228.

39. O'Hara PJ, Borkowski GP, Hertzer NR, O'Donovan PB, Brigham SL, Beven EG. Natural history of periprosthetic air on computerized axial tomographic examination of the abdomen following abdominal aortic aneurysm repair. *J Vasc Surg* 1984;1:429–433.

40. Williams GM. The management of massive ultrafiltration distending the aneurysm sac after abdominal aortic aneurysm repair with a polytetrafluoroethylene aortobiliac graft. *J Vasc Surg* 1998;28:551–555.

41. Chambers ST. Diagnosis and management of staphylococcal infections of vascular grafts and stents. *Intern Med J* 2005;35 (Suppl 2):S72–78.

42. Mark AS, McCarthy SM, Moss AA, Price D. Detection of abdominal aortic graft infection: comparison of CT and in-labeled white blood cell scans. *AJR Am J Roentgenol* 1985;144:315–318.

43. Sapoval MR, Gaux JC, Long AL *et al.* Transient periprosthetic thickening after covered-stent implantation in the iliac artery. *AJR Am J Roentgenol* 1995; 164:1271–1273.

44. Lu MT, Millstine J, Menard MT, Rybicki FJ, Viscomi S. Periaortic lymphoma as a mimic of posttraumatic intramural hematoma. *Emerg Radiol* 2006;13:35–38.

45. Kallis P, Keogh BE, Davies MJ. Pseudoaneurysm of aortocoronary vein graft secondary to late venous rupture: case report and literature review. *Br Heart J* 1993;70:189–192.

46. Bianchi P, Nano G, Cusmai F *et al.* Uninfected para-anastomotic aneurysms after infrarenal aortic grafting. *Yonsei Med J* 2009;50:227–238.

47. Abou-Zamzam AM, Jr, Ballard JL. Management of sterile para-anastomotic aneurysms of the aorta. *Semin Vasc Surg* 2001;14:282–291.

48. Odero A, Arici V, Canale S. [Proximal abdominal aortic aneurysms after infrarenal aortic reconstruction]. *Ann Ital Chir* 2004;75:211–221.

49. Lehnert T, Gruber HP, Maeder N, Allenberg JR. Management of primary aortic graft infection by extra-anatomic bypass reconstruction. *Eur J Vasc Surg* 1993;7:301–307.

50. Edwards MJ, Richardson JD, Klamer TW. Management of aortic prosthetic infections. *Am J Surg* 1988; 155:327–330.

51. Lee WK, Mossop PJ, Little AF *et al.* Infected (mycotic) aneurysms: spectrum of imaging appearances and management. *RadioGraphics* 2008;28:1853–1868.

52. Morgan R. Current treatment methods for postcatheterization pseudoaneurysms. *J Vasc Interv Radiol* 2003;2003:697–710.

53. Soto JA, Múnera F, Morales C *et al.* Focal arterial injuries of the proximal extremities: helical CT arteriography as the initial method of diagnosis. *Radiology* 2001;218:188–194.

54. Pilleul F, Forest J, Beuf O. Magnetic resonance angiography of splanchnic artery aneurysms and pseudoaneurysms. *J Radiol* 2006;87:127–131.

55. Busuttil SJ, Goldstone J. Diagnosis and management of aortoenteric fistulas. *Semin Vasc Surg* 2001;14: 302–311.

56. Limani K, Place B, Philippart P, Dubail D. Aortoduodenal fistula following aortobifemoral bypass. *Acta Chir Belg* 2005;105:207–209.

57. Vu QD, Menias CO, Bhalla S, Peterson C, Wang LL, Balfe DM. Aortoenteric fistulas: CT features and potential mimics. *RadioGraphics* 2009;29:197–209.

58. Hagspiel KD, Turba UC, Bozlar U *et al.* Diagnosis of aortoenteric fistulas with CT angiography. *J Vasc Interv Radiol* 2007;18:497–504.

59. Chuter TA, Lukaszewicz GC, Reilly LM *et al.* Endovascular repair of a presumed aortoenteric fistula: late failure due to recurrent infection. *J Endovasc Ther* 2000;7:240–244.

60. Antoniou GA, Koutsias S, Antoniou SA, Georgiakakis A, Lazarides MK, Giannoukas AD. Outcome after endovascular stent graft repair of aortoenteric fistula: A systematic review. *J Vasc Surg* 2009;49:782–789.

61. Favre JP, Gournier JP, Adham M, Rosset E, Barral X. Aortobronchial fistula: report of three cases and review of the literature. *Surgery* 1994;115:264–270.

62. Foster CL, Kalbhen CL, Demos TC, Lonchyna VA. Aortobronchial fistula occurring after coarctation repair: findings on aortography, helical CT, and CT angiography. *AJR Am J Roentgenol* 1998;171: 401–402.

63. MacIntosh EL, Parrott JC, Unruh HW. Fistulas between the aorta and tracheobronchial tree. *Ann Thorac Surg* 1991;51:515–519.

64. Szolar DH, Riepl T, Stiskal M, Preidler KW. Aortobronchial fistula as a late complication of posttraumatic chronic aortic aneurysm. *AJR Am J Roengenol* 1995; 164:1511.

65. Aidala E, Trichiolo S, Del Ponte S, Di Summa M, Poletti G, Zanetti PP. Aortobronchial fistula after aortic dissection type B. *J Cardiovasc Surg (Torino)* 2000;41:259–262.

66. Holdright DR, Kilner PJ, Somerville J. Haemoptysis from false aneurysm: near fatal complication of repair of coarctation of the aorta using a Dacron patch. *Int J Cardiol* 1991;32:406–408.

67. Garniek A, Morag B, Schmahmann S, Rubinstein ZJ. Aortobronchial fistula as a complication of surgery for correction of congenital aortic anomalies. *Radiology* 1990;175:347–348.

68. Bockler D, Schumacher H, Schwarzbach M, Ockert S, Rotert H, Allenberg JR. Endoluminal stent-graft repair of aortobronchial fistulas: bridging or definitive long-term solution? *J Endovasc Ther* 2004;11: 41–48.

69. Riesenman PJ, Brooks JD, Farber MA. Thoracic endovascular aortic repair of aortobronchial fistulas. *J Vasc Surg* 2009;50:992–998.

Clinical cases

Case 1

A 74-year-old male with an aorto-bi-iliac graft extending from the infrarenal aorta to both external iliac arteries.

Several months after surgery, the patient developed symptoms of graft failure and infection and a CT scan was performed; CTA showed signs of infection (Figure 7.6A–C). Antibiotic therapy was initiated but the patient's condition did not improve. A second angiographic study showed the presence of an important hemorrhage (Figure 7.6D–F) and an endovascular balloon was inserted for temporal hemostasis (Figure 7.6G). The patient was then transferred to the operating theater for removal of the prosthesis.

Teaching point

Radiological findings such as perigraft gas, perianeurysmatic fat infiltration, fluid collection and bone cortical erosion near a vascular graft and within an appropriate clinical setting are highly suspicious of inflammation and infection.

Case 2

Patient with axillo-bifemoral bypass secondary to Leriche's syndrome.

A CT scan was performed as there was suspicion of thrombosis and infection of the graft. The images clearly showed the site and extent of the infection (Figure 7.7A–D). In particular, volume-rendering reconstruction showed subcutaneous graft irregularities and stenotic areas (Figure 7.7D).

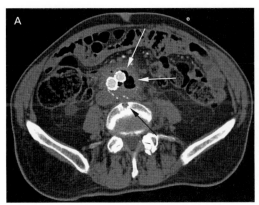
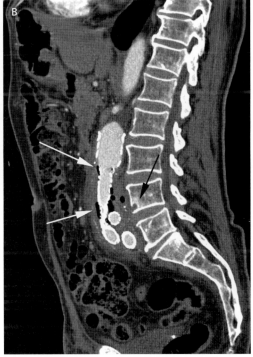

Figure 7.6 (A) Axial CT image showing air inside the aortic aneurysm sac (white arrows) and periaortic fat infiltration, both of which are compatible with graft infection and with L4 anterior cortical erosion (black arrow). (B) Sagittal CT reconstruction shows air inside the sac (white arrows) and the adjacent bone compromise (black arrow). (C) Coronal CT reconstruction shows a pelvic fluid collection (arrows) surrounding the left common iliac artery with an endoprosthesis inside it. (D) Coronal CT reconstruction 1 week after antibiotic treatment shows infection progress, fluid collection surrounding the right limb of the prosthesis and contrast leak adjacent to its distal end (arrows), a finding absent on the earlier CT. (E) Volume-rendering CT image after infrarenal aortic resection, infected endograft retrieval and axillo-bifemoral graft implant (white arrows) shows a pseudo-aneurysm adjacent to the distal aortic stump (yellow arrow). (F) Angiographic study shows important contrast extrasavation, demonstrating important bleeding. (G) Positioning of a balloon for temporal hemostasis.

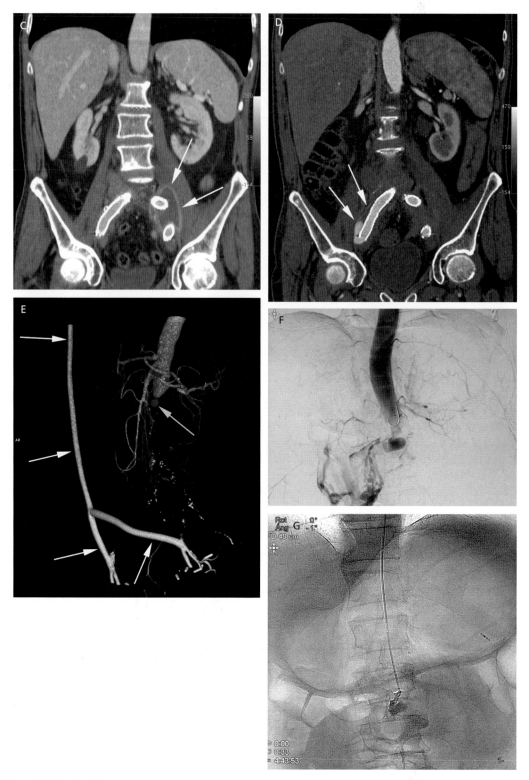

Figure 7.6 (*Continued*)

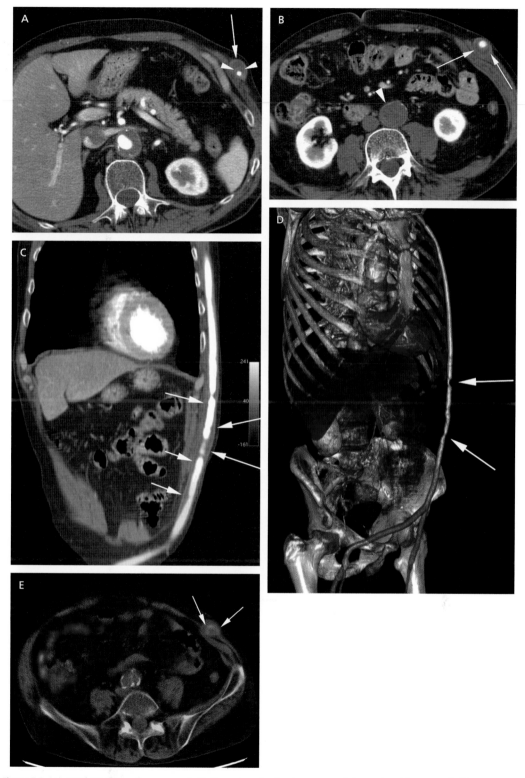

Figure 7.7 (A) Axial CT image shows a partially thrombosed subcutaneous graft (arrowheads) surrounded by a perigraft collection (arrow). (B) Distal axial CT image shows aortic infrarenal occlusion (arrowhead) and extension of the perigraft collection (arrows). (C) Coronal reconstruction shows the perigraft collection (arrows) and graft lumen irregularity. (D) Volume-rendering reconstruction showing subcutaneous graft irregularities and stenotic areas (arrows). (E) PET-TC image showing high tracer uptake in the abscess zone (arrow).

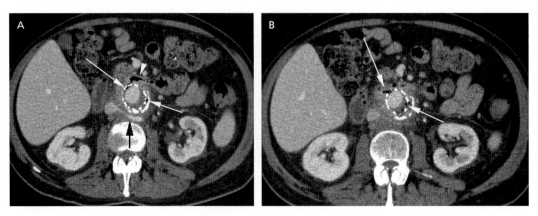

Figure 7.8 (A) Axial CT shows gas bubbles adjacent to the graft (arrows) and in contact with the horizontal portion of the duodenum (arrowhead), consistent with an aortoenteric fistula. Periaortic fat infiltration and a retroaortic left renal vein are seen. (B) Distal axial CT image shows gas bubbles between the duodenum and the graft (long arrow), inside the aneurysm and inside the graft (short arrow). Partial thrombosis of the graft is seen.

The patient was also referred to nuclear medicine for a [18F]fluorodeoxyglucose (FDG)-PET/CT scan and this confirmed the presence of the infection (Figure 7.7E).

Teaching points
• Perigraft fluid collections can extend for long segments around grafts.
• Endoluminal thrombus accompanied by perigraft fluid must suggest infection.
• [18F]FDG-PET can be useful for confirmation of infection in doubtful cases.

Case 3
A 59-year-old male who 3 months previously had had endograft surgery for an abdominal aortic aneurysm. He presented with pain and fever.

A CT scan was performed and showed gas bubbles adjacent to the graft and in contact with the duodenum, consistent with an AEF. Periaortic fat infiltration and retroaortic left renal vein were also detected as well as partial thrombosis of the graft (Figure 7.8).

Teaching point
Fluid and gas around a graft that is adjacent to the duodenum indicates AEF, especially in cases with digestive tract bleeding.

CHAPTER 8

Radiological Imaging of Tuberculosis and Human Immunodeficiency Virus

Jorge Carrillo

Universidad Nacional de Colombia, Bogotá, Colombia

Introduction

It is estimated that billion people around the world (one-third of the world's population) are infected with tuberculosis (TB). Of these, one in every 10 will become actively infected at some point in their lives. The global TB incidence rate is decreasing slowly (>1% each year).

In the 30 years since the start of the human immunodeficiency virus (HIV) syndrome epidemic, 30 million people around the world have died from causes related to this infection. Despite the decrease in the global new infection incidence rate, it is estimated that by the end of 2010, 34 million people worldwide (30.9–36.9 million) were infected with HIV.

The immune system alterations suffered by patients with HIV infection make them highly susceptible to developing TB disease. TB is the main cause of death in people infected by HIV: at least one in every four deaths in those infected with HIV can be attributed to TB.

Basic knowledge of the clinical problem

Estimates of the global burden of disease caused by TB in 2009 were 9.4 million incident cases (range, 8.9–9.9 million) and 14 million prevalent cases (range, 12–16 million). Of the 9.4 million incident cases in 2009, an estimated 1.0–1.2 million (11–13%) were HIV positive. In 2009, 26% of TB patients knew their HIV status (up from 22% in 2008), including 53% of patients in Africa. Of the 1.7 million people who died from TB in 2009, 400 000 (24%) had been living with HIV. There were 33 million people living with HIV and 2.6 million becoming newly infected with HIV. Of the 1.8 million HIV-related deaths in 2009, 400 000 (22%) were due to TB [1].

With the introduction of the highly active antiretroviral therapy (HAART), considerable demographic changes have occurred and the morbidity and mortality associated with HIV infection have decreased dramatically. Also, in nine observational cohort studies in 37 879 patients, the decrease in TB incidence among HIV-infected patients taking HAART was 67% (95% CI 61–37%; range, 54–92%). This percentage decrease is similar among patients from developed countries and from those of low income, and has been seen among patients with different CD4 counts. The most important reduction in absolute risk was found in the most severely immunosuppressed patients [2,3].

The use of isoniazid preventive therapy (IPT) has been shown to be effective in reducing the TB risk in both individuals infected with HIV and those not infected. In a meta-analysis of 11 trials, use of IPT was associated with a TB risk reduction of 60%

Diagnostic Imaging of Infections and Inflammatory Diseases: A Multidisciplinary Approach, First Edition. Edited by Alberto Signore and Ana María Quintero.
© 2014 John Wiley & Sons, Inc. Published 2014 by John Wiley & Sons, Inc.

(95% CI 48–69%) over a follow-up period of at least 2 years. The effect was similar in therapies lasting 6 and 12 months [4].

HIV-negative individuals with *Mycobacterium tuberculosis* infection have a lifetime risk of developing active TB of approximately 10%. In patients co-infected with *M. tuberculosis* and HIV, this risk can exceed 10% each year, depending on the patients' degree of immunodeficiency and the prevailing socioeconomic conditions [5].

HIV-positive patients have a risk of developing TB that ranges between 50 and 200 times higher than that of the general population [6]. Susceptibility to infection is related to the pattern of cytokines produced by T cells. Th1 cells (T helper 1) produce interferon-γ, which is essential in the control mycobacterial infections. When the lymphocytes of HIV-positive patients who are infected with TB are exposed *in vitro* to *M. tuberculosis*, they produce less interferon-γ, but similar amounts of interleukin (IL)-4 and IL-10, compared with HIV-negative patients with TB. This suggests that a reduced Th1 response in HIV-infected patients contributes to their susceptibility to TB infection [7].

Clinical studies have shown the detrimental effects of TB on the course of HIV infection. The risk of death in HIV-infected patients with TB was reported to be twice that in HIV-infected patients without TB, regardless of the CD4 count [8]. *M. tuberculosis* probably increases HIV replication by inducing macrophages to produce tumor necrosis factor, IL-1 and IL-6 [9].

Koening *et al.* published a series that described high mortality in patients diagnosed with TB in the 3 months following the start of HAART. In this group of patients, mortality was 27%, which is three times higher than that among TB and AIDS patients, and is attributed to subclinical TB not being recognized at the time of starting the HAART. They recommend a rigorous screen for TB before starting HAART and empirical treatments in high-risk patients [10].

An immune reconstitution syndrome is described in HIV-infected patients starting antiretroviral therapy, with clinical and radiological worsening of infections present in the host (usually mycobacterial). Recovery of cellular immunity due to the treatment is responsible for this phenomenon and must be distinguished from the progression of the original infection, resistance to treatment, adverse reactions to drugs, or co-morbid infection or neoplastic disease [11,12]. Nevertheless, in an open label, randomized, controlled trial in Durban, South Africa, in individuals with TB and HIV co-infection, the initiation of antiretroviral therapy during TB therapy significantly improved survival [13].

Chest X-ray is not indicated as a screening method for TB. However, in certain populations, the combination of clinical data, conventional radiography and bacilloscopy allow early diagnosis of TB. Clinical manifestations of respiratory infections are common and non-specific (cough and dyspnea) and in an important percentage of patients, diagnostic images play an important role in their initial management. In patients diagnosed with TB, radiographic changes may give an indication of the patient's immune condition and specific findings that suggest bronchogenic or hematogenous dissemination will direct therapy.

The clinical questions

Despite advances in the development of antiretroviral therapies and prophylaxis schemes, pulmonary diseases and particularly respiratory infections are an important cause of morbidity and mortality in HIV-infected patients. Clinicians in their daily practice frequently have to face the following questions:
• Are the respiratory symptoms of patients with retroviral infection related to infectious or non-infectious diseases?
• In patients with suspected infectious pulmonary disease, what is the etiology: bacterial, viral, fungal, or related to mycobacteria?
• In the context of mycobacterial disease, which mycobacterium is involved (TB or non-TB)?
• In patients with TB–AIDS, is the worsening of radiological manifestations related to resistance to treatment or immune reconstitution syndrome?

Methodological considerations

Imaging studies of patients with suspected pulmonary disease associated with retroviral infection must start with conventional radiography. In specific situations, the combination of clinical manifestations, laboratory tests and alterations on conventional radiographs, allows a precise diagnosis without the need for other diagnostic imaging methods.

Indications for computed tomography (CT) in the study of HIV patients with suspected pulmonary disease can be summarized as:

• Evaluation of the patient with respiratory symptoms and a normal radiograph.
• Characterization of non-specific parenchymal changes found on a conventional radiograph.
• Detection and characterization of mediastinal abnormalities, particularly lymph nodes.
• Characterization of chest wall abnormalities.
• Staging of AIDS-related malignancies.
• Planning and performing percutaneous biopsies.

The CT technique depends on the findings found on X-rays. In general, when confirmation or characterization of mediastinal and/or hilar abnormalities is required, or if vascular abnormalities and pleural–parenchymal disease are suspected, the study must be performed with intravenous contrast material. When CT is indicated to characterize a parenchymal abnormality or to evaluate pulmonary parenchyma in patients with respiratory symptoms and a normal X-ray, the study must include reconstructions from a high-resolution protocol. In patients with chest wall abnormalities, multiplanar and 3D reconstructions allow the extension of the lesion to be accurately defined.

Magnetic resonance imaging (MRI) can play a role in the evaluation of mediastinal abnormalities in patients with a history of allergic reactions to iodinated contrast materials and in the study of chest wall abnormalities.

Positron emission tomography (PET)/CT is useful in the staging of bronchogenic carcinoma in potential candidates for surgery due to tumor size, to detect lymph node and metastatic disease, as well as the evaluation of disease activity (see Chapter 15).

Normal findings and artifacts

Chest X-ray analysis must include evaluation of the mediastinum, pulmonary vasculature, airways, pulmonary parenchyma, pleura and chest wall. In the mediastinum, the analysis focuses on the detection of abnormal densities and widening or alteration of the contour of normal anatomical structures. Evaluation of the cardiac silhouette and chambers is of great importance when studying the mediastinum and deserves a detailed consideration. Abnormalities of pulmonary vasculature reflect changes

in a patient's hemodynamics and will be associated with changes in cardiac chambers. Airway disease (central and peripheral) is frequent in HIV patients and the detection of abnormalities in airway size and walls can suggest specific entities. In an important number of cases, pulmonary disease affects the parenchyma. The radiological aspect of normal pulmonary parenchyma corresponds to the density of alveolar air and overlapping arterial and venous pulmonary vessels transporting blood from and to cardiac chambers. Arterial vessels (pulmonary artery branches) are defined as vertically distributed tubular structures, which ramify and decrease in size from the central to peripheral areas. Venous vessels are distributed more horizontally and their aspect is similar to that of arterial structures. In general, the density of pulmonary parenchyma is uniform and the sensitivity of imaging techniques to detect abnormalities is good. Once the parenchymal abnormality is detected, a careful characterization and analysis of the distribution of the abnormalities allows a differential diagnosis to be proposed as well as the need for complementary studies. Observation of the lung periphery, lung apex and dependent part of the pleural cavity (lateral and posterior costophrenic recesses) allows most pleural diseases to be ruled out. Evaluation of thoracic wall structures gives precise knowledge of their radiological anatomy and density of composing structures. In general, the presence of a mass and abnormal densities raises suspicion of pulmonary wall primary entities or secondary involvement of the components of the pulmonary wall due to pulmonary or extrapulmonary diseases.

Interpretation of CT follows similar parameters to those for radiographs regarding the systematic analysis of the different anatomical structures, with variation inherent to the particular technique. Normal pulmonary parenchyma show alveolar air and arterial and venous pulmonary vessels. In high-resolution CT (HRCT), peripheral arterioles and venules can be identified. The former are seen at a distance of 0.5–1 cm from the visceral pleura; they are centrilobular structures and bifurcate at an acute angle. The latter are peripheral structures from the secondary pulmonary lobules, found 2 cm away from the visceral pleura and bifurcating at an obtuse angle. Iodinated contrast resolution allows tissue differentiation and opacification of vascular structures, enabling accurate evaluation of the mediastinum. Spatial resolution and the lack of overlapping anatomical structures are great advantages of CT for precise characterization of pulmonary parenchyma. These same advantages enable detection and characterization of entities that are altering the pleural cavity and chest wall.

Pathological findings and significance

The traditional concept of primary TB and reactivation TB, each with specific radiological manifestations, has been changing based on molecular epidemiological studies that have concluded that radiological manifestations of TB are dependent on the patient's level of immunity and not the timing of infection onset [14].

Radiological alterations are related to the degree of immunosuppression associated with the retroviral infection. Patients with high CD4 levels (>200/mm^3) have radiographic manifestations similar to those of the general population patients with TB, with cavitations predominantly in the apical and posterior segments of the upper lobes and the apical segments of the lower lobes. Patients with advanced immunosuppression frequently have lymph node enlargement, basal parenchymal consolidations, hematogenous dissemination and extrapulmonary TB. These findings have traditionally been considered "atypical" in an adult patient with pulmonary TB. Up to 20% of patients with advanced immunosuppression and TB have chest X-rays described as normal [15–17].

Picon et al. conducted a study in 113 HIV-infected patients with TB and a control group of 118 non-HIV-infected patients with TB, finding a higher frequency of "atypical" presentations in the first group (pulmonary lesions accompanied by intrathoracic lymph node enlargement, hematogenous TB and pulmonary TB together with superficial lymph node enlargement). Patients from the first group had less cavitation than the patients from the second group. No differences were found between HIV-positive patients without AIDS and HIV-negative patients [18].

The study by Busi et al. performed between 1997 and 2001 and comparing radiological patterns between HAART-treated and non-HAART-treated patients with pulmonary TB and HIV, concluded that those receiving HAART had a higher frequency of post-primary or classic TB pattern; these manifestations were probably related to at least partial restoration of the cellular immunity induced by the HAART [19].

Alterations to pulmonary parenchyma in patients with high CD4 counts are similar to those previously described in reactivation TB or post-primary TB. In the early phases, a poorly defined opacity is found ("exudative" lesion) in the apical or posterior segments of the upper lobes or the apical segments of the lower lobes (Figure 8.1). Isolated alteration of the anterior segments of the upper lobes is rare (2–6%). In most patients, initial opacity progresses to coarse reticular opacities and nodules, with distorted pulmonary architecture ("fibroproliferative" lesion). Seventy-five percent of patients have a combination of "exudative" and "fibroproliferative" patterns (Figure 8.2). When these lesions heal they can distort the pulmonary architecture and cause traction bronchiectasis and atelectasis [20].

Cavitations are variable and can be present in 40–87% of patients. These are of variable sizes, single or multiple and can appear isolated or within areas of consolidation. The most common complication of tuberculous cavitations is endobronchial spread. Chest HRCT is more sensitive than chest X-ray in the detection of cavitations and endobronchial spread, which appear as centrilobular nodules and/or ramified linear opacities (tree-in-bud pattern) [21] (Figure 8.3).

Bronchogenic spread of TB may be seen in either primary or post-primary TB and occurs more frequently in HIV-infected individuals than in non-HIV hosts. Bronchitis and bronchiolitis due to TB are common and can be present in HIV patients in the absence of cavitations [16].

The range of differential diagnoses of small airway disease in HIV patients is wide and includes bacterial infection, Mycobacterium avium complex infection, aspergillosis and non-infectious entities such as Kaposi's sarcoma and lymphoma [22]. Airway abnormalities, especially when asymmetric and associated with parenchymal cavitation or enlarged, low density, rim-enhancing mediastinal or hilar nodes, are particularly suggestive of mycobacterial disease [23].

Bronchial stenosis occurs in 10–40% of patients with active TB. Radiological manifestations include persistent lobar or segmental collapse, lobar hyperinflation, obstructive pneumonia and mucous impaction [24].

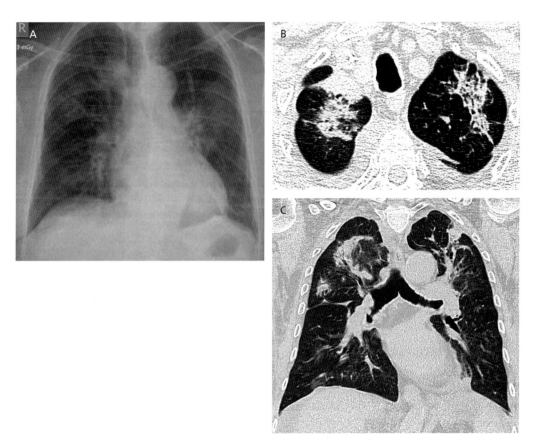

Figure 8.1 (A) Chest X-ray showing bilateral areas of consolidation, mainly apical. (B) Chest axial CT image showing consolidations in the apical segment of the right upper lobe and apicoposterior segment of the left upper lobe. (C) Chest coronal CT reconstruction showing bilateral apical bronchocentric consolidation.

The parenchymal abnormalities in primary TB described above are found in patients with low CD4 counts. The most common presentation of primary TB is unifocal consolidation and any lobule can be affected. In two-thirds of cases, parenchymal abnormalities resolve without sequelae. In 7–9% of patients there can be a round opacity (nodule or mass) known as a tuberculoma, and in these patients it is common to find the consolidation is associated with lymph node enlargement.

Hilar or mediastinal lymphadenopathy has been noted to be more common among those with HIV-related TB than among non-HIV-infected individuals with TB; and of those infected with HIV, lymphadenopathy is more common in patients with findings of advanced immunosuppression [25,26]. The most common location for TB lymphadenopathy is the right para-trachea and hilar (bilateral), but it can be found in any lymph node station in the mediastinum. In contrast-enhanced CT studies, TB lymphadenopathies are characterized by central hypodensity with peripheral rim enhancement and obliteration of the surrounding perinodal fat. Central hypodensity is related to central necrosis and the enhancing ring to vascular, inflammatory, perinodal reaction [27] (Figure 8.4).

Early and limited hematogenous dissemination is common in primary TB, usually without clinical or radiographic manifestations. In around 1–7% of all forms of TB, hematogenous dissemination may have clinical manifestations and can be detected radiographically (miliary TB) [20]. Chest X-rays are characterized by soft tissue density, well-defined nodules of 2–3 mm in diameter. In 85% of cases, nodules are diffusely and symmetrically distributed, more profusely in the lower lobes. HRCT is more sensitive than radiographs in the detection of miliary TB and is characterized by randomly

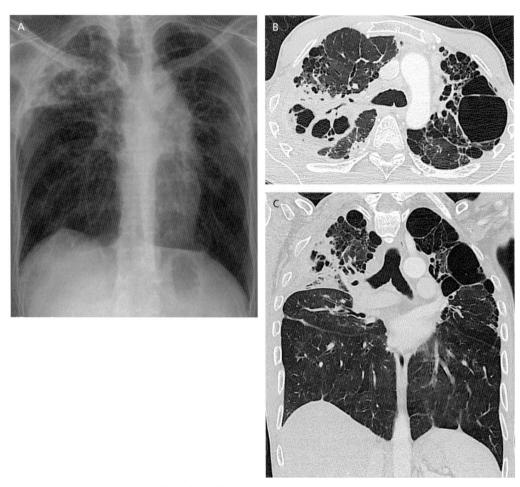

Figure 8.2 (A) Chest X-ray showing bilateral mixed parenchymal opacities and apical radiolucent images in a patient with a left thoracostomy tube. (B) Chest axial CT image and (C) coronal reconstruction showing volume loss in the upper lobes, consolidation in the posterior segment of the right upper lobe and bilateral apical, subpleural thin-walled avascular lesions.

distributed micronodules associated with second-ary pulmonary lobules. Miliary TB is more frequent in immunocompromised hosts [16] (Figure 8.5).

Tuberculous pleuritis is frequently associated with primary TB. In these patients, it is character-ized by variable volumes of free pleural effusion (Figure 8.6), without parenchymal abnormalities. In post-primary disease, pleural effusion is scarce; it can be loculated and is accompanied by paren-chymal disease with cavitation [28]. Pleural effu-sions occur over a wide range of CD4 cell counts. In some series, pleural effusion was more frequent in patients with high CD4 counts, while other series found no significant difference between patients with CD4 counts above or below 200 cells/mm^3 [15,29].

Role for therapy follow-up and patient management

The follow-up of patients being treated for TB is essentially clinical. Imaging follow-up is limited to patients with high risk of relapse, patients treated for some multiresistant infections and patients who did not complete treatment due to drug toxicity. In cases of clinical worsening, complementary imaging studies must be performed. When imaging studies for the follow-up of HIV-infected patients being treated for TB are indicated, the technique of choice is conventional radiography. CT is reserved for patients with non-specific parenchymal involve-ment, mediastinal or chest wall abnormalities, or complicated pleuropulmonary disease.

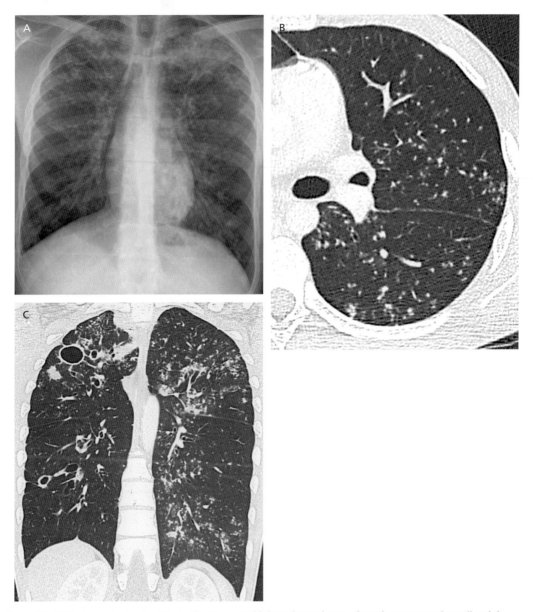

Figure 8.3 (A) Posteroanterior chest X-ray showing apical bilateral mixed parenchymal opacities with small nodular lesions and radiolucent images suggestive of cavitation. (B) Chest CT image showing centrilobular nodules and ramified linear opacities with a tree-in-bud pattern in the apicoposterior segment of the left upper lobe and the apical segment of the left lower lobe. (C) Chest coronal CT reconstruction showing centrilobular nodules, a tree-in-bud pattern, bronchial wall thickening and cystic lesions in the right upper lobe.

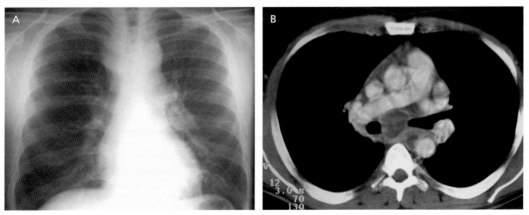

Figure 8.4 (A) Chest X-ray showing mediastinal widening compatible with right para-tracheal lymphadenopathies. (B) Chest CT image showing hypodense subcarinal lymphadenopathies with a ring pattern of contrast enhancement.

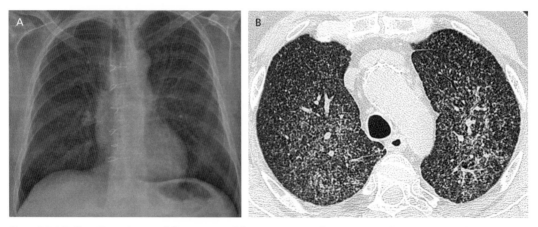

Figure 8.5 (A) Chest X-ray showing diffuse micronodular opacities. (B) Chest CT image showing micronodules of soft tissue density with well-defined margins and random distribution.

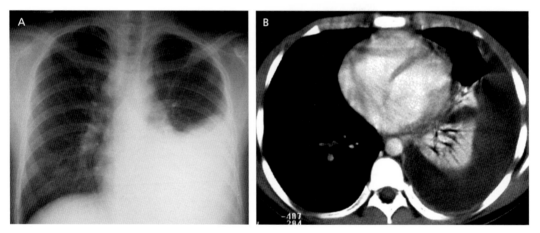

Figure 8.6 (A) Chest X-ray showing left basal opacity with costophrenic angle obliteration due to pleural effusion. (B) Chest CT image showing left free pleural effusion with passive lingular and lower lobe atelectasis.

References

1. WHO. Global tuberculosis control. Report 2010 http://whqlibdoc.who.int/publications/2010/9789241564069eng.pdf

2. Lawn SD, Wood R. Incidence of tuberculosis during highly active antiretroviral therapy in high-income and low-income countries. *Clin Infect Dis* 2005;41:1783–1786.

3. Brinkhof MW, Egger M, Boulle A *et al.* Tuberculosis after initiation of antiretroviral therapy in low-income and high-income countries. *Clin Infect Dis* 2007;45:1518–1521.

4. Lawn SD, Wood R, Cock KM, Kranzer K, Lewis JJ, Churchyard GJ. Antiretrovirals and isoniazid preventive therapy in the prevention of HIV-associated tuberculosis in settings with limited health-care resources. *Lancet Infect Dis* 2010;10:489–498.

5. Corbett EL, Watt CJ, Walker N *et al.* The growing burden of tuberculosis: global trends and interactions with the HIV epidemic. *Arch Intern Med* 2003;163:1009–1021.

6. Markowitz N, Hansen NI, Hopewell PC *et al.* Incidence of tuberculosis in the United States among HIV-infected persons. The pulmonary complications of HIV infection study group. *Ann Intern Med* 1997;126:123–132.

7. Zhang M, Gong J, Iyer DV, Jones BE, Modlin RL, Barnes PF. T cell cytokine responses in persons with tuberculosis and human immunodeficiency virus infection. *J Clin Invest* 1994;94:2435–2442.

8. Whalen C, Horsburgh CR, Hom D, Lahart C, Simberkoff M, Ellner J. Accelerated course of human

immunodeficiency virus infection aftertuberculosis. *Am J Respir Crit Care Med* 1995;151:129–135.

9. Nakata K, Rom WN, Honda Y *et al. Mycobacterium tuberculosis* enhances human immunodeficiency virus-1 replication in the lung. *Am J Respir Crit Care Med* 1997;155:996–1003.

10. Koenig SP, Riviere R, Leger P *et al.* High mortality among patients with AIDS who received a diagnosis of tuberculosis in the first 3 months of antiretroviral therapy. *Clin Infect Dis* 2009;48:829–831.

11. Lawn DS, Bekker LG, Miller RF. Immune reconstitution disease associated with mycobacterial infections in HIV-infected individuals receiving antiretrovirals. *Lancet Infect Dis* 2005;5:361–373.

12. Phillips P, Bonner S, Gataric T *et al.* Nontuberculous mycobacterial immune reconstitution syndrome in HIV-infected patients: spectrum of disease and long-term follow up. *Clin Infect Dis* 2005;41:1483–1497.

13. Abdool Karim SS, Naidoo K, Grobler A *et al.* Effect of initiating antiretroviral therapy during tuberculosis treatment in HIV-infected individuals: results of a randomized controlled trial in TB-HIV co-infected patients in South Africa (SAPiT Study). *N Engl J Med* 2010;362:697–706.

14. Geng E, Kreiswirth B, Burzynski J *et al.* Clinical and radiographic correlates of primary and reactivation tuberculosis. A molecular epidemiology study. *JAMA* 2005;293:2740–2745.

15. Perlman DC, el Sadr WM, Nelson ET *et al.* Variation of chest radiographic patterns in pulmonary tuberculosis by degree of human immunodeficiency virus-related immunosuppression. The Terry Beirn Community Programs for Clinical Research on AIDS (CPCRA). The AIDS Clinical Trials Group (ACTG). *Clin Infect Dis* 1997;25:242–246.

16. Leung AN, Brauner MW, Gamsu G *et al.* Comparison of CT findings in HIV-seropositive and HIV-seronegative patients. *Radiology* 1996;198:667–691.

17. Greenberg SD, Frager D, Suster B *et al.* Active pulmonary tuberculosis in patients with AIDS: spectrum of radiographic findings (including normal appearance). *Radiology* 1994;193:115–119.

18. Picon DL, Avancini ML, Bassanesi SL *et al.* Differences in the clinical and radiological presentation of intrathoracic tuberculosis in the presence or absence of HIV infection. *J Bras Pneumol* 2007;33:429–436.

19. Busi Rizzi E, Schinina V, Palmieri F, Girardi E, Bibbolino C. Radiological patterns in HIV-associated pulmonary tuberculosis: comparison between HAART-treated and non-HAART-treated patients. *Clin Radiol* 2003;58:469–473.

20. Woodring JH, Vandiviere HM, Fried AM, Dillon ML, Williams TD, Melvin IG. Update: the radiographic features of pulmonary tuberculosis. *AJR Am J Roentgenol* 1986;14:497–506.

21. Im J, Itoh H, Shim Y *et al.* Pulmonary tuberculosis: CT findings-early active disease and sequential change with antituberculous therapy. *Radiology* 1993;186:653–660.

22. McGuinness G, Gruden J, Bhalla M, Harkin TJ, Jagirdar J. AIDS-related airway disease. *AJR Am J Roentgenol* 1997:168:67–77.

23. Pastores SM, Naidich DP, Aranda CP, McGuinness O, Rom WN. Intrathoracic adenopathy associated with pulmonary tuberculosis in patients with human immunodeficiency virus infection. *Chest* 1993:103:1433–1437.

24. Lee KS, Kim YH, Kim WS, Hwang SH, Kim PN, Lee BH. Endobronchial tuberculosis: CT features. *J Comput Assist Tomogr* 1991;15:424–428.

25. Batungwanayo J, Taelman H, Dhote R, Bogaerts J, Allen S, Van de Perre P. Pulmonary tuberculosis in Kigali, Rwanda: impact of human immunodeficiency virus infection on clinical and radiographic presentation. *Am Rev Respir Dis* 1992;146:53–56.

26. Shafer RW, Chirgwin KD, Glatt AE, Dahdouh MA, Landesman SH, Suster B. HIV prevalence immunosuppression, and drug resistance in patients with tuberculosis in an area endemic for AIDS. *AIDS* 1991;5:399–405.

27. Im JG, Song KS, Kang HS *et al.* Mediastinal tuberculous lymphadenitis: CT manifestations. *Radiology* 1987;164:115–119.

28. Epstein DM, Kline LR, Albelda SM *et al.* Tuberculous pleural effusions. *Chest* 1987;91:106–109.

29. Jones BE, Young SMM, Antoniskis D, Davidson PT, Kramer F, Barnes PF. Relationship of the manifestations of tuberculosis to CD4 cell counts in patients with pulmonary tuberculosis. *Am Rev Respir Dis* 1993;148:1292–1997.

Clinical cases

Case 1

A 45-year-old HIV-positive female who had been diagnosed with AIDS 5 years previously. The patient had received HAART for the last year. She consulted for a 2-month evolution of cough with mucous sputum, unquantified fever, weight loss and hemoptysis during the last 8 days. The basal CD4 count was 350 cells/mm^3 and sputum culture was positive for acid alcohol-resistant bacilli.

Based on radiographic findings (Figure 8.7) and positive bacilloscopy, the diagnosis of pulmonary TB with bronchogenic dissemination was confirmed.

With conventional antituberculous treatment (supervised short scheme) the patient had a favorable clinical response, with improvement in respiratory symptoms. No control imaging studies were performed during the first 3 months of treatment.

Teaching point

In patients with high CD4 counts, radiological manifestations of TB are similar to those in immunocompetent patients from the general population.

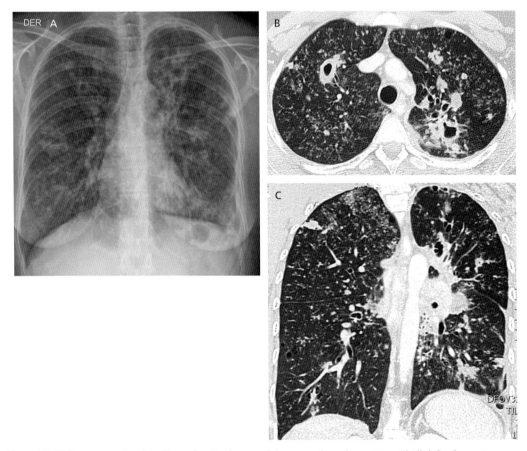

Figure 8.7 (A) Posteroanterior chest X-ray showing large nodular parenchymal opacities with ill-defined margins, cavitation in the upper lobes and bilateral multilobar small nodular opacities with bronchial wall thickening. (B) Chest axial CT image showing cavitated nodules in the apical segment of the right upper lobe and apicoposterior segment of the left upper lobe, centrilobular nodules and ramified linear densities (tree-in-bud pattern). (C) Chest coronal CT reconstruction showing centrilobular nodules and tree-in-bud pattern, ill-defined peribronchovascular nodules of soft tissue density and peribronchovascular interstitium thickening.

Case 2

A 37-year-old male with AIDS diagnosed 3 year previously presented with a 1-month evolution of dry cough and fever. The patient had not been receiving antiretroviral therapy. The CD4 count at admission was 180 cells/mm^3, sputum bacilloscopy was negative and bronchoalveolar lavage (BAL) showed acid alcohol-resistant bacilli. Culture confirmed the presence of *M. tuberculosis*.

Based on radiographic findings (Figure 8.8) and BAL results, pulmonary TB was diagnosed.

The patient showed a good clinical response to the supervised short treatment scheme. Control radiographic studies performed at the end of the treatment showed resolution of parenchymal and hilar abnormalities.

Teaching point

In HIV-positive patients with low CD4 counts, radiographic manifestations of TB are "atypical".

Case 3

A 28-year-old male diagnosed with AIDS 4 years previously. He had a history of Kaposi's sarcoma treated with chemotherapy.

There was worsening of respiratory symptoms 1 month after starting HAART, with new parenchymal opacities seen on chest CT images (Figure 8.9).

Fibrobronchoscopy showed bronchial Kaposi's sarcoma lesions and BAL showed mycobacterial infection. Culture confirmed *M. tuberculosis* infection. HAART therapy was initially interrupted and

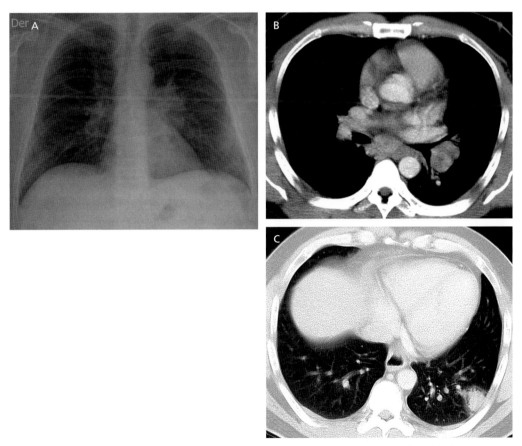

Figure 8.8 (A) Chest X-ray showing altered left hilar contour compatible with lymphadenopathies. (B) Chest CT image showing subcarinal and left hilar lymphadenopathies. (C) Chest CT image showing a subpleural nodule with a ground-glass halo in the left lower lobe.

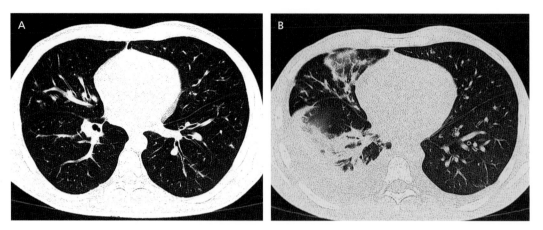

Figure 8.9 (A) Chest CT showing soft tissue density nodules of irregular margins in the left lower lobe. (B) Chest CT showing areas of consolidation in the right middle and lower lobes and right pleural effusion.

treatment for TB started. With clinical improvement, HAART was restarted with an adequate clinical response.

Teaching points
• In patients with AIDS in whom HAART is started and who show worsening of respiratory symptoms, immune reconstitution syndrome must be considered.
• Of the entities associated with this syndrome, *M. tuberculosis* infection must be considered as the first option.

PART III
Nuclear Medicine Imaging

Nuclear Medicine Imaging of Infections: Techniques, Acquisition Protocols and Interpretation Criteria

Alberto Signore

"Sapienza" University, Rome, Italy

Introduction

Several techniques and radiopharmaceuticals are available for imaging infection and inflammation. It is possible to image cells and soluble molecules involved in infections or tissue and function alterations induced by the infection/inflammatory process.

In the past decades, nuclear medicine has developed enormously in this field and in many cases has become an indispensable diagnostic tool for clinicians. Scientists have proposed radiopharmaceuticals for imaging the edema, T and B lymphocytes, monocytes, granulocytes, apoptotic cells, endothelial activation, immune complexes and other inflammation-related processes and, recently, Gram-positive and -negative bacteria, candida, viruses and other microorganisms [1–5]. Some of these radiopharmaceuticals are commercially available, others still in the experimental phase. The nuclear medicine physician has a wide range of tools with which to better answer specific questions posed by clinicians.

When inflammation/infection affects the function of a tissue or an organ, other radiopharmaceuticals can also be used to determine the entity of function impairment. Brain, lung, liver, heart, bowel or bone infections can affect the primary function of the organ, thus requiring that not only are the extent and severity of the infectious process evaluated, but also the functional impairment of the organ.

Nuclear medicine techniques can also facilitate the investigation, *in vivo*, of different pathogenetic events occurring in the natural history of the diseases. In some brain, lung and bowel infections, the presence of lymphomonocytes and related events, which are usually the first mediators of inflammation, can be studied. As mentioned above, the presence of bacteria and granulocytes, which appear when the inflammation becomes septic, as well as the extent of damage in terms of cells undergoing apoptosis can also be studied.

The available radiopharmaceuticals and their clinical roles are summarized in Tables 9.1, 9.2 and 9.3.

In most cases, the choice of the correct radiopharmaceutical is important in answering the clinical question. Sometimes it is the specificity of the appropriate radiopharmaceutical that provides the histological/clinical information; at other times it is the way it is used, and the way images are acquired

Diagnostic Imaging of Infections and Inflammatory Diseases: A Multidisciplinary Approach, First Edition. Edited by Alberto Signore and Ana María Quintero.

Table 9.1 Commercially available radiopharmaceuticals for imaging inflammation/infection

Radiopharmaceutical	Target	Application in molecular imaging of inflammation/infection	Isotopes
Albumin nanocolloids	Non-specific extravasation	Rheumatoid arthritis and other inflammatory lesions	^{99m}Tc
Anti-G mAb (Sulesomab, Leukoscan®) [Murine IgG1 mAb Fab' fragment]	Non-specific cross-reacting antigen 90 (NCA-90) on human granulocytes	Fever of unknown origin, acute inflammatory disorders, osteomyelitis, endocarditis, appendicitis	^{99m}Tc
Anti-G mAb (Besilesomab, (Scintimun®) [Murine IgG1 mAb]	Non-specific cross-reacting antigen 95 (NCA-95) on human granulocytes	Bowel disease, bone infections, lung abscesses, diabetic foot infections	^{99m}Tc
Fluorodeoxyglucose (FDG)	Activated lymphocytes, monocytes and granulocytes	Inflammatory disorders, e.g. lymphoma, vasculitis, sarcoidosis, rheumatoid arthritis, Alzheimer's and Parkinson's disease, etc., and infections, such as osteomyelitis, spondylodiscitis, prosthetic joint infection, etc. in animal models and humans	^{18}F
Ga-citrate	Transferrin receptors (CD71)	Animal tumor model, fever of unknown origin in HIV patients	^{67}Ga
Human autologous white blood cells (leukocytes)	Active migration in inflammatory lesion	Acute inflammation	^{99m}Tc-HMPAO, ^{111}In-oxine, ^{99m}Tc-SnF$_2$
Octreotide (Octreoscan®)	Somatostatin receptor	Granulomatous and chronic inflammation	^{111}In
Human polyclonal immunoglobulin (HIG)	Non-specific	Inflammation/infection	^{99m}Tc

Adapted from Signore and Glaudemans [1], Malviya *et al.* [2], Signore *et al.* [3], Signore *et al.* [4] and Chianelli *et al.* [5].

and interpreted, that are relevant. Indeed, with radiolabeled autologous white blood cells (WBCs), the differential diagnosis between sterile inflammation and infection or even activated bone marrow (if a WBC scan is combined with a nanocolloid scan) can be obtained by using the appropriate acquisition protocol and appropriate image interpretation criteria, despite labeled WBCs not being a bacteria specific radiopharmaceutical. A similar consideration can be made for the use of radiolabeled anti-granulocyte monoclonal antibodies (anti-G mAbs) and for [^{18}F]fluorodeoxyglucose ([^{18}F]FDG).

Techniques for imaging inflammation/infection

In terms of imaging modalities, there are three main types of nuclear medicine instrumentation:

• Anger's gamma cameras [which can acquire planar images of one field or the total body, or three-dimensional images known as single-photon emission computed tomography (SPECT) and now also available in a hybrid version for fused nuclear medicine and radiological imaging (SPECT/CT)]
• Positron emission tomographs [PETs, which can acquire 3D images usually fused with CT or magnetic resonance imaging (MRI): PET/CT and PET/MRI]
• Portable radioactivity detectors for use in operating rooms or at a patient's bedside (which can detect and measure radioactivity without producing images, although they can provide small high-resolution images).

These instruments are designed for radioactivity detection and imaging in man, but similar

Table 9.2 Experimental radiopharmaceuticals for imaging inflammation/infection

Radiopharmaceutical	Target	Application in molecular imaging of inflammation/infection	Isotopes
(R)-N-methyl-N-(1-methylpropyl)-1-(2-chlorophenyl) isoquinoline-3-carboxamide (^{11}C-PK11195)	Peripheral benzo-diazepine receptors (PBR)	HSV encephalitis, Rasmussen's encephalitis, AIDS patients	^{11}C
1D09C3 [Humanized IgG4 mAb]	HLA-DR	Lymphoma (experimental stage)	^{99m}Tc
2′-fluoro-5-[^{124}I]iodo-1-β-D-arabinofuranosyluracil (^{124}I-FIAU)	Herpes simplex virus thymidine kinase (HSVtk)	Herpes virus infection in an animal model	^{124}I
9-[(3-[^{18}F]fluoro-1-hydroxy-2-propoxy)methyl]guanine ([^{18}F] FHPG)	Herpes simplex virus (HSV)	Herpes simplex encephalitis in an animal model	^{18}F
Adalimumab (Humira®) [Fully human IgG1 mAb]	TNF-α	Rheumatoid arthritis	^{99m}Tc
Anti-E-Selectin [Murine IgG1 mAb]	E-Selectin	Rheumatoid arthritis	^{111}In
Anti-G mAb (Sulesomab, Leukoscan®) [Murine IgG1 mAb Fab′ fragment]	Non-specific cross-reacting antigen 90 (NCA-90) on human granulocytes	Fever of unknown origin, acute inflammatory disorders, osteomyelitis, endocarditis, appendicitis	^{111}In
Anti-MIF mAb	MIF	Inflammation in animal model	^{125}I
Basiliximab (Simulect®) [Chimeric IgG1 mAb]	CD25	T-cell leukemia	^{211}At
Complement factor 5a (C5a)	Neutrophils, monocytes	Intramuscular infection in an animal model	^{99m}Tc
Daclizumab (Zenapax®) [Humanized IgG1 mAb]	CD25	T-cell leukemia imaging and therapy	^{18}F, ^{99m}Tc, ^{111}In, ^{125}I, ^{212}Bi, ^{67}Ga
EP1645 [Human anti-CD4 mAb fragment]	CD4 on T lymphocytes	Rheumatoid arthritis	^{99m}Tc
Epidermal growth factor (EGF)	EGF receptor	Metastatic lymph nodes in humans, breast cancer, skin wounds	^{123}I, ^{111}In, ^{125}I
f-Met-Leu-Phe	Formyl-peptide receptor on granulocytes and monocytes	Bacterial infection	^{99m}Tc, ^{111}In
Ga-citrate	Transferrin receptors (CD71)	Animal tumor model, fever of unknown origin in HIV patients	^{68}Ga
Human autologous white blood cells (leukocytes)	Active migration in inflammatory lesion	Acute inflammation	[^{18}F]FDG, ^{64}Cu
Human polyclonal immunoglobulin (HIG)	Non-specific	Inflammation/infection	^{111}In
IFN-γ	Many different cells	Lung inflammatory diseases	^{123}I
IIa–IIIb receptor antagonist (DMP444)	IIa–IIIb	Infective experimental endocarditis	^{99m}Tc
IL-1a/b	IL1RI=B, Mo, N, IL1RII=En, Fi, He, Ke, T	Inflammatory processes in animal models	^{123}I, ^{125}I
IL-12	T, NK	T lymphocytes and lymphocytic infiltrates in animal models	^{125}I

(Contninued)

Table 9.2 (*Continued*)

Radiopharmaceutical	Target	Application in molecular imaging of inflammation/infection	Isotopes
IL-1ra (receptor antagonist)	IL-1 receptor	Rheumatoid arthritis, inflammatory process	^{123}I, ^{125}I
IL-2	T, B, NK	Graves' ophthalmopathy, Type 1 diabetes, celiac disease, Crohn's disease, thyroid autoimmune disease, kidney graft rejection, cutaneous melanoma, kidney allograft, atherosclerosis	^{123}I, ^{125}I, ^{99m}Tc, ^{35}S, ^{18}F
IL-6, IL-10 G-CSF	T, B, Mφ, He, HP, N, phagocytes	Infectious foci in animal model	^{125}I
IL-8	N, Ba, T	Infectious foci, including osteomyelitis, liver abscess and joint prosthesis infection, and soft tissue infections	^{99m}Tc, ^{123}I, ^{125}I, ^{131}I
Infliximab (Remicade®) [Chimeric IgG1 mAb]	TNF-α	Crohn's disease, rheumatoid arthritis	^{99m}Tc
J001X	CD11b, CD14 (macrophages, monocytes)	Arthritis, chronic berilliosis and other inflammatory lesions in an animal model	^{99m}Tc
Leukotriene (LTB$_4$) receptor antagonist (RP517; DPC 11870-11; MB88, fMLFK)	BLT1, BLT2	Inflammation/infection in an animal model	^{99m}Tc, ^{111}In
Liposomes	Cells of reticuloendothelial system	Small animal models of osteomyelitis, experimental colitis and focal infection	^{111}In, ^{99m}Tc
MAX.16H5 [Murine IgG1 mAb]	CD4	Rheumatoid arthritis	^{99m}Tc
MCP-1	Mo, Mφ, Gr	Subacute inflammation in an animal model	^{99m}Tc
Neutrophil elastase inhibitor (EPI-HNE-2/4)	Neutrophil elastase	Inflammation/infection in an animal model	^{99m}Tc
OKT-3 (Muromonab®) [Murine IgG2a mAb]	CD3	Rheumatoid arthritis and renal transplant rejection	^{99m}Tc
Platelet factor (PF4) (P482, P1827)	Human white blood cells (leukocytes)	Bacterial infections	^{99m}Tc
Rituximab (Mabthera®) [Chimeric IgG1 mAb]	CD20 on B lymphocytes	Sentinel lymph node (SLN) and rheumatoid arthritis	^{99m}Tc
Somatostatin analogs	Somatostatin receptor	Granulomatous and chronic inflammation	^{123}I, ^{99m}Tc, ^{68}Ga
SSEA-1 (LeuTech®) [Murine IgM]	CD15 on human granulocytes	Appendicitis imaging	^{99m}Tc
TGF-β	TGF-RI-V, on many different cells	Angiogenesis	^{125}I
Visilizumab (Nuvion®) [Humanized IgG2 mAb]	CD3	T lymphocyte in animal model	^{99m}Tc

B, B lymphocytes; Ba, Basophils; Ep, epithelial cells; En, endothelial cells; Fi, fibroblasts; Gr, granulocytes; He, hematopoietic cells; HP, hematopoietic precursors; Ke, keratinocytes; Lym, lymphocytes; Mo, monocytes; Mφ, macrophage; T, T lymphocytes; N, neutrophils; NC, neoplastic cells; NK, natural killer cells; SMS, smooth cell muscles; IL1RI, IL1RII, receptor types I and II; TGF, tumor growth factor; TNF, tumor necrosis factor.

Adapted from Signore and Glaudemans [1], Malviya *et al.* [2], Signore *et al.* [3], Signore *et al.* [4] and Chianelli *et al.* [5].

Table 9.3 Experimental radiopharmaceuticals for imaging fungi and bacteria

Radiopharmaceutical	Target	Application in molecular imaging of inflammation/infection	Isotopes
Alafosfalin	Bacteria	Bacterial infection	^{99m}Tc
Antimicrobial peptides (UBI 29-41, P483H, HNP1-3, hLF 1-11)	Bacterial and fungal infection	Infection	^{99m}Tc
Bacteriophage	Bacteria	Infection in an animal model	^{99m}Tc
Biotin	Bacteria	Osteomyelitis and endocarditis	^{111}In, ^{99m}Tc
CBT21	Microbial infections	Fungal infection in an animal model	^{99m}Tc
Cefoperazone	Bacteria	Bacterial infection	^{99m}Tc
Ceftizoxime	Bacterial wall	Bacterial infection	^{99m}Tc
Ceftriaxone	Bacteria	Bacterial infection	^{99m}Tc
Cefuroxime	Bacteria	Bacterial infection	^{99m}Tc
Chitinase	Microbial infections	Fungal infection in an animal model	^{123}I
Ciprofloxacin (Infecton™)	Prokaryotic topoisomerase IV and DNA gyrase	Microbial infection	^{99m}Tc, ^{18}F
Enrofloxacin	Bacterial infection	Infection	^{99m}Tc
Ethambutol	Mycobacteria	Mycobacterial infection in an animal model	^{99m}Tc
Fleroxacin	Bacterial infection	Infection in an animal model	^{18}F
Fluconazole	Microbial infections	Fungal infection in an animal model	^{99m}Tc
Isoniazid	Mycobacteria	*Mycobacterium tuberculosis* infection in an animal model	^{99m}Tc
Kanamycin	Bacteria	Bacterial infection	^{99m}Tc
Levofloxacin	Bacterial infection	Infection	^{99m}Tc
Lomefloxacin	Bacterial infection	Infection with PET	^{99m}Tc, ^{18}F
Moxifloxacin	Bacteria	Bacterial infection	^{99m}Tc
Nitrofurantoin	Bacteria	Bacterial infection	^{99m}Tc
Norfloxacin	Microbial infections	Infection	^{99m}Tc
Ofloxacin	Bacterial infection	Infection	^{99m}Tc
PAMA4	Bacteria	Bacterial infection	^{99m}Tc
Pefloxacin	Bacteria	Bacterial infection	^{99m}Tc
Rifampin	Bacteria	Bacterial infection	^{99m}Tc
Sitafloxacin	Bacteria	Bacterial infection	^{99m}Tc
Sparafloxacin	Bacteria	Bacterial infection	^{99m}Tc
Sparfloxacin	Gram-positive and -negative bacteria	Bacterial infection in an animal model	^{99m}Tc
Trovafloxacin	Bacterial infection	Infection in an animal model	^{18}F

Adapted from Signore and Glaudemans [1], Malviya *et al.* [2], Signore *et al.* [3], Signore *et al.* [4] and Chianelli *et al.* [5].

instrumentation is now also available for small animal imaging with incredibly high resolution and efficacy.

Radiolabeled WBCs are the most comonly used radiopharmaceutical for infections and have been applied in a variety of different clinical situations. Nevertheless, it is difficult to draw evidence-based conclusions on the clinical relevance of this technique for most applications. The results of radionuclide imaging for the most important clinical indications are summarized here and the reader is referred to recent meta-analyses of data collected between 1985 and 2005 for a more comprehensive review of the clinical use of radiolabeled WBCs as compared to other available diagnostic techniques [6–9].

Osteomyelitis

The diagnosis of osteomyelitis can be challenging and radionuclide imaging procedures are routinely performed as part of the diagnostic work-up (see also Chapters 3 and 10). Bone scintigraphy is extremely sensitive, ubiquitously available, relatively inexpensive and rapidly completed. The accuracy of the test in unviolated bone exceeds 90% [10]. Many, if not most, patients referred for radionuclide evaluation of osteomyelitis, however, present with pre-existing conditions, including fractures, orthopedic hardware, pedal ulcers, or neuropathic joints. These conditions adversely affect the specificity of the bone scan, necessitating the performance of additional imaging studies to differentiate infection from increased bone mineral turnover. Currently, WBC imaging is the radionuclide procedure of choice for diagnosing osteomyelitis, followed by the use of [^{18}F] FDG and radiolabeled anti-G mAbs. There are, however, some differences between the use of ^{111}In-labeled WBCs and ^{99m}Tc-labeled WBCs. In diabetic foot infections, the sensitivity of ^{111}In-labeled WBC imaging for diagnosing pedal osteomyelitis ranges from 72% to 100% and the specificity from 67% to 100%, whereas the reported sensitivities and specificities of ^{99m}Tc-HMPAO (hexamethylpropylene amine oxime)-labeled WBC imaging for diagnosing diabetic pedal osteomyelitis are generally lower, ranging from 86% to 93% and from 80% to 98%, respectively [11]. Similar differences have been reported for the use of labeled WBCs in IBD, with ^{111}In-labeled WBCs being the more accurate.

In order to maximize the accuracy of labeled WBC imaging, it often needs to be performed in combination with bone marrow imaging using radiolabeled albumin nanocolloids that are taken up by reticuloendothelial cells present in bone marrow. Therefore, although leukocytes usually do not accumulate at sites of increased bone mineral turnover in the absence of infection, they do accumulate in the bone marrow. The normal distribution of hematopoietically active bone marrow is very variable and it may not be possible to determine if a focus of activity on a labeled WBC image represents infection or atypically located, but otherwise normal, bone marrow [12]. This distinction can be made easily and accurately by performing bone marrow imaging using ^{99m}Tc-sulfur colloids or ^{99m}Tc-albumin nanocolloids. Both labeled WBCs and sulfur colloid accumulate in the bone marrow; leukocytes also accumulate in infection, while sulfur colloid does not. The combined study is positive for infection when activity is present on the labeled WBC image without corresponding activity on the sulfur colloid marrow image. The overall accuracy of combined WBC/marrow imaging is approximately 90% and this imaging is especially useful in the evaluation of prosthetic joint and neuropathic joint infections [13–16].

It is important to note that in contrast to other sites in the skeleton, labeled WBC imaging is not useful for detecting spinal osteomyelitis or spondylodiscitis (infection of two adjacent vertebral bodies and their intervertebral disc), and in these cases the use of [^{18}F]FDG or ^{111}In-biotin, a vitamin easily and avidly taken up by bacteria, is suggested (see Chapters 4 and 11). Although increased uptake is virtually diagnostic of the disease, 50% or more of cases show areas of decreased, or absent, activity. Photopenia is not specific for vertebral osteomyelitis and is associated with a variety of non-infectious conditions, including tumor, infarction and previously treated osteomyelitis [17].

Osteomyelitis can also be a complication of joint replacement surgery. With increasing numbers of implantations, infections and loosening of the prostheses have become more common. The risk of infection is highest during the first 2 years after implantation. Nevertheless, very acute infections, occurring within 1–2 weeks after surgery and not usually requiring nuclear medicine to be diagnosed, can be distinguished from late (with 2 years) and chronic infections. The duration and extent of surgery are important determinants of infection, and the patient's age and immune status are also critical to the successful outcome of the implantation. Differentiating infection from aseptic loosening is difficult because the clinical presentation and the histopathological changes in both entities are remarkably similar, but their differentiation is extremely important because their treatment is different. Non-specific markers of inflammation, such as the erythrocyte sedimentation rate (ESR) and C-reactive protein (CRP) level, may be elevated in both loosening and infection. Joint aspiration with Gram stain and culture is considered the definitive diagnostic test; its sensitivity, however, is variable, ranging from 28% to 92%; specificity is more consistent, ranging from 92% to 100%. Plain radiographs are neither sensitive nor specific and cross-sectional imaging modalities, such as CT and MRI, are limited by hardware-induced artifacts. Radionuclide imaging, reflecting physiological rather than anatomical changes, is not affected by metallic hardware and plays an important role in the diagnosis of prosthetic joint infection.

The current imaging procedure of choice for evaluating suspected joint replacement infection is combined WBC and bone marrow imaging, which has an overall accuracy ranging from 88% to 98%. Although inflammation may be present in both the infected and aseptically loosened device, neutrophils, which are invariably present in infection, are usually absent in aseptic loosening. The success of labeled WBC imaging is highly dependent on the presence of a neutrophil response, and this critical histological difference between infection and aseptic loosening accounts for the high sensitivity and specificity of combined WBC/marrow imaging for diagnosing prosthetic joint infection [18]. The administered radiolabeled WBCs migrate to the spleen, liver and, to a lesser extent, the lungs and bones. This biodistribution persists over time but, in the presence of an infected focus, radiolabeled cells migrate from the lung, spleen and bone marrow to accumulate progressively in the infected site. Therefore, the increased accumulation of labeled cells with time in suspected areas is the main criterion for the correct diagnosis of infection. Cells radiolabeled with ^{99m}Tc-HMPAO present in the liver tend to lose the radiopharmaceutical from their cytoplasm and it is subsequently excreted via the bile into the bowel. Therefore, some physiological activity in the bowel, increasing with time, can also be observed and should not be confused with an infection.

Inflammatory bowel disease

Inflammatory bowel disease (IBD) is a group of idiopathic, chronic disorders, of uncertain etiology, including Crohn's disease and ulcerative colitis.

Crohn's disease is a transmural, aspecific, chronic inflammatory disease that most frequently affects the terminal part of the small bowel (the ileum) and the colon, but it can be localized in any region of the bowel. The disease is pathologically characterized by the presence of architectural distortion with transmural or superficial patchy granulomatous infiltration and/or the presence of acute inflammatory cells. The disease may be complicated by perforations of the bowel wall with abscess development, fistula and bowel bleeds.

Ulcerative colitis is a chronic inflammatory disease of the colon, restricted to the mucous and submucous wall of the colon. The disease can be limited to the rectal region (proctitis) or can extend to the sigmoid region (proctosigmoiditis) until the left flexure of the colon (colitis) or even the right flexure (subtotal colitis). Pathologically, the disease is characterized by diffuse mucosal inflammation and the presence of acute inflammatory cells. The symptoms are more or less the same as in Crohn's disease. Complications are perforations, fistula and abscess formation. In cases of large ulcerative processes, the toxic damage to the muscle tissue can induce the loss of neuromuscular function with progressive dilatation of the colon (toxic megacolon).

In IBD, US, CT and particularly MRI, are helpful to evaluate the presence of extramural complications such as abscesses, fistula and perforations in addition to evaluate the extent and activity of the diseases (see Chapters 6 and 13). Scintigraphic imaging allows additional information to be obtained about the activity of disease. The first imaging modality is certainly MRI as this provides a clear, broad characterization of bowel diseases. Labeled WBC imaging is a useful adjunct to MRI, particularly in three situations: to better define the activity of the disease in a given segment; for the differential diagnosis between fibrotic and inflammatory strictures; and for the early detection of asymptomatic disease relapse in patients in clinical remission, particularly after surgery, or in patients whose physical presentation and laboratory tests are discordant. It can also be used as a screening test to identify patients who need further investigation and to monitor response to treatment. Although early studies were performed with ^{111}In-labeled WBCs, it is now agreed that ^{99m}Tc-labelled WBCs also can be used if imaging is limited to within 3 hours due to bowel excretion of ^{99m}Tc-HMPAO. Imaging at multiple time points and SPECT maximize the sensitivity of the test [19].

There are some limitations to labeled WBC imaging in IBD. The test cannot define anatomical changes such as strictures, which are best delineated with endoscopy and contrast radiography. It is less sensitive for upper than for lower gastrointestinal tract disease. The sensitivity of the test also may be affected adversely by corticosteroid administration [19].

Fever of unknown origin

The most common causes of fever of unknown origin (FUO) are infections, malignancies, autoimmune diseases and collagen vascular diseases. In a significant number of cases (30%), the origin remains unknown. Diagnosis is often made by a good anamnestic investigation (with special attention to occupational and recreational exposure to pathogens, recent travel history and drug abuse). A thorough physical examination (searching for skin eruptions or lesions, lymphoadenopathy and hepatosplenomegaly) is required, as well as the following blood tests: whole blood count, inflammatory markers such as ESR and CRP, immune system profile, etc. Microbiological cultural examinations include blood, urine, spinal fluid cultures, viral titers and a Mantoux test (for tuberculosis).

Radiological imaging modalities, such as US, CT and MRI, may be helpful for diagnosis in FUO, but in the majority of cases the origin of the FUO remains uncertain.

Scintigraphic imaging with labeled WBCs and PET imaging with [18F]FDG are accurate modalities to evaluate patients with FUO (see Chapter 16). WBC imaging can contribute useful information about infection in patients with FUO, particularly if there is a high suspicion of an occult infection (elevated CRP, ESR and WBC count). A negative study virtually excludes infection/inflammation as the cause of the fever [11,20]. In contrast, it is suggested that when patients with FUO have a low probability of infection (low ESR, WBC count and CRP), an [18F]FDG-PET scan should first be performed.

Postoperative infections

Radionuclide imaging is a useful adjunct to morphological imaging and can facilitate the differentiation of abscesses from other fluid collections, tumor and normal postoperative changes. [67]Gallium (^{67}Ga)-citrate can detect intra-abdominal infections, but the presence of variable large bowel activity can obscure foci of infection. The need to wait for 48 hours or more between injection and imaging is another disadvantage. ^{67}Ga-citrate accumulates in infections and tumors, as well as in normal healing surgical incisions. Labeled WBCs, in contrast, rarely accumulate in uninfected neoplasms and do not, with few exceptions, accumulate in normally healing surgical incisions. Consequently, WBC imaging is the preferred radionuclide

test for the evaluation of postoperative infections [21–23]. The role of radiological imaging and nuclear medicine imaging is described in Chapters 5 and 12.

Cardiovascular infections

In cases of suspected cardiovascular infections, echocardiography is readily available and accurately diagnoses bacterial endocarditis. Radionuclide imaging methods play a very limited role in the diagnostic work-up of this entity. Echocardiography is less sensitive, however, for detecting myocardial abscesses, infected emboli and device-associated infections. WBC imaging accurately detects these infections, but SPECT/CT images are mandatory [24]. [18F]FDG can also be used successfully for imaging device-associated infections, for which an early (1-hour) and a late (3-hour) acquisition is suggested to improve sensitivity and specificity. Prosthetic vascular graft infections, though uncommon, are very serious complications of vascular surgery. Imaging studies are routinely used to confirm or exclude a vascular graft infection. CT is usually the initial imaging modality used (see Chapter 7). WBC imaging with either ^{99m}Tc or ^{111}In is a useful complement, particularly if SPECT/CT acquisitions can be made. The sensitivity of WBC imaging for diagnosing prosthetic vascular graft infection ranges from 58% to 100%, although in most series it has been reported to be higher than 90%. A long duration of the symptoms or pretreatment with antibiotics does not adversely affect the study results. The specificity of WBC imaging is more variable, ranging from 53% to 100%. Causes of false-positive results include perigraft hematoma, bleeding, graft thrombosis, pseudoaneurysms and graft endothelialization, which occur 1–2 weeks after placement [25–31]. [18F]FDG-PET/CT is a valid alternative for imaging vascular graft infections (see Chapters 7 and 14).

Lung infections

Although pulmonary uptake of labeled WBCs is a normal physiological event during the first few hours after their injection, after 24 hours such uptake is abnormal. Focal pulmonary uptake that is segmental or lobar in appearance is usually associated with bacterial pneumonia (see Chapters 8, 15 and 17). This pattern is also seen in patients with cystic fibrosis and is due to leukocyte accumulation in pooled secretions in bronchiectatic regions of the lungs. Non-segmental focal pulmonary uptake is caused by technical problems during labeling or re-infusion, and is not usually associated with infection.

Diffuse pulmonary activity on images obtained more than 4 hours after re-injection of labeled cells is associated with opportunistic infections, radiation pneumonitis, pulmonary drug toxicity and adult respiratory distress syndrome. Diffuse pulmonary activity is also seen in septic patients with normal chest radiographs who have no clinical evidence of respiratory tract inflammation or infection. Circulating neutrophils, activated by cytokines, easily pool in the pulmonary circulation. Cytokines presumably also activate pulmonary vascular endothelial cells, causing increased adherence of leukocytes to the cell walls, further retarding their transit through the pulmonary vasculature. Finally, it is important to note that while diffuse pulmonary activity on labeled WBC images is associated with numerous conditions, it is almost never seen in bacterial pneumonia [32,33].

Central nervous system infections

In the central nervous system (CNS) the differential diagnosis of a contrast-enhancing brain lesion identified on CT or MRI includes abscess, tumor, cerebrovascular accident and even multiple sclerosis. WBC scintigraphy provides valuable information about contrast-enhancing brain lesions. A positive study indicates that the origin of the brain lesion is almost assuredly infectious; a negative result rules out infection with a high degree of certainty. Faint uptake in brain tumors has been observed and false-negative results in patients receiving high-dose steroids have been reported [34–36].

[^{18}F]FDG has been particularly used for imaging encephalitis and Creutzfelt–Jakob diseases [37].

Radiolabeled WBCs are also indicated for imaging extracranial infections and to monitor the efficacy of antibiotic therapy, such as in malignant necrotizing otitis and sinusitis, and soft tissue infections of the face (periorbital or labial and zygomatic as a complication of dermal filler injection for cosmetic reasons). Dental abscesses are also of interest [38] as well as focal infections of the salivary glands, brachial cysts and thyroid. Finally, an interesting field of application of nuclear medicine technique is the successful use of radiolabeled somatostatin analogs in the evaluation of disease activity in autoimmune exophthalmos.

HIV-associated infections

WBC imaging has a very limited role in the evaluation of AIDS-related infections in contrast with [^{18}F]FDG-PET imaging that helps in evaluating lung infections, brain infections and other HIV-associated inflammatory/infective processes. WBCs are not sensitive for detecting the opportunistic infections that often involve the lungs and lymph nodes of these patients. This is not surprising because most opportunistic infections do not incite a neutrophilic inflammatory response and the HIV-infected patient may have only a few competent leukocytes (see Chapter 15). The test is useful, however, for detecting colonic infections in the HIV-positive patient [39,40].

Preimaging considerations and patient preparation

Image acquisition protocols and image interpretation criteria may vary from institution to institution and depend also on the experience of physicians and institutions. It may vary also according to the type of equipment available (single- or double-head cameras, SPECT and SPECT/CT), the technique used and the radioactivity injected. It is therefore extremely difficult to suggest the "best" protocol.

As for all studies using labeled blood products, it is essential that measures are in place for correct patient identification, to avoid the administration of labeled cells to the wrong patient. And as for all nuclear medicine studies, pregnancy should be excluded in all female patients in their reproductive years. Patients who are breast-feeding must be informed about the correct procedures to follow, e.g. the period of interruption of breast-feeding, the importance of limiting the contact dose and the possibility of collecting some breast-milk for use during the period that the baby should not be breast-fed [41–43]. If the risk of providing unsterile milk is deemed larger than a small radiation risk due to a radionuclide in milk with a short half-life, it may be advisable not to recommend interruption of breast-feeding. For females with active menstrual bleeding, it is preferable to delay the investigation until after the active bleeding period. If this is not possible, the patient should be carefully informed about the fact that sanitary towels or tampons may become radioactive and are therefore considered contaminated waste.

Patients should preferably be fasting at the time of sampling so that interference from the possible interaction of high levels of cholesterol and glucose in the blood does not have to be considered.

A careful history must be obtained from the referring physician to ensure that the procedure applied, e.g. the use of [111]In- or ^{99m}Tc-labeled WBCs, and the type and time of acquisition are correct. The blood results for the patient have to be checked to identify if infection parameters in the blood are elevated and there are enough white blood cells for labeling. Further, the possibility of the interference of some drugs and antibiotics with cell labeling must be considered. Several authors describe no interference between such treatment and the accuracy of WBC scanning. Others advise delaying the scan until 2 weeks after therapy withdrawal, or in the case of a doubtful scan performed on a patient on antibiotics, repeated 2 weeks later. At present it is not possible "*a priori*" to exclude patients who are receiving antibiotic treatment.

As far as [18F]FDG is concerned, the major goal of patient preparation is to minimize tracer uptake in normal issues, such as the myocardium and skeletal muscle, while maintaining uptake in the target tissues.

In the case of a diagnostic procedure in a patient who is known or suspected to be pregnant, the International Committee for Radiation Protection (ICRP) reports that the administration of 259 MBq (7 mCi) of [18F]FDG results in an absorbed radiation dose by the non-gravid uterus of 4.7 mGy (i.e. 1.8×10^{-2} mGy/MBq) [44]. The ICRP does not recommend interruption of breast-feeding following [18F]FDG administration since very little [18F]FDG is excreted in the milk. However, it can be suggested that contact between mother and child should be limited for 12 hours following injection of [18F]FDG to reduce infant radiation dose from exposure to the mother.

It has been advocated that high glucose levels may interfere with the target sites of inflammation/infection due to competitive inhibition of [18F]FDG uptake by D-glucose. Following sporadic reports of the successful study of patients with glucose levels higher than 0.2 g/dL (1.0 mmol/L), it has been recently demonstrated in a series including 123 cases with suspected infection that neither diabetes nor hyperglycemia at the time of the study have any significant impact on the false-negative rate in this particular clinical scenario. This is slightly different from the situation for tumor imaging, especially the imaging of pancreatic and lung cancers, for which reduced [18F]FDG uptake is already observed at glucose levels of 0.14 g/dL (0.8 mmol/L). Patients must fast (although intake of non-caloric beverages, e.g. water or coffee, is allowed) for 4 hours before [18F]FDG imaging and should be actively encouraged to drink sufficient water to ensure hydration and promote diuresis. A blood glucose test must be performed and the result recorded in the patient file.

Necessary medications are allowed and must be recorded. The patient should be advised to avoid strenuous physical exercise during the 24 hours preceding injection. Strategies to reduce unwanted [18F]FDG accumulation, particularly in children and adolescents, include warming of blankets and the uptake room during localization, as this can decrease brown fat activity. Children younger than 5 years should be sedated and pre-medication for anxiety given to other patients if indicated. A quiet uptake room will help to reduce anxiety. Patients should be well hydrated and must void prior to positioning on the PET/CT table [45].

Image acquisition protocols for WBCs and anti-G mAbs

While labeled WBCs and antibodies have a very different biodistribution *in vivo*, their accumulation at infection sites has similar kinetics and, therefore, these radiopharmaceuticals can be considered together.

For the image acquisition with a gamma-camera, a large-field-of-view camera with a low-energy high-resolution collimator is usually preferred for technetium (140 keV using a 15–20% window) and a medium-energy collimator for indium.

When ^{99m}Tc-HMPAO-labeled WBCs are used, early imaging of lungs is suggested for quality control, as well as of the pelvis and abdomen, because normal bowel activity is seen in 20–30% of children at 1 hour and 2–6% of adults at 3–4 hours after injection. Lung images at 30 minutes (also called "early images") are therefore suggested together with a whole-body image at 3–4 hours (also called "delayed images") and at 20–24 hours (also called "late images"). Images of the regions of interest must also be obtained for at least $5–8 \times 10^5$ counts/view (fixed-count images) or, better, 5–10 minutes/view (fixed-time images), including a region of normal bone marrow as a reference (iliac bone, sternum or head bone). However, this method is recommended only to readers with considerable experience since images may need to be "normalized" to bone marrow. The alternative to fixed-count or fixed-time images is to acquire images for a time corrected according to isotope decay time (time-corrected images) (Table 9.4) (i.e. 200 seconds at 3 hours and 2000 seconds at 23 hours for ^{99m}Tc; 400 seconds at 3 hours and 500 seconds at 23 hours for ^{111}In). The basis for this kind of "time-corrected acquisition mode" is illustrated in Figure 9.1.

Images are presented, not as a percentage of maximum uptake, but all with the same range of activity in row counts (Figures 9.2 and 9.3). This method reduces operator interference in the final image interpretation and an objective increase over time in activity or area of activity in the suspected site can be considered to indicate an infection. This approach also makes quantitative analysis more accurate. If early and delayed images are acquired with the same numbers of counts, delayed images should be corrected for the radioisotope half-life. A limited study to evaluate a specific region of the body is acceptable in selected cases.

SPECT or SPECT/CT images are mandatory in selected indications (e.g. endocarditis, vascular prosthesis, head and neck infections). SPECT or SPECT/CT scans at 3–6 hours should be acquired using a 15 second/step protocol with a 64×64 or 128×128 matrix, and with a 90–120 seconds/step

Table 9.4 Calculation of acquisition time for images corrected for isotope decay. (A) ^{99m}Tc and (B) ^{111}In

A								λ/t	$exp(-\lambda/t)$
	Min post 1st acquisition	Hours post 1st acquisition	Corrected acquisition time (s)						
Early images	0	0	100	150	200	250			
	90	1.5	119	178	238	297		0.173	0.841
	120	2	126	189	252	315		0.231	0.794
Delayed images	150	2.5	133	200	267	334		0.289	0.749
	180	3	141	212	283	354		0.347	0.707
	210	3.5	150	225	300	375		0.404	0.667
	1170	19.5	951	1426	1902	2377		2.252	0.105
	1200	20	1007	1511	2015	2519		2.310	0.099
Late images	1230	20.5	1067	1601	2135	2668		2.368	0.094
	1260	21	1131	1696	2262	2827		2.426	0.088
	1290	21.5	1198	1797	2396	2995		2.483	0.083

B								λ/t	$exp(-\lambda/t)$
Early images	0	0	100	150	200	250			
	90	1.5	102	152	203	254		0.016	0.985
	120	2	102	153	204	255		0.021	0.980
Delayed images	150	2.5	103	154	205	257		0.026	0.974
	180	3	103	155	206	258		0.031	0.969
	210	3.5	104	156	207	259		0.036	0.964
	1170	19.5	122	184	245	306		0.202	0.817
	1200	20	123	184	246	307		0.207	0.813
Late images	1230	20.5	124	185	247	309		0.212	0.809
	1260	21	124	186	249	311		0.217	0.805
	1290	21.5	125	187	250	312		0.222	0.801

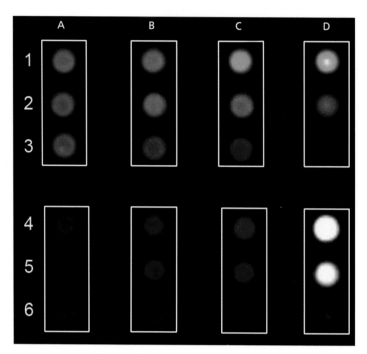

Figure 9.1 A ^{99m}Tc phantom example to illustrate the importance of acquiring images with time corrected for decay rather than for a fixed number of time or counts. Here spot activities in column A were acquired at time 0, spots in column B after 3 hours, spots in column C after 6 hours and spots in column D after 20 hours. In rows 1 and 4, spots have an increasing activity with time (50 µCi in A, 60 µCi in B, 75 µCi in C and 100 µCi in D), simulating a huge active recruitment of labeled leukocytes in the target region. In rows 2 and 5, spots have the same activity at each time point (50 µCi) and simulate an active recruitment of labeled leukocytes in the target region thus keeping activity constant. In rows 3 and 6, spots initially have an activity of 50 µCi in A and this decays with time, simulating leukocytes that early migrate but do not accumulate any more with time in the target region. Therefore rows 1 and 4 are comparable to an acute infection; rows 2 and 5 to a low grade or chronic infection; rows 3 and 6 to a sterile inflammation or to bone marrow activity. Spot activities in rows 1, 2 and 3 were acquired all together for a fixed number of counts at each time point (100 000 counts). Spot activities in rows 4, 5 and 6 were also acquired all together at each time point, but for a time corrected for ^{99m}Tc decay (100 seconds for A4, A5 and A6; 141 seconds for B4, B5 and B6; 200 seconds for C4, C5 and C6; 1007 seconds for D4, D5 and D6, as shown in Table 9.4). In the images acquired with a "fixed-count-acquisition mode", an increase in activity with time (row 1) is correctly seen as an increase with time, but an activity that remains constant with time (row 2) is wrongly visualized as decreasing with time, and a constant activity that decays with time (row 3) is seen as decreasing with time. In contrast, in the images acquired with a "time-decay corrected acquisition mode" an increase in activity with time (row 4) is correctly seen as an increase with time, as well as an activity that remains constant with time (row 5) which is also clearly seen as an increase with time, and a constant activity that decays with time (row 3) is seen as a constant activity with time. This must be taken into consideration in image interpretation in dynamic studies with radiolabeled WBCs.

protocol at 16–20 hours when using ^{99m}Tc, and a 20–30 seconds/step at 3–4 hours and a 30–40 seconds/step protocol at 16–20 hours for ^{111}In, according to isotope decay (as in Table 9.4).

Whole body images should also be acquired with speed adjusted to isotope decay in order to easily compare WBS acquired at 3–4 h and 20–24 h. For osteomyelitis, the suggested time points for images are 30 minutes, 2–3 hours and 20–24 hours. The

basis of this procedure is illustrated in Figure 9.4, which highlights how activity is stable with time in bone marrow and decreases with time in sterile inflammation but increases with time in acute and subacute infections.

When using ^{99m}Tc-HMPAO-labeled WBCs in cases of abdominal infections and IBD, images should only be acquired at 30 minutes and 2–3 hours after injection of the labeled WBCs. This is because ^{99m}Tc-

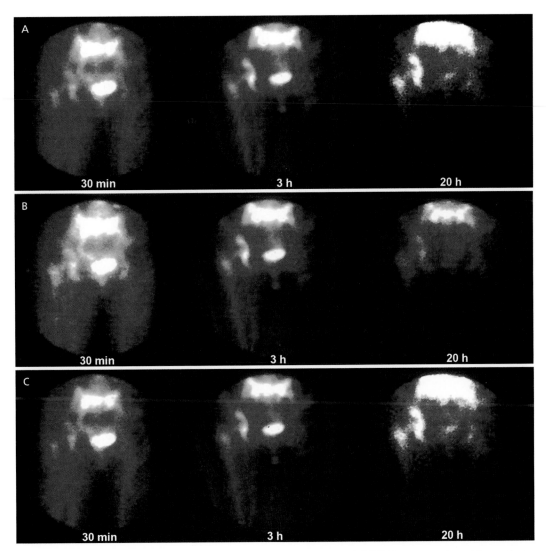

Figure 9.2 A ^{99m}Tc-HMPAO-WBC scan acquired with a "count-acquisition mode" (700 kcounts per image) in a patient with suspected infection of a left hip prosthesis. Posterior images were acquired at 30 minutes, 3 hours and 20 hours after ^{99m}Tc-labeled WBC administration. (A) Images appear as they were acquired and each image is normalized for its maximal activity. (B) The intensity scale of the images has been intentionally modified to make the result negative (activity in the prosthesis decreases with time). (C) The intensity scale of images has been intentionally modified to make the result positive (activity in the prosthesis increases with time). It is difficult to know if the scan is really positive or negative as image correction is operator-dependent and there is a different bladder activity at each time point.

HMPAO is released by WBCs with time and taken up by the liver and excreted via the bowel, thus producing false-positive images at later time points. This problem does not occur if ^{99m}Tc-anti-G mAbs or ^{111}In-labeled WBCs are used and these are preferable for studying abdominal infections. For the same reason, when using ^{99m}Tc-labeled WBCs, vascular graft infections of abdominal vessels (aorto-bi-siliac grafts) should be imaged within 3 hours of their administration. An early dynamic acquisition (one image every 5 seconds for 150 seconds) soon after injection of labeled cells may help to map the vascular structures and detect obstructions or aneurysms.

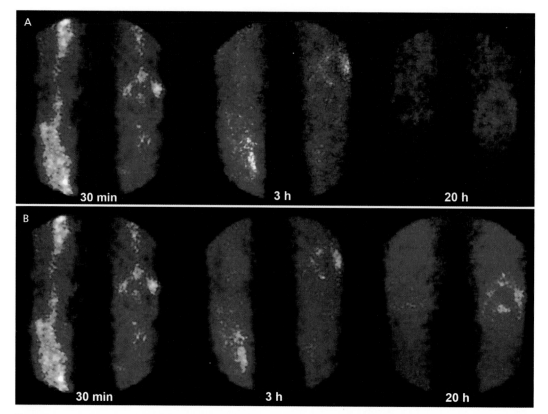

Figure 9.3 A WBC scan of a patient with a suspected infection of a left knee prosthesis. Anterior images were acquired using a "fixed-time" protocol, after ^{99m}Tc-labeled WBC administration. (A) All images were acquired for 100 seconds (158 kcounts, 103 kcounts and 17 kcounts) and the study appears negative. (B) Images are correctly acquired with a "time-decay corrected" acquisition protocol (105 seconds at 30 minutes, 141 seconds at 3 hours and 1007 seconds at 20 hours; 158 kcounts, 145 kcounts and 175 kcounts, respectively) and the intensity scale of all images has been normalized to the same activity range (as it must be when using the "time-decay corrected" acquisition protocols) and the study is clearly positive. This analysis is operator-independent and not influenced by bone marrow activity, bladder activity, intestinal activity or blood pool activity.

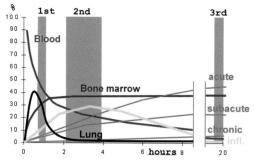

Figure 9.4 Modification of activity with time in bone marrow, lungs, blood, sterile inflammation and infections (acute, subacute and chronic). Based on these kinetics, it is understandable why three images (early, delayed and late) need to be acquired to discriminate between bone marrow activity, sterile inflammation and infection. The gray bars show the timeframes in which early, delayed and late images are acquired.

Interpretation criteria for WBCs and anti-G mAbs

Accurate interpretation of labeled WBC scintigraphy requires knowledge of the normal and abnormal variants of WBC localizations. The diagnosis of an infection is made by comparing early and delayed images. The images are classified as negative if there is no uptake or a significant decrease in uptake from early to delayed images; positive when uptake is seen in both early and delayed images and increases over time; and equivocal when uptake in the early and delayed images is the same or slightly decreasing.

After visual assessment, semi-quantitative evaluation may also be performed. The purpose is to evaluate whether quantification of uptake can help to differentiate infection from non-specific uptake. Regions of interest (ROIs) are drawn over the region with the greatest activity and copied to a presumed normal reference tissue (e.g. anterosuperior iliac crest, unaffected proximal, distant or contralateral bone, etc.). The mean counts per pixel in these ROIs are recorded to calculate lesion-to-reference (L/R) ratios both in early and delayed images (L/R$_{early}$ and L/R$_{late}$, respectively). When the L/R ratio increases with time (L/R$_{late}$ > L/R$_{early}$), the scan is considered indicative of infection; when the L/R$_{late}$ is similar or slightly decreased with respect to L/R$_{early}$, the examination is classified as equivocal; and when L/R$_{late}$ is significantly decreased compared to L/R$_{early}$, the examination is classified as negative for infection.

If SPECT/CT images are used, delineation of the site of increased radiopharmaceutical uptake may be calculated using a 50% isocontour on a single transaxial slice with the hottest activity (lesion) and the reference tissue (e.g. anterorsuperior iliac crest). The same criteria as described above may be used for imaging classification.

Criteria for positivity
• L/R ratios in delayed and late images are calculated as described above.
• The antero-superior iliac crest or the contralateral region should be used as the reference region.

Qualitative analysis
• Images must be evaluated without operator modifications of single frames.
• Iliac bone uptake should be used as the reference region for bone marrow (or sternum or skull) whenever possible.

Semi-quantitative analysis
• L/R ratios in delayed and late images are calculated as described above.
• The antero-superior iliac crest or the contra-lateral region should be used as the reference region.

Additional investigations based upon the imaging results
Fusion of WBC images with CT or MR images of the part of the body that is suspected to be infected or inflamed may be helpful for a more accurate localization of WBC uptake, particularly when differentiating soft tissue uptake from bone uptake (e.g. in the diabetic foot). In the diabetic foot, superficial/soft tissue infections often show a decrease in activity between the 3-hour and 24-hour images, but osteo-myelitis always shows an increase in activity with time. SPECT/CT also helps in the differential diagnosis. In Charcot foot, an additional scan with colloids for bone marrow imaging is mandatory to differentiate between expanded bone marrow (a common finding in Charcot foot) and osteomyelitis.

When using ^{111}In-labeled WBCs for IBD evaluation, stool collection and counting at early and late time points may indicate the presence of radiolabeled cells migrating from infected mucosa to the lumen, an indirect sign of an infected bowel. Planar acquisition of the pelvis in the "sitting" position (sitting the patient above the gamma camera) may better discriminate between rectal and bladder activity in cases of suspected rectosigmoidal extent of IBD.

In vascular grafts, oblique views may help to differentiate between uptake in the graft itself and in the surrounding tissue.

Pitfalls and artifacts
Regardless of which tracer is used, uptake of labeled WBCs depends on intact chemotaxis, the number and types of cells labeled, and the cellular component of a particular inflammatory response. Labeling of WBCs, now a routine procedure, does not affect their chemotactic response. A total white count of at least 2000/μL is needed to obtain satisfactory images. In most clinical settings, a mixed leukocyte population is labeled. Hence, the majority of cells labeled are neutrophils and the procedure is most useful for identifying neutrophil-mediated inflammatory processes, such as bacterial infections. The procedure is less useful for those diseases in which the predominant cellular response is not neutrophilic, i.e. opportunistic infections, tuberculosis and sarcoidosis. Although pulmonary uptake of labeled WBCs is a normal physiological event during the first few hours after injection, 24 hours after injection such pulmonary uptake is abnormal. Focal pulmonary uptake that is segmental or lobar in appearance is usually associated with infection. Non-segmental focal pulmonary uptake, however, is caused by technical problems during labeling or reinfusion and is generally not associated with infection.

[111]In-labeled WBCs do not accumulate in normal bowel. Bowel activity is always abnormal and is seen in antibiotic-associated colitis, pseudomembranous colitis, infectious colitis, IBD, ischemic colitis and gastrointestinal bleeding.

Radiolabeled WBCs do not accumulate in normally healing surgical wounds, so the presence of such activity indicates infection. There are, however, certain exceptions. Granulating wounds that heal by secondary intention can appear as areas of intense activity on WBC images even in the absence of infection. Examples include stomies (tracheostomies, ileostomies, feeding gastrostomies, etc.) and skin grafts. Vascular access lines, dialysis catheters and even lumbar punctures can all produce false-positive results in the absence of appropriate clinical history.

Interpretation criteria for FDG

The evaluation of $[^{18}F]$FDG imaging should take into consideration the clinical question raised by the clinician, the physiological distribution of $[^{18}F]$ FDG, the individual variations in the specific patient evaluated and the intensity of $[^{18}F]$FDG uptake [standardized uptake value $(SUV)_{max}$ or SUV_{mean}].

In addition, it is important to evaluate the presence of potential causes of false-negative results:
• Lesion size
• Low metabolic rate
• Hyperglycemia
• Lesions masked by adjacent high physiological uptake
• Concomitant drug use interfering with the uptake, e.g. ongoing steroid therapy in systemic disorders.
and potential causes of false-positive results:
• Artifacts: injection artifacts and external contamination; reconstruction artifacts from attenuation correction (e.g. chest movement and liver uptake, metallic devices)
• Physiological uptake (muscular activity; myocardial uptake; uptake in the oropharyngeal tract and vocal cords, stomach and intestine; post-therapy uptake in bone marrow and spleen, and thymus in young patients)
• Pathological uptake not related to infection/inflammation (e.g. finding an unsuspected cancer).

Care should be taken in the interpretation of PET data corrected for attenuation using a low-dose CT (particularly when metallic material/implants are present). Assessment of both attenuation corrected and non-corrected images is recommended.

There are no general criteria published for all inflammatory and infectious disorders. Most research articles on the subject have defined interpretation criteria for the purposes of the specific study described. Some authors have reported specific interpretation criteria that can be used more generally, although no definitive consensus has been agreed upon.

For joint prostheses, the most relevant criteria have been proposed by Reinhartz *et al.* [46] for painful hip arthroplasties. They propose five main patterns corresponding to no loosening (patterns 1–3), mechanical loosening (pattern 4) and infection (pattern 5, corresponding to uptake of $[^{18}F]$FDG in the periprosthetic soft tissue). They reported an overall accuracy of 95% with use of these criteria, but this has not been confirmed by others. In any event, visual interpretation using these criteria is more reliable than quantitative (SUV) analysis, which is not recommended. Kobayashi *et al.* also proposed a qualitative classification for prosthetic joint infections of the hip, based on the pattern of $[^{18}F]$ fluoride uptake around the prosthesis [47]. Despite Reinhartz *et al.* [46] and Kobayashi *et al.* [47] using different radiopharmaceuticals, it is interesting to note that different criteria have been used and different areas around the prosthesis seem to be involved in infection, but, in conclusion, $[^{18}F]$FDG cannot yet be used in prosthetic joint infections to discriminate between sterile inflammation and infection.

In cases of diabetic foot infection, recently Familiari and Signore [48] applied a protocol with dual-time imaging (at 1 hour and 2 hours post injection) and calculated the SUV_{max} in the suspected region of infection. They then proposed an interpretation criterion similar to that currently used for WBC scanning to differentiate between sterile inflammation and infection, based on the SUV_{max} increase with time always being greater than 2. Using this criterion, the accuracy of $[^{18}F]$FDG for osteomyelitis was very low and no other qualitative or quantitative criteria could be defined to achieve an accuracy comparable to that for the WBC scan, which can distinguish well between infected and non-infected bones and also between soft tissue infection and osteomyelitis.

Keijsers *et al.* however reported that a high parenchymal lung uptake (with elevated SUV) was predictive of severe sarcoidosis, especially if the mediastinum/hilum SUV_{max} was low [49]. Conversely, the same authors reported that the absence of metabolic activity in the lung parenchyma was related to low-activity disease and justified a wait-and-see policy [50].

Vascular prostheses are a potential field of application of [^{18}F]FDG instead of WBC scan. However, since physiological uptake is often visible in vascular prostheses, patterns of interpretation have to be carefully analyzed. It is now accepted that linear, diffuse and homogeneous uptake is not likely to represent infection, whereas focal and/or heterogeneous uptake with projection on the vessel on CT is highly suspicious [51].

There is increasing evidence that [^{18}F]FDG is strongly indicated in the evaluation of vasculitides. Hautzel *et al.* [52] and Meller *et al.* [53] proposed criteria for the diagnosis of active giant-cell arteritis. The Meller criteria are qualitative and compare uptake in the aorta with that in the liver or brain, but they have yet to be used. Hautzel defined an optimal aorta-to-liver ratio cut-off of 1.0 using ROC curve analysis to differentiate giant-cell arteritis patients from normal patients. Although this resulted in good diagnostic performance, this parameter also has not been further evaluated by other authors.

Conclusion

The main indications of nuclear medicine procedures for diagnosis of infection have been reviewed. Emphasis has been given to the choice of the correct radiopharmaceutical depending on the clinical question, but also to the correct methodology of the examination and to the correct image interpretation. Nuclear medicine techniques in most cases are complementary to radiological techniques and efforts are ongoing in the scientific community to define common diagnostic flow charts for effective diagnosis of infections, reducing unnecessary costs and optimizing available resources.

Acknowledgements

The author wishes to thank his collaborators, students (Marco Chianelli, Ida Sonni, Anna Rapisarda, Ivan Baldazzi, Marta Pacilio, Tiziana Lanzolla, Christophe van de Wiele and Rudi Dierckx) and PhD students (Kelly Luz Anzola, Lisa Bodei, Valentina Di Gialleonardo, Filippo Galli, Andor Glaudemans, Paola Erba, Francesca Grippaudo, Elena Lazzeri, Francesca Maccioni and Gaurav Malviya) who have significantly contributed to the development of the principles described in this chapter. The author is also grateful to the members of the Committee on Infection/Inflammation of the European Association of Nuclear Medicine (EANM), other colleagues who have greatly contributed to the progress of nuclear medicine in this field (Ora Israel, Francois Jamar, Josè Martin-Comin, Erik de Vries, Manel Roca, Elena Lazzeri, Paola Erba, Velimir Ivanchevich, Johannes Meller and John Buscombe) and to all those who have contributed to useful discussions in meetings and congresses at national and international level. The contribution of international societies such as the International Society of Radiolabelled Elements (ISORBE), the International Research Group on Immuno-Scintigraphy and Therapy (IRIST) and Nuclear Medicine Discovery (NuMeD) is also greatly appreciated. The knowledge of the author has grown enormously thanks to their meetings and conferences, thanks to continuous discussion with their members and thanks to their generous support for research on this topic. Generous thanks is also due to the pharmaceutical companies and industries that have contributed to the development of this field and in particular to AAA, Alliance Medical, Bioscan, Comecer, Covidien, Excel Diagnostics, General Electric, Genzyme, GI-pharma, Hermes, Keosys, IBA, IBD Holland, ImaginAb, ITECO, LiTech, Mallinckrodt, Nordion, Novartis, NSA, OcreoPharm, OMNIA, PBI, Philips, Ridgeway, Roche, Siemens, and Zeiss.

Particular thanks go to Presidents of the EANM, the Italian Association of Nuclear Medicine (AIMN), the American Society of Nuclear Medicine (SNM) and the International Atomic Energy Agency (IAEA) who, by nominating the author to be coordinator of task groups and committees, have allowed him to realize this project of worldwide standardization of nuclear medicine techniques for imaging infection and inflammation towards the important task of defining common diagnostic flow charts in collaboration with the European Society of Radiology (ESR), the European Study Group of Implant Associated Infections (ESGIAI), the European Society of Clinical Microbiology and Infective Diseases (ESCMID), the European Society of Vascular Surgery (ESVS), the European Crohn's and Colitis Organization (ECCO), the European Society of Gastrointestinal and Abdominal Radiology (ESGAR), the European Association for Study of

Diabetes (EASD) and the European Society of Cardiology (ESC).

References

1. Signore A, Glaudemans AW. The molecular imaging approach to image infections and inflammation by nuclear medicine techniques. *Ann Nucl Med* 2011;25: 681–700.

2. Malviya G, Galli F, Sonni I, Pacilio M, Signore A. Targeting T and B lymphocytes with radiolabelled antibodies for diagnostic and therapeutic applications. *Q J Nucl Med Mol Imaging* 2010;54:654–676.

3. Signore A, Prasad V, Malviya G. Monoclonal antibodies for diagnosis and therapy decision making in inflammation/infection. Foreword. *Q J Nucl Med Mol Imaging* 2010;54:571–573.

4. Signore A, Mather SJ, Piaggio G, Malviya G, Dierckx RA. Molecular imaging of inflammation/infection: nuclear medicine and optical imaging agents and methods. *Chem Rev* 2010;110:3112–3145.

5. Chianelli M, Boerman OC, Malviya G, Galli F, Oyen WJ, Signore A. Receptor binding ligands to image infection. *Curr Pharm Des* 2008;14:3316–3325.

6. Annovazzi A, Bagni B, Burroni L, D'Alessandria C, Signore A. Nuclear medicine imaging of inflammatory/infective disorders of the abdomen. *Nucl Med Commun* 2005;26:657–664.

7. Prandini N, Lazzeri E, Rossi, B, Erba P, Parisella MG, Signore A. Nuclear medicine imaging of bone infections. *Nucl Med Commun* 2006;27:633–644.

8. Cascini GL, De Palma D, Matteucci F *et al*. Fever of unknown origin, infection of subcutaneous devices, brain abscesses and endocarditis. *Nucl Med Commun* 2006;27:213–222.

9. Capriotti G, Chianelli M, Signore A. Nuclear medicine imaging of diabetic foot infection: results of meta-analysis. *Nucl Med Commun* 2006;27:757–764.

10. Palestro CJ, Love C. Radionuclide imaging of musculoskeletal infection: conventional agents. *Semin Musculoskelet Radiol* 2007;11:335–352.

11. Palestro CJ, Love C, Bhargava KK. Labeled leukocyte imaging: current status and future directions. *Q J Nucl Med Mol Imaging* 2009;53:105–123.

12. Palestro CJ, Love C, Tronco GG, Tomas MB, Rini JN. Combined labeled leukocyte and technetium-99m sulfur colloid marrow imaging for diagnosing musculoskeletal infection: principles, technique, interpretation, indications and limitations. *RadioGraphics* 2006;26:859–870.

13. Palestro CJ, Kim CK, Swyer AJ, Capozzi JD, Solomon RW, Goldsmith SJ. Total hip arthroplasty: periprosthetic ^{111}In labeled leukocyte activity and complementary ^{99m}Tc sulfur colloid imaging in suspected infection. *J Nucl Med* 1990;31:1950–1955.

14. Palestro CJ, Swyer AJ, Kim CK, Goldsmith SJ. Infected knee prosthesis: diagnosis with In-111-leukocyte, Tc-99m-sulfur colloid and Tc-99m-MDP imaging. *Radiology* 1991;179:645–648.

15. Love C, Marwin SE, Tomas MB *et al*. Diagnosing infection in the failed joint replacement: a comparison of coincidence detection fluorine-18 FDG and indium-111-labelled leukocyte/technetium-99m-sulfur colloid marrow imaging. *J Nucl Med* 2004;45: 1864–1871.

16. Palestro CJ, Mehta HH, Patel M *et al*. Marrow versus infection in the Charcot joint: indium-111 leukocyte and technetium-99m sulfur colloid scintigraphy. *J Nucl Med* 1998;39:346–350.

17. Palestro CJ, Kim CK, Swyer AJ, Vallabhajosula S, Goldsmith SJ. Radionuclide diagnosis of vertebral osteomyelitis: indium-111-leukocyte and technetium-99m-methylene diphosphonate bone scintigraphy. *J Nucl Med* 1991;32:1861–1865.

18. Gemmel F, Van den Wyngaert H, Love C, Welling MM, Gemmel P, Palestro CJ. Prosthetic joint infections: radionuclide state-of-the-art imaging. *Eur J Nucl Med Mol Imaging* 2012;38:892–909.

19. Palestro CJ, Tomas MB, Love C. Infection and inflammation in pediatrics. In: Treves ST (ed). *Pediatric Nuclear Medicine/PET*, 3rd edn. New York: Springer, 2007, pp. 419–445.

20. Seshadri N, Solanki CK, Balan K. Utility of 111In-labeelled leukocyte scintigraphy in patients with fever of unknown origin in an era of changing disease spectrum and investigational techniques. *Nucl Med Commun* 2008;29:277–282.

21. Ascher NL, Ahrenholz DH, Simmons RL *et al*. Indium-111 autologous tagged leukocytes in the diagnosis of intraperitoneal sepsis. *Arch Surg* 1979; 114:386–392.

22. Coleman RE, Black RE, Welch OM, Maxwell JG. Indium-Ill labeled leukocytes in the evaluation of suspected abdominal abscesses. *Am J Surg* 1980;139: 99–104.

23. Palestro CJ, Love C, Tronco GG, Tomas MB. Role of radionuclide imaging in the diagnosis of postoperative infection. *RadioGraphics* 2000;20:1649–1660.

24. Cerqueira MD, Jacobson AF. Indium-111 leukocyte scintigraphic detection of myocardial abscess formation in patients with endocarditis. *J Nucl Med* 1989;30:703–706.

25. Brunner MC, Mitchell RS, Baldwin JC *et al*. Prosthetic graft infection: limitations of indium white blood cell scanning. *J Vasc Surg* 1986;3:42–48.

26. Fiorani P, Speziale F, Rizzo L *et al*. Detection of aortic graft infection with leukocytes labeled with techne-

tium 99m-hexametazime. *J Vasc Surg* 1993;17: 87–96.

27. Krznaric E, Nevelsteen A, Van Hoe L *et al.* Diagnostic value of ^{99}Tc^m-d,l-HMPAO-labelled leukocyte scintigraphy in the detection of vascular graft infections. *Nucl Med Commun* 1994;15:953–960.

28. Prats E, Banzo J, Abós MD *et al.* Diagnosis of prosthetic vascular graft infection by technetium-99m-HMPAO-labeled leukocytes. *J Nucl Med* 1994;35: 1303–1307.

29. Palestro CJ, Vega A, Kim CK, Vallabhajosula S, Goldsmith SJ. Indium-111-labeled leukocyte scintigraphy in hemodialysis access-site infection. *J Nucl Med* 1990;31:319–324.

30. Liberatore M, Iurilli AP, Ponzo F *et al.* Aortofemoral graft infection: the usefulness of 99m-Tc-HMPAO-labelled leukocyte scan. *Eur J VascEndovasc Surg* 1997;14 (Suppl A):27–29.

31. De la Cueva L, Plancha MC, Reyes MD *et al.* Vascular thromboses: 99mTc-HMPAO leukocyte scintigraphy false positive result in diagnosis of infection. *Eur J Vasc Endovasc Surg* 2005;30:109.

32. Love C, Tomas MB, Palestro CJ. Pulmonary uptake on labeled leukocyte images: uptake patterns and their significance. *Nucl Med Commun* 2002;23:559–563.

33. Love C, Opoku-Agyemang P, Tomas MB, Pugliese PV, Bhargava KK, Palestro CJ. Pulmonary activity on labeled leukocyte images: physiologic, pathologic, and imaging correlations. *RadioGraphics* 2002;22: 1385–1393.

34. Palestro C, Swyer AJ, Kim CK, Muzinic M, Goldsmith SJ. Role of111In-Iabeled leukocyte scintigraphy in the diagnosis of intracerebral lesions. *Clin Nucl Med* 1991;16:305–308.

35. Schmidt KG, Rasmussen JW, Frederiksen PB, Kock-Jensen C. Pedersen NT. Indium-Ill-granulocyte scintigraphy in brain abscess diagnosis: Limitations and pitfalls. *J Nucl Med* 1990;31:1121–1127.

36. Kim DG, Lee JL, Lee DS, Lee MC, Choi KS, Han DH. 99mTc-HMPAO labeled leukocyte SPECT in intracranial lesions. *Surg Neuro* 1995;44:338–345.

37. Engler H, Lundberg PO, Ekbom K *et al.* Multitracer study with positron emission tomography in Creutzfeldt-Jakob disease. *Eur J Nucl Med Mol Imaging* 2003;30:85–95.

38. Kao CH, Wang SJ. Spread of infectious complications of odontogenic abscess detected by Technetium-99m-HMPAO-labeled WBC scan of occult sepsis in the intensive care unit. *J Nucl Med* 1992;33:25–45.

39. Fineman D, Palestro CJ, Kim CK *et al.* Detection of abnormalities in febrile AIDS patients with In-111-labeled leukocyte and GA-67 scintigraphy. *Radiology* 1989;170:677–680.

40. Palestro CJ, Goldsmith SJ. The use of gallium and labeled leukocyte scintigraphy in the AIDS patient. *Q J Nucl Med* 1995;39:221–230.

41. Ahlgren L, Ivarsson S, Johansson L *et al.* Excretion of radionuclides in human breast milk after the administration of radiopharmaceuticals. *J Nucl Med* 1985;26:1085–1090.

42. Mountford PJ, Coakley AJ. A review of the secretion of radioactivity in human breast milk: data, quantitative analysis and recommendations. *Nucl Med Commun* 1989;10:15–27.

43. Rubow S, Klopper J, Wasserman H *et al.* The excretion of radiopharmaceuticals in human breast milk: additional data and dosimetry. *Eur J Nucl Med* 1994;21: 144–153.

44. ICRP. Radiation dose to patients from radiopharmaceuticals. Addendum 3 to ICRP Publication 53. ICRP Publication 106. Approved by the Commission in October 2007. *Ann ICRP* 2008;38:1–197.

45. Jamar F, Buscombe J, Chiti A, *et al.* EANM/SNMMI Guideline for 18F-FDG use in inflammation and infection. *J Nucl Med* 2013 Apr;54(4):647–658.

46. Reinartz P, Mumme T, Hermanns B *et al.* Radionuclide imaging of the painful hip arthroplasty: positron-emission tomography versus triple-phase bone scanning. *J Bone Joint Surg Br* 2005;87:465–470.

47. Kobayashi N, Inaba Y, Choe H, Ike H, Fujimaki H, Tezuka T. Use of F-18 fluoride PET to differentiate septic from aseptic loosening in total hip arthroplasty patients. *Clin Nucl Med* 2011;36:e156–161.

48. Familiari D, Glaudemans AW, Vitale V *et al.* Can sequential ^{18}F-FDG PET/CT replace WBC imaging in the diabetic foot? *J Nucl Med* 2011;52:1012–1019.

49. Keijsers RG, Grutters JC, van Velzen-Blad H, van den Bosch JM, Oyen WJ, Verzijlbergen FJ. (18)F-FDG PET patterns and BAL cell profiles in pulmonary sarcoidosis. *Eur J Nucl Med Mol Imaging* 2010;37:1181–1188.

50. Keijsers RG, Verzijlbergen EJ, van den Bosch JM *et al.* ^{18}F-FDG PET as a predictor of pulmonary function in sarcoidosis. *Sarcoidosis Vasc Diffuse Lung Dis* 2011;28: 123–129.

51. Fukuchi K, Ishida Y, Higashi M *et al.* Detection of aortic graft infection by fluorodeoxyglucose positron emission tomography: comparison with computed tomographic findings. *J Vasc Surg* 2005;42:919–925.

52. Hautzel H, Sander O, Heinzel A, Schneider M, Müller HW. Assessment of large-vessel involvement in giant cell arteritis with ^{18}F-FDG PET: introducing an ROC-analysis-based cutoff ratio. *J Nucl Med* 2008;49: 1107–1113.

53. Meller J, Strutz F, Siefker U *et al.* Early diagnosis and follow-up of aortitis with [(18)F]FDG PET and MRI. *Eur J Nucl Med Mol Imaging* 2003;30:730–706.

CHAPTER 10

Nuclear Medicine Imaging of Osteomyelitis: White Blood Cell, Monoclonal Antibody, or Bacterial Imaging?

Christopher J. Palestro

Hofstra North Shore-LIJ School of Medicine, Hempstead, NY and
North Shore Long Island Jewish Health System, Manhasset & New Hyde Park, NY, USA

Introduction

The diagnosis of osteomyelitis can be challenging. Symptoms such as erythema, edema and pain are non-specific; the differential diagnosis includes fractures, septic arthritis, cellulitis and even bone infarction. Laboratory tests such as the erythrocyte sedimentation rate (ESR) and C-reactive protein (CRP) are not specific and cannot be used alone to make the diagnosis of osteomyelitis. Thus, it is not surprising that imaging tests, both morphological and functional, frequently are used to confirm the diagnosis. This chapter reviews the role of *in vitro* labeled white blood cells (WBCs; leukocytes), monoclonal antibodies (mAbs) and bacterial imaging in the diagnosis of osteomyelitis.

Basic knowledge of the clinical problem

Osteomyelitis is an infectious process of the bone and is caused by bacteria, viruses and fungi. The infection may be localized or may involve the periosteum, cortex, marrow and cancellous tissue. Acute osteomyelitis can arise either hematogenously or via direct or contiguous inoculation.

Acute hematogenous osteomyelitis, which is caused by seeding of organisms within the bone that are transported by the blood from a remote source, occurs most often in children. The highly vascular metaphyses are the most commonly affected parts of the bone, presumably because slowed blood flow predisposes the metaphyseal vessels to thrombosis and the bone itself to localized necrosis and infection [1].

Direct or contiguous inoculation osteomyelitis is secondary to spread of organisms from direct trauma, a contiguous focus of infection, or sepsis following surgery. Conditions that predispose to osteomyelitis include diabetes mellitus, sickle cell disease, intravenous drug abuse, alcoholism and immunosuppression. Open fractures, recent orthopedic surgery and joint prostheses also are risk factors for osteomyelitis [1].

The clinical questions

The diagnosis of osteomyelitis is not always obvious and imaging procedures routinely are performed as part of the diagnostic work-up. There are a myriad of imaging tests from which to choose: radiographs,

Diagnostic Imaging of Infections and Inflammatory Diseases: A Multidisciplinary Approach, First Edition. Edited by Alberto Signore and Ana María Quintero.

computed tomography (CT), magnetic resonance imaging (MRI), radionuclide bone, gallium and *in vitro* and *in vivo* labeled WBC studies. None of these tests is equally useful in all situations; the particular test to be selected depends on the circumstances of a given patient. Radiographs, which are relatively inexpensive and widely available, should be the initial imaging procedure performed in all patients suspected of having osteomyelitis, regardless of the situation. Even when not diagnostic, radiographs are useful because they provide an anatomical overview of the region of interest and any pre-existing conditions that potentially could influence both the selection and interpretation of subsequent procedures [2].

Methodological considerations

In vitro labeled WBC imaging is the radionuclide test of choice for diagnosing complicated osteomyelitis. Although a variety of labeling techniques have been used, the most commonly employed procedures make use of the lipophilic compounds ^{111}In-oxyquinolone and ^{99m}Tc-exametazime. The labeling procedure takes about 2–3 hours. Approximately 40–60 mL of whole blood is withdrawn from the patient into an anticoagulant-containing syringe. Since all blood cells can be labeled, the WBCs must be separated from erythrocytes and platelets prior to labeling. After withdrawal, therefore, the syringe containing the blood is kept upright for about 1–2 hours to promote erythrocyte sedimentation. Sedimentation can be facilitated by the addition of hydroxyethyl starch or by performing hypotonic lysis of the red cells. After the erythrocytes have been separated, the WBC-rich plasma is centrifuged and the WBC "pellet" at the bottom of the tube is removed, incubated with the radiolabel, washed and re-injected into the patient. The usual dose of ^{111}In-labeled WBCs is 10–18.5 MBq (300–500 μCi); the usual dose of ^{99m}Tc-exametazime-labeled WBCs is 185–370 MBq (5–10 mCi). When using ^{111}In-labeled WBCs, imaging typically is performed about 24 hours after injection of labeled cells. When using ^{99m}Tc-labeled WBCs, imaging usually is performed within 3–4 hours and 20–24 hours after injection [3].

Although *in vitro* labeled WBC imaging is very accurate, there are significant limitations to the procedure. The labeling process is labor intensive,

not always available and requires direct contact with blood products. Labeling a sufficient number of WBCs to obtain images of diagnostic quality may not be possible in severely leukopenic or very young patients. Image quality, especially when using ^{111}In as the radiolabel, is suboptimal. For musculoskeletal infection, the need to perform complementary bone marrow imaging adds complexity and expense to the procedure. Considerable effort, therefore, has been devoted to developing *in vivo* methods of labeling WBCs, including antigranulocyte monoclonal antibodies (anti-G mAbs) and antibody fragments, peptides and chemokines.

BW 250/183 (besilesomab) is a murine monoclonal G1 immunoglobulin that binds to the NCA-95 antigen present on WBCs [4]. About 10% of the injected activity is neutrophil bound at 45 minutes after injection with 20% of the activity circulating freely in the blood [5]. The free activity presumably localizes in inflammatory foci through non-specific, non-antigen related uptake and increased vascular permeability [6]. Studies usually become positive by 6 hours after injection, although delayed, next day imaging, may increase sensitivity. Up to 40% of the injected dose accumulates in the bone marrow, potentially obscuring small foci of infection [7]. A significant disadvantage to BW 250/183 is the high incidence of dose-dependent human antimurine antibody (HAMA) response, which has been reported to be more than 30% in patients receiving repeated injections. To minimize the likelihood of a HAMA response, the recommended dose is no more than 250 μg of antibody per injection [7].

Fanolesomab is a 900-kDa M class immunoglobulin that exhibits a high affinity (association constant $K_d = 10^{-11}$ M) for the carbohydrate moiety 3-fucosyl-N-acetyl lactosamine contained in the CD15 antigen expressed on human WBCs. This antibody binds to neutrophils in greater proportion than to any other cell type. Binding increases proportionately with increasing numbers of circulating neutrophils and is up-regulated with neutrophil activation. The normal distribution of ^{99m}Tc-fanolesomab includes the reticuloendothelial system, urinary tract and blood pool. Small bowel activity appears within 4 hours, colonic activity by 24 hours. Accumulation in infection is via two mechanisms: binding to circulating neutrophils that migrate to the infection and binding to neutrophils and CD-15 containing neutrophil debris already sequestered in the infection [8]. Imaging usually is performed about 2 hours after injection. As a result of reports of serious adverse events, including two fatalities, following its administration, ^{99m}Tc-fanolesomab is no longer available [8].

Antibody fragments are attractive because, unlike the whole antibody, they do not induce a HAMA response. Sulesomab is a 50-kDa fragment antigen-binding (Fab') portion of a murine mAb of the IgG1 class that binds to normal cross-reactive antigen-90 (NCA-90) present on WBCs. NCA-90 also is present on the macrophage–monocyte cell lineage in normal colonic mucosa and in colonic adenocarcinoma. Approximately 3–6% of the injected activity is associated with circulating neutrophils; by 24 hours after injection, about 35% of the activity remaining in the body is in the bone marrow. Initial investigations suggested that in addition to binding to circulating neutrophils that subsequently migrate to foci of infection, sulesomab also crosses permeable capillary membranes and binds to WBCs already present at the site of infection [7]. Work by Skehan et al. [9] however, suggests that sulesomab does not bind to circulating WBCs and that it is cleared into infection non-specifically through increased capillary membrane permeability. Imaging sequences depend to some extent on the indication for the test.

While most of the techniques that have been developed for labeling WBCs in vivo make use of anti-G mAbs, recent investigations have focused on cytokines, low molecular weight proteins (>20 kDa) that interact with specific cell-surface receptors on specific cell populations. Binding affinities, usually in the nanomolar range, are high [10].

One cytokine that has generated considerable interest is interleukin 8 (IL-8), a member of the CXC subfamily of chemokines, or chemotactic cytokines, that binds with high affinity to the CXC type I (IL-8 type A) and CXC type II (IL-8 type B) receptors expressed on neutrophils and monocytes [10]. Side effects of IL-8 are limited and are dose related. Administration of IL-8 in doses of 10–100 μg/kg in animals resulted in a transient decrease in the number of circulating granulocytes, which normalized within 30 minutes, followed by an increase in the number of circulating granulocytes, which peaked at about 2 hours [11,12]. Administration of 40 ng/kg −1 μg/kg of IL-8 produced a temporary

decrease in the number of circulating granulocytes, without subsequent granulocytosis [11,13]. Administration of ^{131}I-IL-8 at doses of 50–100 μg to 11 patients with infections resulted in a transient decrease in the number of WBCs, with complete normalization by 1 hour [14]. Imaging sequences have not been established for this agent.

Among the myriad of radionuclide imaging tests currently available, none is truly specific for infection and the search continues for new and better agents.

Radiolabeled antibiotics are one group of compounds that has been investigated for their potential as infection-specific tracers. One of the first, and certainly the most extensively investigated, of these compounds is the radiolabeled 4-fluoroquinolone antibiotic, ^{99m}Tc-ciprofloxacin (Infecton). Ciprofloxacin is a broad-spectrum antibiotic that inhibits the actions of DNA gyrase in Gram-negative bacteria and type IV topoisomerase in Gram-positive bacteria, resulting in rapid bacterial death. ^{99m}Tc-ciprofloxacin presumably is incorporated into and metabolized by bacteria present in the infectious focus and, assuming that the uptake is proportional to the number of microorganism present, the measured radioactivity would accurately and specifically localize infection. Although the concept is intriguing, there is considerable controversy about ^{99m}Tc-ciprofloxacin as an infection-specific tracer. Siaens et al. [15] compared ^{99m}Tc-ciprofloxacin to another radiolabeled fluroquinolone, ^{99m}Tc-enrofloxacin, in rats with abscesses and sterile inflammations. They observed that infectious foci were best seen on 1-hour images, with subsequent wash-out over time, and that neither tracer demonstrated significant differences in abscess-to-muscle ratios among the various infections and inflammations studied. They found no evidence of specific bacterial binding by either tracer.

Antimicrobial peptides play a critical role in the biological defense system of multicellular organisms. They are produced by various cells, including phagocytes and endothelial and epithelial cells, and bind to the bacterial cell membrane. Their expression may be constant or induced on contact with microbial organisms; they also may be transported to sites of infection by WBCs [16]. Radiolabeled synthetic fragments of ubiquicidin (UBI), a naturally occurring human antimicrobial peptide that targets bacteria, possess the ability to differentiate infection from sterile inflammation. Imaging usually is completed within 1–2 hours after injection [17–20].

Selecting the appropriate tracer

At the present time, there appears to be little, if any, role for radiolabeled antibiotics for diagnosing infection, musculoskeletal or otherwise. The concept of radiolabeled antibiotics as infection-specific imaging agents is enticing, but flawed. It was presumed, in early investigations, that once inside, the agent would be retained within the bacterium, while unbound activity would be cleared, and radionuclide images would identify high concentrations of radiolabeled bacteria, i.e. foci of infection. More recent data have shown that this is not the case and much of the original enthusiasm for radiolabeled antibiotics as a diagnostic tool has waned.

The results for radiolabeled antimicrobials are encouraging, but these tracers are not yet available for routine clinical use. Thus, the choice left is between *in vitro*-labeled WBCs and anti-G mAbs/antibody fragments. The data suggest that, for diabetic foot infections, the accuracies of *in vitro*-labeled WBC and anti-G mAb imaging are comparable and the choice is governed by personal preference and availability. For diagnosing prosthetic joint infection, however, *in vitro*-labeled WBC imaging is superior to anti-G mAb imaging, primarily because of higher specificity and when available, should be used.

Normal findings and artifacts

Although the normal distribution of labeled WBCs varies to some degree with the method used for labeling, the labeled cells invariably accumulate in the bone marrow. As a result, labeled WBC imaging often must be performed in conjunction with bone marrow imaging to maximize the accuracy of the test. The reason for this is as follows. Although WBCs do not usually accumulate at sites of increased bone mineral turnover in the absence of infection, they do accumulate in the bone marrow. The normal distribution of hematopoietically active bone marrow in adults is variable. Systemic diseases such as sickle cell and Gaucher's disease produce generalized alterations in marrow distribution; fractures, orthopedic hardware, neuropathic joints and even calvarial hyperostosis can cause localized alterations. In children, the normal distribution of

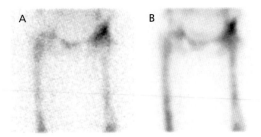

Figure 10.1 Old trauma left femur. There is increased activity in the left femoral head on the labeled WBC image (A) and the test could easily be interpreted as consistent with osteomyelitis. (B) The bone marrow image, however, is virtually identical to the WBC image and the combined study is negative for osteomyelitis.

hematopoietically active marrow varies with age. As a result, it is not always possible to determine if activity on a WBC image is due to infection or to bone marrow. This differentiation can be made easily and accurately by performing ^{99m}Tc-sulfur colloid bone marrow imaging. Both WBCs and sulfur colloid accumulate in the bone marrow; WBCs also accumulate in infection, while sulfur colloid does not. WBC/marrow imaging is positive for infection when activity is present on the WBC image without there being corresponding activity on the marrow image (Figures 10.1 and 10.2) [21].

WBC/marrow imaging can be performed in various ways; the precise methodology varies from institution to institution. Regardless of the protocol used, patients should be injected with 370 MBq (10 mCi) of freshly prepared ^{99m}Tc-sulfur colloid. Using preparations that are more than 1–2 hours old may result in a persistent blood pool, urinary bladder activity and decreased marrow uptake, all of which degrade image quality. The interval between injection and imaging should be at least 30 minutes. When using both ^{99m}Tc-labeled WBCs and ^{99m}Tc-labeled anti-G mAbs, because of potentially confounding activity on both WBC and marrow images, the two tests should be performed 48–72 hours apart [21].

WBC/marrow imaging has certain limitations and pitfalls. If WBCs do not migrate to the focus of infection, marrow imaging does not contribute any additional information. WBC accumulation in lymph nodes produces incongruent WBC/marrow images, even in the absence of infection. Careful examination of the images, however, usually reveals

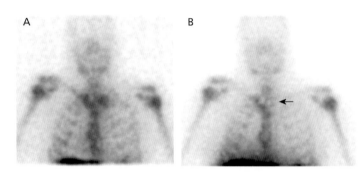

Figure 10.2 Sternoclavicular osteomyelitis. The labeled WBC image (A) is unremarkable. (B) On the bone marrow image there is a photopenic defect in the left half of the sternal manubrium and medial aspect of the left clavicle (arrow) and the combined study is positive for osteomyelitis. Intensity of uptake is not a useful criterion for diagnosing osteomyelitis on labeled WBC images.

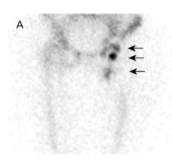
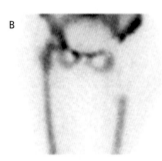

Figure 10.3 Lymph node activity. Nodal activity (arrows) can result in spatially incongruent WBC/marrow images and should not be misinterpreted as indicative of infection. Nodal activity usually is round and discrete, and may be unifocal or multifocal.

that the incongruent areas are round, discrete and often multiple (Figure 10.3) [21].

Animal data suggest that the marrow image becomes photopenic within about 1 week after the onset of the infection. Although this has not proven to be a problem when evaluating joint prostheses or the neuropathic joint, there are no human data that show how soon after the onset of osteomyelitis the marrow image becomes photopenic. Consequently, these studies should be interpreted cautiously in the acute setting [21,22].

Pathological findings and significance

Peripheral osteomyelitis

The sensitivity of combined WBC/marrow imaging for diagnosing osteomyelitis is about 90%. King et al. [23] studied 20 patients with combined WBC/marrow imaging and reported that the test accurately confirmed or excluded infection in all of them. Palestro et al. [24] performed combined WBC/marrow imaging on 73 patients with suspected musculoskeletal infection and reported that the test was 100% sensitive, 94% specific and 96% accurate for diagnosing osteomyelitis. Seabold et al. [25],

using albumin colloid for the bone marrow imaging component, reported that in 97 patients with previous surgical intervention, the sensitivity and specificity of combined WBC/marrow imaging was 88% and 92%, respectively. Achong and Oates [26], using a computer subtraction technique, reported a sensitivity, specificity and accuracy of 95%, 93% and 94%, respectively, for diagnosing osteomyelitis with combined WBC/marrow imaging.

The overall sensitivity of the AGA BW 250/183 for diagnosing osteomyelitis ranges from 69% in the hips to 100% in the lower leg and ankle [5,27]. Available data suggest that ^{99m}Tc-fanolesomab accurately diagnoses musculoskeletal infection (Figure 10.4). In one investigation it was compared to three-phase bone and ^{111}In-labeled WBC imaging [28]. Bone scintigraphy was sensitive (100%) but not specific (38%). ^{99m}Tc-fanolesomab was sensitive (91%), moderately specific (69%) and comparable to ^{111}In-labeled WBCs (91% sensitivity, 62% specificity).

The role of sulesomab for diagnosing musculoskeletal infection has been investigated extensively. Becker et al. [29] prospectively compared ^{99m}Tc-sulesomab and ^{99m}Tc-labeled WBCs, and

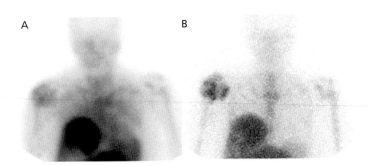

Figure 10.4 Septic arthritis right shoulder. (A) At 4 hours after injection of ^{99m}Tc-fanolesomab, there is abnormal activity in the right shoulder. (B) At 24 hours, the abnormal accumulation is more intense.

found that the sensitivity, specificity and accuracy of the radiolabeled antibody fragment, 91%, 90% and 91%, respectively, were slightly better than those of ^{99m}Tc-labeled WBCs (89%, 84% and 86%, respectively). Vicente et al. [30] reported that the test was 75% sensitive, 95% specific and 87% accurate for diagnosing acute osteomyelitis. Ivančević et al. [31] performed ^{99m}Tc-sulesomab imaging in 30 patients with previous bone injuries and possible "low-grade" bone infection. They found that although the test was very sensitive (100%), it was not specific (58%), and concluded that this agent was reliable for excluding but not for proving the presence of infection. Ryan [32] retrospectively reviewed ^{99m}Tc-sulesomab imaging in 55 patients with suspected orthopedic infection and came to similar conclusions. Devillers et al. [33] prospectively compared ^{99m}Tc-sulesomab to ^{99m}Tc-labeled WBCs in 23 patients with possible osteomyelitis. These investigators found that it was less sensitive (86% vs. 93%) and less specific (72% vs. 100%) than ^{99m}Tc-labeled WBCs. Von Rothenburg et al. [34] retrospectively evaluated 30 patients with suspected osteomyelitis and reported a sensitivity of 95% and a specificity of 65% for ^{99m}Tc-sulesomab.

There are limited data on the role of ^{99m}Tc-IL-8 for diagnosing musculoskeletal infection. In a rabbit model of acute osteomyelitis, ^{99m}Tc-IL-8 clearly showed the area of osteomyelitis. Although absolute uptake of ^{99m}Tc-IL-8 in the focus of infection was significantly lower than that of ^{99m}Tc-methyl diphosphonate (MDP) and ^{67}Ga-citrate, the target-to-background ratio was higher with the radiolabeled cytokine due to its rapid background clearance [35].

Published data indicate that single-photon emission CT (SPECT)/CT improves the accuracy of the radionuclide studies used for diagnosing osteomyelitis, primarily through improved localization of

tracer accumulation. The contribution of SPECT/CT in patients suspected of having osteomyelitis, including 21 who underwent ^{67}Ga-citrate imaging and 11 who underwent ^{111}In-labeled WBC imaging, was studied by Bar Shalom et al. [36]. In this investigation SPECT/CT was helpful in about half the patients, primarily by providing precise anatomical localization and delineation of the extent of the infection. Horger et al. [37], using a ^{99m}Tc-labeled anti-G mAb, studied 27 patients with a history of trauma and superimposed bone infection. The accuracy of scintigraphy including SPECT was 59%. The accuracy of SPECT/CT was 97%. SPECT/CT was especially useful for distinguishing soft tissue infection from osteomyelitis in the appendicular skeleton. In another investigation, Horger et al. [38] compared SPECT/CT to SPECT in three-phase bone imaging performed on 31 patients, nine of whom had osteomyelitis. Although the sensitivities of the three-phase bone with SPECT and SPECT/CT both were 78%, SPECT/CT was significantly more specific than bone scintigraphy with SPECT (86% vs. 50%, p < 0.05). The CT component improved specificity by excluding active bone infection and by identifying causes besides infection that were responsible for increased tracer accumulation.

Filippi et al. [39] compared ^{99m}Tc-exametazime-labeled WBC imaging with SPECT and SPECT/CT in 28 patients with suspected musculoskeletal infection, and reported that the accuracy improved from 64% for scintigraphy with SPECT to 100% for SPECT/CT. SPECT/CT altered study interpretation in more than one-third of the patients. The CT component of the test improved localization of labeled WBC activity, making it possible to exclude osteomyelitis in seven patients and to provide more precise delineation of the extent of infection in three patients.

Diabetic foot infection

A diabetic foot infection is defined as an inframalleolar infection in a person with diabetes mellitus. These infections, which are common, complex and costly, cause substantial morbidity, are responsible for the largest number of diabetes-related hospital bed-days and are the most common cause of non-traumatic lower extremity amputations. The major predisposing factor to infection in the diabetic foot is the mal perforans ulcer, which results from trauma or excessive pressure on a foot lacking protective sensation. Once the cutaneous integument is breached, the wound may become actively infected and, by contiguous extension, infection can involve deeper tissues, including the bone [40].

Diabetic patients with a significant foot infection may lack pain and fail to mount a systemic inflammatory response, and the diagnosis of osteomyelitis often is overlooked [40]. Imaging studies therefore, are an important part of the diagnostic evaluation of these individuals. The sensitivity of ^{111}In-labeled WBC imaging for diagnosing pedal osteomyelitis in diabetics ranges from 72% to 100% and the specificity from 67% to 100% [40–46]. Newman et al. [45], in one of the largest prospective investigations reported, evaluated 41 foot ulcers in 35 diabetic patients. Final diagnoses were based on histolopathological and microbiological analysis of bone specimens in all cases. Patients underwent imaging at 4 and 24 hours after injection of labeled cells. Focally increased activity of approximately the same intensity on the dorsal and plantar views was the criterion for osteomyelitis (Figure 10.5). Osteomyelitis was present in 28 (68%) of the 41 ulcers. The sensitivity of 24-hour ^{111}In-labeled WBC imaging was 89% and the specificity was 69%.

Twenty-four hour ^{111}In-labeled WBC imaging was the most accurate (82%) test for diagnosing pedal osteomyelitis in this investigation. It was more sensitive (89% vs. 69%) and more specific (69% vs. 39%) than three-phase bone scintigraphy. Palestro et al. [46], in a prospective investigation of 25 patients, using the criterion of Newman et al. [45], reported a sensitivity and specificity of 80% and 67%, respectively for ^{111}In-labeled WBC imaging.

The reported sensitivities and specificities of [99mTc]-labeled WBC imaging for diagnosing diabetic pedal osteomyelitis are similar to those reported for ^{111}In-labeled WBC imaging, ranging from 86% to 93% and from 80% to 98%, respectively [40]. Familiari et al. [47], in an intraindividual comparison of 13 patients, reported that planar [99mTc]-labeled WBC imaging was more accurate than [^{18}F]FDG-PET/CT for diagnosing pedal osteomyelitis in diabetics.

Most diabetic patients who undergo evaluation for pedal osteomyelitis present with an ulcer in the distal forefoot. A less frequent complication that usually develops in the mid or hind foot is the neuropathic, or Charcot, joint. Repetitive stress on an insensitive foot leads to bone and joint disruption, deformity and instability, which lead to degeneration, subluxation and destruction of the joint, resulting in a grossly deformed foot. Although infection is a relatively uncommon complication, differentiating between infection and the neuropathic joint, or diagnosing infection superimposed on the neuropathic joint, can be challenging. It is important to recognize that labeled WBCs accumulate in the uninfected neuropathic joint. This uptake is due, at least in part, to the presence of hematopoietically active marrow. As with other sites in the

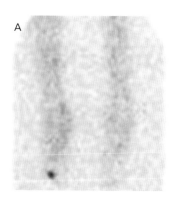
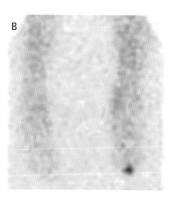

Figure 10.5 Osteomyelitis of the right great toe. Using focally increased activity on (A) dorsal and (B) plantar views as the criterion for osteomyelitis, the accuracy of labeled WBC imaging for diagnosing osteomyelitis of the distal forefoot in diabetics with pedal ulcers is about 80%.

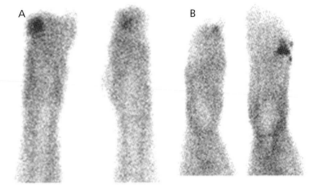

Figure 10.6 Pedal osteomyelitis. There is focally increased activity in the first digit of the right foot and the fourth and fifth digits of the left foot, on both (A) dorsal and (B) plantar views of a study acquired 1 hour after injection of the anti-G mAb ^{99m}Tc-fanolesomab.

skeleton, performing complementary marrow imaging facilitates the differentiation of WBC uptake in bone marrow from uptake in infection [40,48].

WBC images lack anatomical detail and it has been suggested that the addition of bone scintigraphy facilitates the differentiation of soft tissue and bone infection. Published data, however, suggest that any improvement in accuracy is marginal. Keenan et al. [41] reported that for diagnosing pedal osteomyelitis, the accuracies of ^{111}In-labeled WBC imaging alone or in combination with bone scintigraphy were identical: 87%. Johnson et al. [44] reported that the accuracy of ^{111}In-labeled WBC imaging rose from 86% (19/22) when interpreted alone, to 91% (20/22) when interpreted together with the bone scan. Palestro et al. [46] reported that the accuracy of ^{111}In-labeled WBC imaging alone was 72% (18/25). When combined with bone imaging, the accuracy of the test was 80% (20/25). The addition of bone imaging changed ^{111}In-labeled WBC image interpretation in only two (8%) of 25 patients. In the remaining 23 (92%) patients, the bone scan did not affect ^{111}In-labeled WBC interpretation. It has been our experience that the bone scan is not useful in the evaluation of diabetic foot infections and we stopped performing this test several years ago.

In an investigation of 25 diabetic patients, Dominguez-Gadea et al. [49] reported that the radiolabeled anti-G mAb, BW 250/183, was 93% sensitive, 78% specific and 84% accurate for diagnosing pedal osteomyelitis, similar to what has been reported for *in vitro*-labeled WBC imaging.

In another investigation, 25 diabetic patients with pedal ulcers underwent ^{99m}Tc-fanolesomab,

[111]In-labled WBC and three-phase bone imaging [46]. The sensitivity, specificity and accuracy of ^{99m}Tc-fanolesomab were 90%, 67% and 76%, respectively, comparable to those obtained with ^{111}In-labeled WBC imaging: 80%, 67% and 72%, respectively (Figure 10.6). ^{99m}Tc-fanolesomab was as sensitive as and significantly more specific than (p = 0.004) three-phase bone imaging.

Harwood et al. [50] performed ^{99m}Tc-sulesomab imaging on 122 diabetic patients with foot ulcers and reported 91% sensitivity, 56% specificity and 80% accuracy for the test. In a subgroup of patients who also underwent WBC imaging, the accuracy of ^{99m}Tc-sulesomab was comparable to that of WBC imaging (81% vs. 75%) (Figure 10.7). It was significantly more specific than bone scintigraphy (50% vs. 21%; p < 0.05) in patients who underwent both tests. Delcourt et al. [51] prospectively compared combined ^{99m}Tc-sulesomab/bone and bone/^{67}Ga-citrate imaging in 25 diabetic patients with 31 sites of suspected pedal osteomyelitis. The sensitivity, specificity and accuracy of ^{99m}Tc-sulesomab/bone imaging were 67%, 85% and 74% and of bone/^{67}Ga-citrate imaging were 44%, 77% and 58%, respectively. Rubello et al. [52] found that the specificity of the test for diagnosing pedal osteomyelitis in diabetics improved from 75% to 88%, without any loss in sensitivity (91%) by performing imaging at 4 and 24 hours, rather than just at 4 hours.

In eight diabetic patients with foot infections ^{131}I-IL-8 rapidly accumulated within foci of infection but not in treated infections or degenerative joint disease [14].

Data on the role of radiolabeled antibiotics and antimicrobials in the evaluation of diabetic foot infections are lacking.

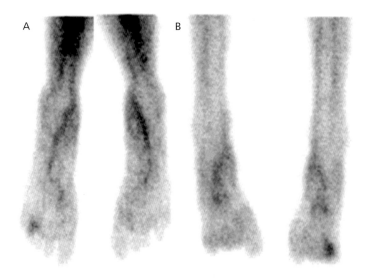

Figure 10.7 Pedal osteomyelitis. There is focally increased activity in the fourth digit of the left foot, on both (A) plantar and (B) dorsal views of a study acquired 1 hour after injection of the anti-G mAb fragment ^{99m}Tc-sulesomab.

Heiba *et al.* [53] reported on the value of combined SPECT/CT imaging using ^{111}In-labeled WBCs, bone scintigraphy and, when necessary, bone marrow imaging, for diagnosis and localization of diabetic foot infections. Dual-isotope SPECT/CT imaging was performed 24 hours after tracer injection. These investigators found that simultaneous dual-isotope (^{111}In-labeled WBC + ^{99m}Tc-MDP) SPECT/CT was significantly more accurate than planar imaging. They also observed that dual-isotope SPECT/CT was significantly more accurate than single-isotope (bone or labeled WBC) SPECT/ CT. The authors found that, because of the poor resolution in ^{111}In-labeled WBC imaging and the small structures being evaluated, it was not always possible, even with the CT component, to distinguish between soft tissue and bone infection. In their experience, the addition of bone SPECT/CT permitted precise localization of labeled WBC accumulation, improving both accuracy and confidence of diagnosis. Although these results demonstrate the incremental value of performing an additional nuclear medicine procedure, there are practical matters, such as patient convenience, cost and additional radiation that must be considered and likely will limit acceptance of this procedure. An alternative and perhaps more practical approach is to use ^{99m}Tc- rather than ^{111}In-labeled WBCs. Image resolution is substantially better and both labeling and imaging can be performed on the same day. Filippi *et al.* [54] studied the contribution of SPECT/CT to

^{99m}Tc-exametazime-labeled WBC imaging of diabetic foot infections. Seventeen patients with 19 clinically suspected sites of infection were included. Planar imaging was performed at 30 minutes, 4 hours and 24 hours. SPECT/CT was performed at 6 hours. Abnormal labeled WBC accumulation was present in 16 of the 19 sites. SPECT/CT changed the interpretation of the planar and SPECT images in 10 of the 19 (53%) sites, excluding osteomyelitis in six cases, identifying osteomyelitis in one site and better defining the extent of disease (osteomyelitis plus soft tissue infection) in three sites. SPECT/CT did not significantly contribute to the evaluation of patients with negative scan results. The authors concluded that ^{99m}Tc-exametazime-labeled WBC imaging with SPECT/CT is a potentially useful test for diagnosing diabetic foot infection by differentiating bone and soft tissue involvement, and by more precisely defining the extent of disease, thereby facilitating treatment planning and avoiding more invasive procedures.

Prosthetic joint infection

More than one million lower extremity arthroplasties are performed annually throughout the world. Although results in most cases are excellent, implants do fail. Differentiating aseptic loosening, the most common cause of prosthetic joint failure, from infection can be challenging. Clinical signs of infection often are absent; laboratory tests are neither sensitive nor specific. Joint aspiration with

Gram stain and culture is the definitive diagnostic test, with specificity in excess of 90%: the sensitivity of the test is more variable, however, ranging from 28% to 92%. Plain radiographs are neither sensitive nor specific and cross-sectional imaging modalities, such as CT and MRI, are limited by hardware-induced artifacts (see Chapter 3). Radionuclide imaging is not affected by orthopedic hardware and is the current imaging modality of choice for diagnosing suspected joint replacement infection [55].

Bone scintigraphy is sensitive for identifying the failed joint replacement, but cannot determine the cause of failure and is best used as a screening test, or in combination with other radionuclide studies. Sequential bone/^{67}Ga-citrate imaging, with an accuracy of 65–80%, offers only modest improvement over the 50–70% accuracy of bone scintigraphy alone [55].

WBC/marrow imaging has an accuracy of about 90% and is the radionuclide procedure of choice for diagnosing prosthetic joint infection (Figures 10.8 and 10.9) [55–63]. Mulamba *et al.* [56] reported a sensitivity of 92% and a specificity of 100% for diagnosing infected hip replacements with WBC/marrow imaging. Palestro *et al.* [57] investigated WBC/marrow imaging in 50 painful total hip replacements and found that the study was 100% sensitive and 97% specific for diagnosing infection. These investigators found that ^{111}In-labeled WBC/marrow imaging was equally satisfactory for the evaluation of painful knee prostheses and was superior to bone scintigraphy (including three-phase) alone, ^{111}In-labeled WBC imaging alone and combined ^{111}In-labeled WBC/bone imaging [58]. In an investigation of 59 failed lower extremity joint replacements, all with surgically, histopathologi-

cally and microbiologically confirmed diagnoses, Love *et al.* [59] reported that the sensitivity, specificity and accuracy of ^{111}In-labeled WBC/marrow imaging for diagnosing prosthetic joint infection were 100%, 91% and 95%, respectively. Love *et al.* [60] presented data on 150 failed joint prostheses with surgically, histopathologically and microbiologically confirmed final diagnoses. In this investigation the sensitivity, specificity and accuracy of WBC/marrow imaging were 96%, 87% and 91%, respectively. The test was significantly more accurate than bone (50%), bone/^{67}Ga-citrate (66%) and WBC/bone (70%) in their series.

Pelosi *et al.* [63] reported that acquiring WBC images at multiple time points may serve as a surrogate and obviate the need for marrow scintigraphy. Presumably, early images reflect WBC uptake in marrow, while late images reflect WBC uptake in infection. Incongruence between early and late

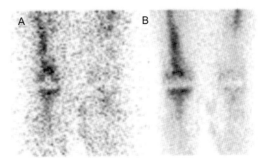

Figure 10.8 Aseptically loosened right knee replacement. There is intensely increased periprosthetic activity on the labeled WBC image (A). The distribution of activity on the bone marrow image (B) is spatially congruent, however, and the combined study is negative for infection.

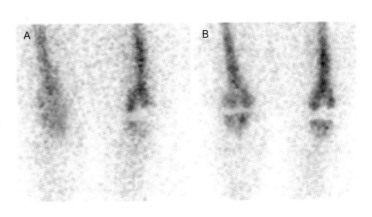

Figure 10.9 Infected right knee replacement. The distribution of activity on the labeled WBC (A) and bone marrow (B) images is spatially incongruent and the combined study is positive for infection. Note the striking periprosthetic activity around the asymptomatic left knee replacement on both the labeled WBC and marrow images.

images is indicative of infection. Using visual analysis, the accuracy of this dual time-point imaging was only about 75%; using semi-quantitative analysis, the accuracy improved to about 95%.

The results of BW 250/183 for diagnosing prosthetic joint infection have been variable. Boubaker et al. [64], in an investigation of 78 hip prostheses, reported a sensitivity and specificity of 67% and 75%, respectively, when the study was interpreted alone. Interpreted together with bone scintigraphy, specificity improved to 84%, while sensitivity was unchanged at 67%. Gratz et al. [65] reported a sensitivity, specificity and accuracy of 91%, 66% and 80%, respectively, for the anti-G mAb alone. When interpreted together with bone scintigraphy, sensitivity, specificity and accuracy improved to 94%, 88% and 89%, respectively. Klett et al. [66] reported that sensitivity and specificity of the test for diagnosing prosthetic hip infection improved from 86% and 57%, respectively, to 100% and 93%, respectively, when semi-quantitative analysis was used. Klett et al. [67] obtained similar results in an investigation of knee replacements.

Several investigators have studied the role of ^{99m}Tc-sulesomab in the evaluation of prosthetic joint infection (see clinical case 2 below). Von Rothenburg et al. [68] evaluated ^{99m}Tc-sulesomab imaging in 38 patients with lower extremity joint replacements, 15 of which were infected. They reported a sensitivity of 93% and a specificity of 65%, and concluded that a negative result reliably excludes infection, while a positive result requires additional investigation. Iyengar et al. [69], in an investigation of 38 upper and lower extremity prosthetic joints, also found the test to be more sensitive (91%) than specific (81%), and like von Rothenberg et al. [68] concluded that a negative result reliably excludes infection. Pakos et al. [70] reported that ^{99m}Tc-sulesomab was only 75% sensitive, 86% specific and 79% accurate for diagnosing prosthetic joint infection. Rubello et al. [52,71] reported that the specificity could be improved by performing early (4-hour) and late (20–24-hour) imaging. In an investigation of 78 knee prostheses, the specificity improved from 78% for early imaging alone to 100% for dual time-point imaging with no change in sensitivity, which was 93% [71]. Gratz et al. [72] reported that quantitative evaluation of time–activity curves significantly improved the accuracy

of the test for diagnosing moderate and mild prosthetic joint infections.

Larikka et al. [73] reported that ^{99m}Tc-ciprofloxacin was 86% sensitive and 78% specific for diagnosing prosthetic knee infection. These investigators reported that the specificity was maximized by obtaining delayed, next-day imaging. In an investigation of 30 painful hip prostheses, Larikka et al. [74] reported that, using next-day imaging, ^{99m}Tc-ciprofloxacin was more accurate than ^{99m}Tc-labeled WBCs (97% vs. 90%) for diagnosing infection. In an animal investigation, Sarda et al. [75] reported that ^{99m}Tc-ciprofloxacin was sensitive but not specific for diagnosing prosthetic joint infection.

Sarda-Mantel et al. [76] evaluated an animal model of prosthetic joint infection with ^{99m}Tc-UBI 29-41 and observed that while all six infected devices were positive on day nine, only four of the six were positive on day 20. They hypothesized that decreased sensitivity over time may have been related to the effects of the protective biofilm or glycocalyx secreted by the bacteria. These data suggest that this agent would be of limited value in the clinical setting, since patients typically are symptomatic for some time before undergoing radionuclide evaluation of their prosthetic joint.

Few data are available about the role of SPECT/CT in the evaluation of prosthetic joint infection. Kasidis et al. [77] evaluated septic loosening of hip prostheses with anti-G mAb scintigraphy and reported that SPECT/CT corroborated the anti-G mAb scintigraphy results in three patients. Graute et al. [78] studied 31 cases of suspected lower extremity prosthetic joint infection with both planar and SPECT/CT imaging using the ^{99m}Tc-radiolabeled anti-G mAb, BW 250/183. Sensitivity, specificity and accuracy of planar imaging alone were 66%, 60% and 61%, respectively. When planar images were interpreted together with SPECT, sensitivity increased to 89%, but specificity decreased to 45% and accuracy fell to 58%. When planar images were interpreted together with SPECT/CT, sensitivity remained at 89% and specificity and accuracy increased to 73% and 77%, respectively. Although SPECT/CT improved the accuracy of the test, the 77% accuracy reported by the authors is no better than what other investigators have reported for planar imaging alone with the same antibody and considerably less than the 90% accuracy of combined planar WBC/marrow imaging for the same indication [55,64–67].

Sternal wound infections

Median sternotomy wound complications vary from sterile wound dehiscence to suppurative mediastinitis. Mediastinal, or sternal, wound infections are characterized by clinical or microbiological evidence of infected presternal tissue and sternal osteomyelitis, with or without mediastinal sepsis and with or without unstable sternum. Superficial sternal wound infection is confined to the subcutaneous tissue. Deep wound infection, or mediastinitis, is associated with sternal osteomyelitis with or without retrosternal space infection [79].

Although the incidence of sternal wound infection in patients undergoing median sternotomy is less than 1%, its associated mortality rate varies from 14% to 47%. The classic symptoms and signs of acute infection are infrequently encountered and can be obscured by associated postoperative pain or concomitant infection. Wound discharge, the most common presentation, is present in up to 70–90% of cases; local symptoms include wound pain, tenderness and sternal instability. Daily clinical evaluation of patients in the immediate postoperative period and a high index of suspicion are the most important factors in ensuring early diagnosis. Blood cultures should be performed in patients with a temperature above 38 °C that persists for more than 48 hours after surgery. Chest radiographs rarely are helpful. CT with mediastinal aspiration provides useful information both for diagnosis and management [79].

Radionuclide imaging also contributes useful information in patients with suspected sternal wound infection [80–86]. Cooper *et al.* [82] studied ^{99m}Tc-labeled WBC imaging in 29 patients with suspected sternal wound infections. They found that the test was 100% sensitive and 89% specific for diagnosing deep sternal wound infection, and suggested that labeled WBC imaging is a useful adjunct when clinical examination fails to confirm the diagnosis or when deep sternal aspirates of a sternal wound infection are not diagnostic. Bessette *et al.* [83] compared CT and dual-isotope SPECT (^{99m}Tc-MDP/^{111}In-labeled WBC) in 32 patients with possible postoperative sternal osteomyelitis following

median sternotomy. These authors found that the radionuclide test was more accurate than CT for differentiating soft tissue inflammation from sternal osteomyelitis.

Quirce *et al.* [84] prospectively investigated planar scintigraphy and ^{99m}Tc-labeled WBC SPECT in 41 patients with clinically suspected deep sternal infection. Nine patients had deep sternal infection, ten had superficial sternal infection and 22 had no infection. Planar imaging failed to detect any of the deep sternal infections at either 4 or 20 hours. SPECT correctly identified eight of nine deep sternal infections at 4 hours and all of them at 20 hours, with no false-positive results. Planar imaging identified 16 of 18 superficial sternal infections at 4 hours and all of them at 20 hours. SPECT identified 17 of 18 infections at 4 hours and all of them at 20 hours. Other infections unrelated to the sternotomy were identified in seven patients. The authors concluded that labeled WBC imaging reliably diagnoses sternal infection after median sternotomy and SPECT facilitates the differentiation of superficial from deep sternal infection. The test also detects other sites of infection, providing alternative diagnoses.

Bitkover *et al.* [85] investigated the anti-G mAb, BW 250/183, for diagnosing sternal infection in 29 patients who had undergone median sternotomy, including five patients with a normal postoperative course who served as controls. SPECT was performed 4 and 20 hours after injection. Twenty-three patients underwent imaging at both time points; six underwent only early imaging. Seven of eight infections were detected. The one false-negative scan occurred in a patient who had early imaging only. All five controls had negative studies. The authors concluded that SPECT reliably distinguishes between superficial and deep sternal infection and that early and late imaging should be performed for optimal results.

Role for therapy follow-up and patient management

It often has been suggested that nuclear medicine procedures are useful for monitoring response to therapy. Substantive data, however, are scant. Palestro *et al.* [24], as part of larger series, reported on three patients with musculoskeletal infection who underwent labeled WBC imaging before and after antibiotic therapy. In two patients the post-therapy studies reverted to normal. At subsequent surgery, both patients were confirmed to be free of infection. One patient had a persistently abnormal study following therapy and operative cultures grew *Staphylococcus aureus*. Newman *et al.* [45] performed follow-up labeled WBC imaging on 21 diabetic patients with pedal osteomyelitis. Intensity of uptake decreased with increasing duration of antibiotic therapy and eventually normalized in 19 of the 21 patients. One of the two patients with a persistently abnormal study was diagnosed with recurrent osteomyelitis; the other patient expired during the investigation. The authors concluded that image intensity on labeled WBC studies parallels the clinical course during antibiotic treatment and may be useful for monitoring patients early in the course of therapy.

Determining the ability of a test to accurately monitor response to treatment in the patient with infection is a complex process. First and foremost the test must be able to diagnose the initial infection accurately. Equally important to the assessment of the accuracy of follow-up studies is the ability to differentiate between persistent or recurrent and new infection. If the organisms are different, it can be assumed that the infection is new. Suppose the organisms are the same, is the infection persistent/recurrent or is it new? Though an interesting concept, there currently are few data available to substantiate the value of radionuclide studies in monitoring therapeutic response in infection.

References

1. Osman DR. Diagnosis and management of musculoskeletal infection. In: Fitzgerald RH, Haufer H, Malkani RL (eds). *Orthopedics*. St. Louis: Mosby, 2002, pp. 695–707.

2. Palestro CJ, Love C, Miller TT. Imaging of musculoskeletal infections. *Best Pract Res Clin Rheumatol* 2006;20:1197–1218.

3. Love C, Palestro CJ. Radionuclide imaging of infection. *J Nucl Med Tech* 2004;32:47–57.

4. Duncker CM, Carrió I, Berná L *et al.* Radioimmune imaging of bone marrow in patients with suspected bone metastases from primary breast cancer. *J Nucl Med* 1990;31:1450–1455.

5. Weiner RE, Thakur ML. Imaging infection/inflammations. *Q J Nucl Med* 1999;43:2–8.

6. Becker W, Goldenberg DM, Wolf F. The use of monoclonal antibodies and antibody fragments in the imaging of infectious lesions. *Semin Nucl Med* 1994; 24:142–153.

7. Love C, Palestro CJ. ^{99m}Tc-fanolesomab palatin technologies. *IDrugs* 2003;6:1079–1085.

8. Love C, Tronco GG, Palestro CJ. ^{99m}Tc-Fanolesomab: A new agent for imaging infection and inflammation. *Q J Nucl Med Mol Imaging* 2006;50:113–120.

9. Skehan SJ, White JF, Evans JW *et al.* Mechanism of accumulation of ^{99m}Tc-sulesomab in inflammation. *J Nucl Med* 2003;44:11–18.

10. Rennen HJJM, Boerman OC, Oyen WJG *et al.* Specific and rapid scintigraphic detection of infection with ^{99m}Tc-Labeled interleukin-8. *J Nucl Med* 2001;42: 117–123.

11. Van der Laken CJ, Boerman OC, Oyen WJ *et al.* The kinetics of radiolabelled interleukin-8 in infection and sterile inflammation. *Nucl Med Commun* 1998;19: 271–281.

12. Laterveer L, Lindley IJ, Heemskerk DP *et al.* Rapid mobilization of hematopoietic progenitor cells in rhesus monkeys by a single intravenous injection of interleukin-8. *Blood* 1996;87:781–788.

13. Van Zee KJ, Fischer E, Hawes AS *et al.* Effects of intravenous IL-8 administration in nonhuman primates. *J Immunol* 1992;148:1746–1752.

14. Gross MD, Shapiro B, Fig LM *et al.* Imaging of human infection with (131)I-labeled recombinant human interleukin-8. *J Nucl Med* 2001;42:1656–1659.

15. Siaens RH, Rennen HJ, Boerman OC *et al.* Synthesis and comparison of 99mTc-enrofloxacin and ^{99m}Tc-ciprofloxacin. *J Nucl Med* 2004;45:2088–2094.

16. Lupetti A, Pauwels EKJ, Nibbering PH *et al.* 99mTc-antimicrobial peptides: promising candidates for infection imaging. *Q J Nucl Med* 2003;47:238–245.

17. Welling MM, Paulusma-Annema A, Balter HS *et al.* Technetium-99m labelled anti-microbial peptides discriminate between bacterial infections and sterile inflammations. *Eur J Nucl Med* 2000;27: 292–301.

18. Welling MM, Lupetti A, Balter HS *et al.* ^{99m}Tc-labeled antimicrobial peptides for detection of bacterial and Candida albicans infections. *J Nucl Med* 2001;42: 788–794.

19. Lupetti A, Welling MM, Mazzi U *et al.* Technetium-99m labelled fluconazole and antimicrobial peptides for imaging of *Candida albicans* and *Aspergillus fumigatus* infections. *Eur J Nucl Med Mol Imaging* 2002;29: 674–679.

20. Welling MM, Mongera S, Lupetti A *et al.* Radiochemical and biological characteristics of ^{99m}Tc-UBI 29-41 for imaging of bacterial infections. *Nucl Med Biol* 2002;29:413–422.

21. Palestro CJ, Love C, Tronco GG *et al.* Combined labeled leukocyte and technetium-99m sulfur colloid marrow imaging for diagnosing musculoskeletal infection:

principles, technique, interpretation, indications and limitations. *RadioGraphics* 2006;26:859–870.

22. Palestro CJ, Love C. Radionuclide imaging of musculoskeletal infection: conventional agents. *Semin Musculoskelet Radiol* 2007;11:335–352.

23. King AD, Peters AM, Stuttle AW *et al.* Imaging of bone infection with labelled white blood cells: role of contemporaneous bone marrow imaging. *Eur J Nucl Med* 1990;17:148–151.

24. Palestro CJ, Roumanas P, Swyer AJ *et al.* Diagnosis of musculoskeletal infection using combined In-111 labeled leukocyte and Tc-99m SC marrow imaging. *Clin Nucl Med* 1992;17:269–273.

25. Seabold JE, Nepola JV, Marsh JL *et al.* Postoperative bone marrow alterations: potential pitfalls in the diagnosis of osteomyelitis with In-111-labeled leukocyte scintigraphy. *Radiology* 1991;180:741–747.

26. Achong DM, Oates E. The computer-generated bone marrow subtraction image: a valuable adjunct to combined In-111 WBC/Tc-99m in sulfur colloid scintigraphy for musculoskeletal infection. *Clin Nucl Med* 1994;19:188–193.

27. Becker W. The contribution of nuclear medicine to the patient with infection. *Eur J Nucl Med* 1995;22:1195–1211.

28. Palestro CJ, Kipper SL, Weiland FL *et al.* Osteomyelitis: Diagnosis with ^{99m}Tc-labeled antigranulocyte antibodies compared with diagnosis with indium-111-labeled leukocytes-initial experience. *Radiology* 2002;223:758–764.

29. Becker W, Palestro CJ, Winship J *et al.* Rapid imaging of infections with a monoclonal antibody fragment (LeukoScan). *Clin Orthop Relat Res* 1996;329:263–272.

30. Vicente AG, Almoguera M, Alonso JC *et al.* Diagnosis of orthopedic infection in clinical practice using Tc-99m sulesomab (antigranulocyte monoclonal antibody fragment Fab'2). *Clin Nucl Med* 2004;29:781–785.

31. Ivančević V, Perka C, Hasart O *et al.* Imaging of low-grade bone infection with a technetium-99m labelled monoclonal anti-NCA-90 Fab' fragment in patients with previous joint surgery. *Eur J Nucl Med Mol Imaging* 2002;29:547–551.

32. Ryan PJ. Leukoscan for orthopaedic imaging in clinical practice. *Nucl Med Commun* 2002;23:707–714.

33. Devillers A, Garin E, Polard JL *et al.* Comparison of Tc-99m-labelled antileukocyte fragment Fab' and Tc-99m-HMPAO leukocyte scintigraphy in the diagnosis of bone and joint infections: a prospective study. *Nucl Med Commun* 2000;21:747–753.

34. Von Rothenburg T, Schaffstein J, Ludvig J *et al.* Imaging osteomyelitis with Tc-99m-labeled antigranulocyte antibody Fab' fragments. *Clin Nucl Med* 2003;28:643–647.

35. Gratz S, Rennen HJ, Boerman OC *et al.* (99m) Tc-interleukin-8 for imaging acute osteomyelitis. *J Nucl Med* 2001;42:1257–1264.

36. Bar-Shalom R, Yefremov N, Guralnik L *et al.* SPECT/CT using 67Ga and 111In-labeled leukocyte scintigraphy for diagnosis of infection. *J Nucl Med* 2006;47:587–594.

37. Horger M, Eschmann SM, Pfannenberg C *et al.* The value of SPET/CT in chronic osteomyelitis. *Eur J Nucl Med Mol Imaging* 2003;30:1665–1673.

38. Horger M, Eschmann SM, Pfannenberg C *et al.* Added value of SPECT/CT in patients suspected of having bone infection: preliminary results. *Arch Orthop Trauma Surg* 2007;127:211–221

39. Filippi L, Schillaci O. Usefulness of hybrid SPECT/CT in ^{99m}Tc-HMPAO-labeled leukocyte scintigraphy for bone and joint infections. *J Nucl Med* 2006;47:1908–1913.

40. Palestro CJ, Love C. Nuclear medicine and diabetic foot infections. *Semin Nucl Med* 2009;39:52–65.

41. Keenan AM, Tindel NL, Alavi A. Diagnosis of pedal osteomyelitis in diabetic patients using current scintigraphic techniques. *Arch Intern Med* 1989;149:2262–2266.

42. Larcos G, Brown ML, Sutton R. Diagnosis of osteomyelitis of the foot in diabetic patients: value of 111In-leukocyte scintigraphy. *AJR Am J Roentgenol* 1991;157:527–531.

43. Maurer AH, Millmond SH, Knight LC *et al.* Infection in diabetic osteoarthropathy: Use of indium-labeled leukocytes for diagnosis. *Radiology* 1986;151:221–225.

44. Johnson JE, Kennedy EJ, Shereff MJ *et al.* Prospective study of bone, indium-111-labeled white blood cell, and gallium-67 scanning for the evaluation of osteomyelitis in the diabetic foot. *Foot Ankle Int* 1996;17:10–16.

45. Newman LG, Waller J, Palestro CJ *et al.* Unsuspected osteomyelitis in diabetic foot ulcers. Diagnosis and monitoring by leukocyte scanning with indium In111 oxyquinoline. *JAMA* 1991;266:1246–1251.

46. Palestro CJ, Caprioli R, Love C *et al.* Rapid diagnosis of pedal osteomyelitis in diabetics with a technetium-99m labeled monoclonal antigranulocyte antibody. *J Foot Ankle Surg* 2003;42:2–8.

47. Familiari D, Glaudemans AW, Vitale V *et al.* Can sequential ^{18}F-FDG PET/CT replace WBC imaging in the diabetic foot? *J Nucl Med* 2011;52:1012–1019.

48. Palestro CJ, Mehta HH, Patel M *et al.* Marrow versus infection in the Charcot joint: Indium-111 leukocyte and technetium-99m sulfur colloid scintigraphy. *J Nucl Med* 1998;39:346–350.

49. Dominguez-Gadea L, Martin-Curto LM, de la Calle H *et al.* Diabetic foot infections: scintigraphic evaluation with 99Tcm-labelled anti-granulocyte antibodies. *Nucl Med Commun* 1993;14:212–218.

50. Harwood SJ, Valdivia S, Hung GL et al. Use of Sulesomab, a radiolabeled antibody fragment, to detect osteomyelitis in diabetic patients with foot ulcers by leukoscintigraphy. *Clin Infect Dis* 1999; 28:1200–1205.

51. Delcourt A, Huglo D, Prangere T et al. Comparison between Leukoscan® (Sulesomab) and gallium-67 for the diagnosis of osteomyelitis in the diabetic foot. *Diabetes Metab* 2005;31:125–133.

52. Rubello D, Casara D, Maran A et al. Role of anti-granulocyte Fab′ fragment antibody scintigraphy (LeukoScan) in evaluating bone infection: acquisition protocol, interpretation criteria and clinical results. *Nucl Med Commun* 2004;25:39–47.

53. Heiba SI, Kolker D, Mocherla B et al. The optimized evaluation of diabetic foot infection by dual isotope SPECT/CT imaging protocol. *J Foot Ankle Surg* 2010; 49:529–536.

54. Filippi L, Uccioli L, Giurato L et al. Diabetic foot infection: usefulness of SPECT/CT for ^{99m}Tc-HMPAO-labeled leukocyte imaging. *J Nucl Med* 2009;50: 1042–1046.

55. Love C, Marwin SE, Palestro CJ. Nuclear medicine and the infected joint replacement. *Semin Nucl Med* 2009;39:66–78.

56. Mulamba L'AH, Ferrant A, Leners N et al. Indium-111 leucocyte scanning in the evaluation of painful hip arthroplasty. *Acta Orthop Scand* 1983;54: 695–697.

57. Palestro CJ, Kim CK, Swyer AJ et al. Total hip arthroplasty: periprosthetic indium-111-labeled leukocyte activity and complementary technetium-99m-sulfur colloid imaging in suspected infection. *J Nucl Med* 1990; 31:1950–1955.

58. Palestro CJ, Swyer AJ, Kim CK et al. Infected knee prostheses: diagnosis with In-111 leukocyte, Tc-99m sulfur colloid, and Tc-99m MDP imaging. *Radiology* 1991;179:645–648.

59. Love C, Marwin SE, Tomas MB et al. Diagnosing infection in the failed joint replacement: a comparison of coincidence detection fluorine-18 FDG and indium-111-labeled leukocyte/technetium-99m-sulfur colloid marrow imaging. *J Nucl Med* 2004; 45: 1864–1871.

60. Love C, Tronco GG, Yu AK et al. Diagnosing lower extremity (LE) prosthetic joint infection: Bone, gallium & labeled leukocyte imaging. Presented at the 2008 SNM Meeting, New Orleans, LA, June 14–18, 2008.

61. El Esper I, Blondet C, Moullart V et al. The usefulness of ^{99m}Tc sulfur colloid bone marrow scintigraphy combined with ^{111}In leucocyte scintigraphy in prosthetic joint infection. *Nucl Med Commun* 2004;25: 171–175.

62. Fuster D, Duch J, Soriano A et al. [Potential use of bone marrow scintigraphy in suspected prosthetic hip infection evaluated with (99m)Tc-HMPAO-leukocytes]. *Rev Esp Med Nucl* 2008;27:430–435.

63. Pelosi E, Baiocco C, Pennone M et al. 99mTc-HMPAO-leukocyte scintigraphy in patients with symptomatic total hip or knee arthroplasty: improved diagnostic accuracy by means of semiquantitative evaluation. *J Nucl Med* 2004;45:438–444.

64. Boubaker A, Delaloye AB, Blanc CH et al. Immuno-scintigraphy with antigranulocyte monoclonal anti-bodies for the diagnosis of septic loosening of hip prostheses. *Eur J Nucl Med* 1995;22:139–147.

65. Gratz S, Höffken H, Kaiser JW et al. Nuclear medical imaging in case of painful knee arthroplasty. *Radiologe* 2009;49:59–67.

66. Klett R, Steiner D, Puille M et al. Antigranulocyte scintigraphy of septic loosening of hip endoprosthesis: effect of different methods of analysis. *Nuklearmedizin* 2001;40:75–79.

67. Klett R, Kordelle J, Stahl U et al. Immunoscintigraphy of septic loosening of knee endoprosthesis: a retrospective evaluation of the antigranulocyte antibody BW 250/183. *Eur J Nucl Med Mol Imaging* 2003;30: 1463–1466.

68. Von Rothenburg T, Schoellhammer M, Schaffstein J et al. Imaging of infected total arthroplasty with Tc-99m-labeled antigranulocyte antibody Fab′ fragments. *Clin Nucl Med* 2004;29:548–551.

69. Iyengar KP, Vinjamuri S. Role of ^{99m}Tc Sulesomab in the diagnosis of prosthetic joint infections. *Nucl Med Commun* 2005;26:489–496.

70. Pakos EE, Fotopoulos AD, Stafilas KS et al. Use of (99m)Tc-sulesomab for the diagnosis of prosthesis infection after total joint arthroplasty. *J Int Med Res* 2007;35:474–481.

71. Rubello D, Rampin L, Banti E et al. Diagnosis of infected total knee arthroplasty with anti-granulocyte scintigraphy: the importance of a dual-time acquisition protocol. *Nucl Med Commun* 2008;29:331–335.

72. Gratz S, Behr TM, Reize P et al. (99m)Tc-fab′ fragments (sulesomab) for imaging septically loosened total knee arthroplasty. *J Int Med Res* 2009;37: 54–67.

73. Larikka MJ, Ahonen AK, Niemelä O et al. ^{99m}Tc-ciprofloxacin (Infecton) imaging in the diagnosis of knee prosthesis infections. *Nucl Med Commun* 2002; 23:167–170.

74. Larikka MJ, Ahonen AK, Niemelä O et al. Comparison of ^{99m}Tc ciprofloxacin, ^{99m}Tc white blood cell and three-phase bone imaging in the diagnosis of hip prosthesis infections: improved diagnostic accuracy with extended imaging time. *Nucl Med Commun* 2002;23:655–661.

75. Sarda L, Saleh-Mghir A, Peker C *et al*. Evaluation of (99m)Tc-ciprofloxacin scintigraphy in a rabbit model of Staphylococcus aureus prosthetic joint infection. *J Nucl Med* 2002;43:239–245.

76. Sarda-Mantel L, Saleh-Mghir A, Welling MM *et al*. Evaluation of ^{99m}Tc-UBI 29-41 scintigraphy for specific detection of experimental *Staphylococcus aureus* prosthetic joint infections. *Eur J Nucl Med Mol Imaging* 2007;34:1302–1309.

77. Kaisidis A, Megas P, Apostolopoulos D *et al*. SPECT scan with ^{99m}Tc-labeled monoclonal antibodies. *Orthopade* 2005;34:462–469.

78. Graute V, Feist M, Lehner S *et al*. Detection of low-grade prosthetic joint infections using ^{99m}Tc-antigranulocyte SPECT/CT: initial clinical results. *Eur J Nucl Med Mol Imaging* 2010;37:1751–1759.

79. Oakley RM, Wright JE. Postoperative mediastinitis: classification and management. *Ann Thorac Surg* 1996;61:1030–1036.

80. Browdie DA, Bernstein RW, Agnew R *et al*. Diagnosis of poststernotomy infection: comparison of three means of assessment. *Ann Thorac Surg* 1991;51:290–292.

81. Oates E, Payne DD. Postoperative cardiothoracic infection: diagnostic value of indium-111 white blood cell imaging. *Ann Thorac Surg* 1994;58:1442–1446.

82. Cooper JA, Elmendorf SL, Teixeira JP *et al*. Diagnosis of sternal wound infection by technetium-99m-leukocyte imaging. *J Nucl Med* 1992;33:59–65.

83. Bessette PR, Hanson MJ, Czarnecki DJ *et al*. Evaluation of postoperative osteomyelitis of the sternum comparing CT and dual Tc-99m MDP bone and In-111 WBC SPECT. *Clin Nucl Med* 1993;18:197–202.

84. Quirce R, Carril JM, Gutiérrez-Mendiguchía C *et al*. Assessment of the diagnostic capacity of planar scintigraphy and SPECT with ^{99m}Tc-HMPAO-labelled leukocytes in superficial and deep sternal infections after median sternotomy. *Nucl Med Commun* 2002;23:453–459.

85. Bitkover CY, Gardlund B, Larsson SA. Diagnosing sternal wound infections with ^{99m}Tc-labeled monoclonal granulocyte antibody scintigraphy. *Ann Thorac Surg* 1996;62:1412–1417.

86. Hauet JR, Barge ML, Fajon O *et al*. Sternal infection and retrosternal abscess shown on Tc-99m HMPAO-labeled leukocyte scintigraphy. *Clin Nucl Med* 2004;29:194–195.

Clinical cases

Case 1
Patient 1: A 67-year-old female with 12-year-old bilateral hip replacements, presented with left hip pain for 6 months. Laboratory studies and plain radiographs were not contributory. On the ^{111}In-labeled WBC image (Figure 10.10A) there is intensely increased activity around the femoral component of the left hip replacement. The distribution of periprosthetic activity on the marrow scan (Figure 10.10B) is virtually identical and the combined study is negative for infection. An aseptically loosened prosthesis was revised at surgery.

Patient 2: A 76-year-old female with a 21-year-old right total hip replacement presented with right hip pain and bacteremia. Plain radiographs were inconclusive. On the ^{111}In-WBC image (Figure 10.11A), periprosthetic activity around the femoral component is unremarkable. When compared with the marrow scan (Figure 10.11B), however, the distribution of activity is spatially incongruent in the region of the femoral head and the combined study is positive for infection.

Teaching points
• The intensity of uptake in infection and normal labeled WBC distribution are variable and diagnosing osteomyelitis with this technique is problematic.
• Complementary ^{99m}Tc-sulfur colloid marrow imaging, as these cases illustrate, overcomes limitations inherent in labeled WBC imaging.

Case 2
Patient 1: A 50-year-old man with a 3-year-old painful cemented left total knee replacement was referred for evaluation of possible infection. Both ESR and CRP levels were elevated. Plain radiographs were suggestive of loosening. An anterior image of the knees (Figure 10.12) performed about 2 hours after injection of ^{99m}Tc-sulesomab demonstrates increased periprosthetic activity. The ^{111}In-labeled WBC scan and bone marrow image (Figure 10.13) also are abnormal. At surgery, an infected prosthesis was removed. Operative cultures grew *S. aureus*.

Patient 2: A 63-year-old woman with a 5-year-old painful cemented left total knee replacement was referred for evaluation of possible infection.

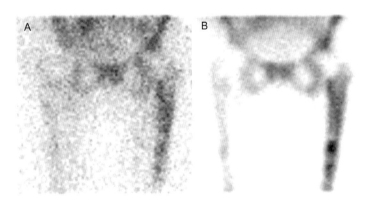

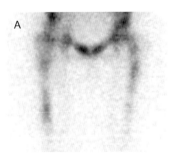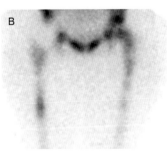

Figure 10.10 Anterior image of the hip acquired 20 hours after (A) ^{111}In-labeled WBC injection and (B) colloid injection for bone marrow imaging in a patient with left hip prosthesis. There are no signs of infection.

Figure 10.11 Anterior image of the hip acquired 20 hours after (A) ^{111}In-labeled WBC injection and (B) colloid injection for bone marrow imaging in a patient with a right hip prosthesis. There is evidence of an infected prosthesis.

ESR was elevated and the CRP level was normal. Plain radiographs were unremarkable. An anterior image of the knees (Figure 10.14), performed about 4 hours after injection of ^{99m}Tc-sulesomab, demonstrates increased periprosthetic activity. The ^{111}In-labeled WBC scan and bone marrow scan (Figure 10.15), however, are negative for infection. At surgery, an aseptically loosened prosthesis was revised.

Teaching points
• Although sensitive, ^{99m}Tc-sulesomab is not specific for diagnosing prosthetic joint infection (at least when only early images are acquired).

• As these cases illustrate, *in vitro*-labeled WBC/bone marrow imaging is the radionuclide test of choice for this purpose.

Case 3
Patient 1: A 62-year-old female with a painful 5-year-old cemented right total hip replacement was referred for evaluation of possible infection. Both ESR and CRP level were elevated and plain radiographs indicated loosening. An anterior image (Figure 10.16) of the thighs obtained about 4 hours

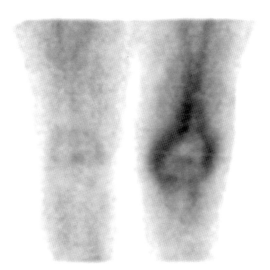

Figure 10.12 Infected left knee replacement. There is diffusely increased activity around the left knee replacement on an image acquired about 3 hours after injection of the antigranulocyte antibody fragment ^{99m}Tc-sulesomab.

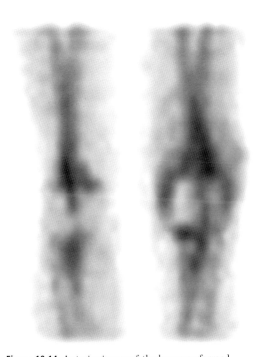

Figure 10.14 Anterior image of the knees performed about 4 hours after injection of ^{99m}Tc-sulesomab.

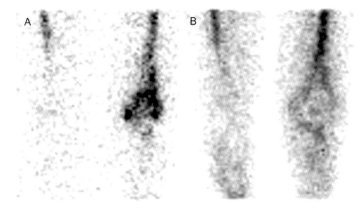

Figure 10.13 (A) ^{111}In-WBC and (B) colloid scan for bone marrow in the same patient as in Figure 10.12.

after injection of ^{99m}Tc-ciprofloxacin is unremarkable, except for slightly asymmetric vascular activity. Periprosthetic activity is indistinguishable from background. At surgery an infected prosthesis was removed. Operative cultures grew *Staphylococcus epidermiidis*.

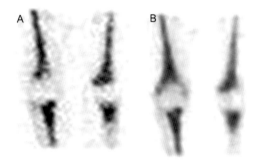

Figure 10.15 (A) ^{111}In-labeled WBC and (B) colloid scan for bone marrow in the same patient as in Figure 10.14.

Patient 2: A 55-year-old male with a painful 3-year-old cemented left total knee replacement was referred for evaluation of possible infection. Both ESR and CRP level were elevated; plain radiographs suggested loosening. An anterior image (Figure 10.17) of the knees obtained about 4 hours after injection of ^{99m}Tc-ciprofloxacin demonstrates intense activity around the prosthesis. At surgery an aseptically loosened prosthesis was revised.

Teaching points
• At one time it was thought that radiolabeled antibiotics would be truly infection-specific imaging agents.
• More recent data, as these cases illustrate, have shown that this is not the case and much of the original enthusiasm for radiolabeled antibiotics as a diagnostic tool has waned.

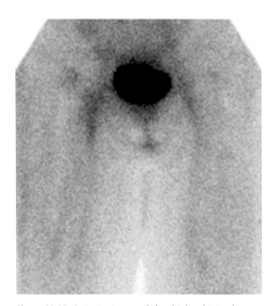

Figure 10.16 Anterior image of the thighs obtained about 4 hours after injection of ^{99m}Tc-ciprofloxacin in a patient with suspected infection of a right hip prosthesis. Periprosthetic activity is indistinguishable from background.

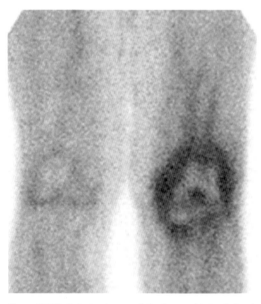

Figure 10.17 Anterior image of the knees obtained about 4 hours after injection of ^{99m}Tc-ciprofloxacin in a patient with suspected infection of a left knee prosthesis. The images demonstrate intense periprosthetic activity.

CHAPTER 11

Nuclear Medicine Imaging of Spondylodiscitis: The Emerging Role of PET

Elena Lazzeri, Paola Anna Erba, Martina Sollini and Giuliano Mariani

University of Pisa, Medical School, Pisa, Italy

Introduction

Spine infections include vertebral osteomyelitis (infection of the vertebral body), discitis (infection of the intervertebral disk) and spondylodiscitis (infection of two adjacent vertebral bodies and their intervertebral disk). Spondylodiscitis is classified as anterior or posterior, and of the spinal canal or bone site, according to anatomical location of the infectious process [1]. The infectious process may extend into the adjacent tissues in different directions; posterior extension can result in epidural or subdural abscess or in meningitis, while anterior or lateral extension can result in paravertebral, retropharyngeal, mediastinal or retroperitoneal abscess (according to the level of infection in the spine). Bacteria represent the prevailing etiology of spondylodiscitis, followed by mycobacterium or, more rarely, mycotic infection. There are many predisposing factors, such as diabetes mellitus, immunodeficiency syndromes [e.g. acquired immune deficiency syndrome (AIDS)], chronic renal failure and alcoholism. The most frequent site of vertebral infection is the lumbar spine (45%) followed by the dorsal (35%) and the cervical tract (20%) [2]. The clinical classification of spondylodiscitis is based on the mechanism by which microorganisms generate the infection in the vertebral site. In particular, spondylodiscitis is classified as primary (when bacterial growth follows hematogenic spread) or secondary, most frequently consequent to surgical procedures or associated with other pathological conditions. Men are affected more frequently than women (3.1:1.5).

Basic knowledge of the clinical problem

Primary spondylodiscitis (of bacterial or mycotic etiology) represents 2–4% of all bone infections. The most frequently isolated bacterium is *Staphylococcus aureus* (55–80%), followed by coagulase-negative staphylococci and by *Enterobacter* (*Salmonella* spp., *Escherichia coli*, *Klebsiella* spp., *Serratia* spp.). *Pseudomonas aeruginosa* is frequently isolated in drug-addicted individuals, while yeast-like microorganisms, such as *Candida* spp., are responsible for infection in drug-addicted patients and those with vascular devices [3–7]. The most common predisposing conditions are AIDS and decompensated diabetes. The incidence of primary spondylodiscitis is higher in patients older than 50 years.

Back pain is always present in spondylodiscitis; motor deficits (in 70% of cases), elevated levels of C-reactive protein (CRP) and increased erythrocyte

Diagnostic Imaging of Infections and Inflammatory Diseases: A Multidisciplinary Approach, First Edition. Edited by Alberto Signore and Ana María Quintero.

sedimentation rate (ESR) (64%) may be present, as well as fever and spinal tenderness (in variable percentages) [3,8].

In adults, primary spine infections are initially localized in the anterior part of the vertebral body, which is more abundantly vascularized [9,10]; at a more advanced stage, the infection usually extends into the adjacent tissues (intervertebral disc and adjacent vertebrae). Spondylodiscitis caused by *Mycobacterium tuberculosis* (vertebral tuberculosis or Pott's disease) begins in the anterior part of the vertebral body and usually involves the subcondral region, and subsequently the cortical bone and adjacent disc. The diffusion of tubercular infection frequently involves the soft paravertebral tissues. Pain accompanied by raised ESR and CRP levels, yet with normal or moderately increased white blood cell (WBC) counts, is the most common clinical presentation [11,12]. Multiorgan pathology is often present, with a high frequency of pulmonary localization that can sometimes mask other symptoms [13].

Secondary spondylodiscitis is caused by direct contamination with microorganisms following a variety of invasive procedures, such as local infiltration of analgesics and, most importantly, surgical procedures for slipped disc, spondylolysis and spondylolisthesis [2,9,10,14,15]. *S. aureus* is predominantly responsible for this type of spondylodiscitis, followed by *Staphylococcus epidermidis*; coagulase-negative Gram-negative bacteria (*E. coli, Enterobacter* spp., *Serratia* spp., *P. aeruginosa* and *Acinetobacter* spp.) are instead more often responsible for vertebral infection in AIDS and drug-addicted patients [1].

The incidence of secondary spondylodiscitis varies according to the type of surgical procedure: less than 1% for discectomy, 1–5% for spinal fusion without instrumentation [15], 2.6–4.4% for spinal fusion with instrumentation [16,17] and up to 6.9% for surgery for scoliosis [18–21].

Microorganisms of low virulence are typically present in intraoperative cultures of infections associated with a spinal implant; their slow-growth pattern can hamper the microbiological diagnosis, since it is often necessary to prolong the culture for more than 1 week [21]. In fact, the presence of pus around spinal implants may represent a foreign body reaction consisting of non-infectious granulomatosis and caused by the metallic debris produced by implant micromotion. Intraoperative identification of this condition confirms the presence of an extensive glycocalyx surrounding the entire spinal hardware without evidence of bacterial growth, similar to that observed in aseptic loosening of a joint prosthesis [22].

Spine involvement may be present in different infective conditions, e.g. septic emboli originating in endocarditis. The actual incidence of this type of spondylodiscitis may be underestimated because of the clinical importance of the primary disease. Clinical manifestations of secondary spondylodiscitis, as well as of the primary condition, are pain, motor deficits and fever accompanied by raised ESR, CRP and WBC count.

The course of spondylodiscitis, either primary or secondary, is strongly affected by a timely diagnosis, which allows early initiation of antibiotic treatment [23]. The diagnosis of spondylodiscitis is based on clinical symptoms, laboratory and imaging findings, and isolation of the responsible microorganism, either directly (by intraoperative cultures of the wound, bone or spinal implants) or indirectly (by blood cultures) [24]. Unfortunately, for every direct sampling procedure, the risk of non-pathogen contamination leading to incorrect diagnosis must be taken into account [25]; on the other hand, blood culture can be negative despite the presence of bacterial infection [26]. Computed tomography (CT)-guided biopsy followed by bacterial culture has a high diagnostic specificity, but its sensitivity has been reported to range between 70% and 91% in patient populations of which a small proportion had vertebral infections [27,28]; whereas in two series of patients suspected of having a spine infection, the diagnostic performance has been reported to be lower (43–47%) [29,30]. Thus, this invasive procedure is not routinely used in patients with suspected spondylodiscitis.

Magnetic resonance imaging (MRI) is currently considered the modality of choice for the evaluation of suspected spine infections [31], with high sensitivity and specificity also in the early phase of primary spondylodiscitis; furthermore, the high spatial resolution of MRI allows the extent of infection to be clearly defined [32] (see Chapter 4). Nevertheless, this technique suffers from some limitations, particularly in patient follow-up during antibiotic therapy and for postoperative infections [33–38].

The clinical questions

A multidisciplinary approach is crucial to establishing a prompt diagnosis and selecting appropriate therapy, remembering that diagnosis is often delayed by poor symptom specificity and that delay of appropriate therapy can lead to irreversible neurological impairment and even to death. Radionuclide imaging procedures are particularly important for the correct diagnosis of secondary spondylodiscitis, because of the lower diagnostic accuracy of radiological imaging in this condition. In cases of suspected primary spondylodiscitis, radionuclide imaging is indicated only when the results of radiological imaging (MRI and/or CT) are uncertain.

The main clinical questions in the management of patients with suspected and/or established spondylodiscitis are:

• Can infection be confirmed/ruled out?
• What is the real extent of the infectious process?
• When can antibiotic therapy safely be discontinued?

Methodological considerations

A gold standard has yet to be established and vertebral infection can be diagnosed by several different nuclear medicine techniques. Studies with ^{18}F-fluorodeoxyglucose positron emission tomography ([^{18}F]FDG-PET) in patients with vertebral infection have shown high sensitivity but variable specificity (35.8–88%) [39–46]. Overall, [^{18}F]FDG seems to be the best commercially available radiopharmaceutical for the diagnosis of spondylodiscitis and especially for therapy follow-up [47,48]. In this condition, the semiquantitative analysis of the PET images, by calculating standardized uptake values (SUVs), allows verification of the treatment response in terms of reduction of hypermetabolic activity in the site of infection [49]. Unfortunately, its use may have limitations in distinguishing complicated bone healing from osteomyelitis; moreover, false positives due to bone metastases are possible [50].

Scintigraphy with autologous labeled leukocytes (WBCs), although highly accurate in many infection pathologies [51,52], is not always useful in the case of vertebral infection because in these patients the WBC scan often shows a photopenic area (cold spot) corresponding to the involved vertebral body, a pattern which is not specific for infection [51] since a vertebral crush may also show a similar appearance. Rarely, an increased uptake of the radiolabeled WBCs at the site of vertebral infection has been described and correlated, to some extent, with the short duration of symptoms; in fact, less than 25% of patients who are symptomatic for more than 2 weeks show a high vertebral WBC uptake [53]. On the other hand, WBC scintigraphy of other pathologies (e.g. Paget's disease or tumors) show areas of reduced WBC uptake [53–61], thus making the presence of a cold area suggestive but nonspecific for vertebral infection. WBC scintigraphy can be performed when it is necessary to evaluate the extent of an infectious process in paravertebral soft tissues.

Other techniques proposed to supplement the diagnostic value of MRI include bone scintigraphy with ^{99m}Tc-methyl diphosphonate (MDP) or ^{99m}Tc-hydroxymethylene diphosphonate (HDP) and ^{67}Ga-citrate [62,63]. Although these techniques allow the diagnosis of a vertebral infection, their specificity is low and therefore they are not routinely used, other than in some selected cases to answer specific clinical questions. Furthermore, a limitation of ^{67}Ga-citrate in particular is its high radiation burden and long acquisition time.

Other newer radiopharmaceuticals, such as radiolabeled PEG-liposomes and interleukin (IL)-8 [64,65] have shown high potential value for diagnosing infection, but they need further evaluation in the clinical setting.

Radiolabeled antimicrobial peptides, reported in experimental animal models to distinguish infection from sterile inflammation [66,67], have been used to diagnose the presence of infectious foci in patients with fever of unknown origin [68] and the presence of vertebral infection; although this procedure has shown very high sensitivity and satisfactory specificity in this clinical setting [68,69], it remains to be further validated in patients with postsurgical spondylodiscitis. ^{99m}Tc-ciprofloxacin, originally used for imaging peripheral bone infection [70,71], has shown discordant results in patients with spine infections, with high sensitivity but quite low specificity, especially when evaluating patients early in the postoperative period [72].

[111]In-biotin is another radiophamaceutical for the diagnosis and therapy follow-up of spondylodiscitis [73,74], although it is not yet commercially available. Biotin, also called vitamin H (molecular

weight about 224 Da), is a water-soluble vitamin of the B-complex group of vitamins, and its mechanism of uptake by infectious processes may be related to the fact that it is a growth factor for many bacteria. In particular, pyruvate carboxylase, a key metabolic pathway for producing energy by ATP cleavage, is biotin-dependent and bacterial acetyl-coA carboxylase is a biotin-dependent enzyme implicated in the first step of fatty acid synthesis [75,76].

Normal and pathological findings and artifacts

Commercially available radiopharmaceuticals

^{99m}Tc-MDP/HDP scintigraphy

Considering that the uptake of radiolabeled diphosphonates by bone is directly correlated with the degree of local osteoblastic activity, areas with vertebral infection show up as "hot" with respect to healthy bone tissues. Nevertheless, even if the bone scan with ^{99m}Tc-MDP/HDP shows high sensitivity, its specificity is very low [62,63].

^{67}Ga-citrate scintigraphy

The clinical usefulness of ^{67}Ga-citrate for the diagnosis of spine infection is based on its high affinity for transferrin and lactoferrin (which are present at sites of infection/inflammation, as well as in tumors) and bacterial siderophores. In spondylodiscitis the uptake of ^{67}Ga-citrate is higher than in healthy bone tissues. Unfortunately, malignant tissue also accumulates ^{67}Ga-citrate and this radiopharmaceutical cannot differentiate spine infection from tumor involvement of the vertebral region [62,63].

^{99m}Tc-MDP/HDP + ^{67}Ga-citrate scintigraphy

It is advised to compare scintigraphic images with labeled diphosphonates and with ^{67}Ga-citrate. If the uptake of ^{67}Ga-citrate is higher than ^{99m}Tc-MDP uptake, the diagnosis of spine infection is highly probable. By contrast, if the uptake of ^{99m}Tc-MDP is higher than ^{67}Ga-citrate uptake, an osteoarthritic or traumatic bone pathology is more likely [62,63].

Labeled white blood cells

WBC scintigraphy often shows a photopenic area (cold spot) corresponding to the involved vertebral body when a spondylodiscitis is present, but increased uptake of the radiolabeled WBCs at the site of vertebral infection can be seen if the infective process is very recent (usually <2 weeks after diagnosis) or if soft tissues are involved.

[^{18}F]FDG-PET/CT

Increased [^{18}F]FDG uptake by infectious processes is due to the high energy demand (and therefore intensive glucose consumption) of mononuclear cells and activated granulocytes [40]. [^{18}F]FDG uptake, due to the presence of medullary cells, is normally seen in the healthy spine. Thus, [^{18}F]FDG-PET/CT is compatible with infection when the uptake of [^{18}F]FDG at the suspected site of vertebral infection is higher than in other healthy vertebral regions. There are no data on the cut-off SUV above which spinal disease is indicated, although published reports show that an SUV of greater than 5 is likely associated with infection, whereas an SUV between 3 and 5 is considered doubtful. The FDG distribution is also important. In the early phases of the infection process, the pathological uptake of FDG is localized to the anterior part of the vertebral body according to the pathophysiology of the disease. In late stages, the pathological uptake may involve the adjacent bone tissues and/or the paravertebral soft tissues. Unfortunately, inflammatory bone processes without bacterial infection are also in a highly activated state of cell metabolism and glucose consumption, thus mimicking infection on [^{18}F]FDG-PET images [44]. Therefore, it is quite difficult to differentiate sterile inflammation from infection on [^{18}F]FDG-PET/CT imaging in patients with suspected hematogenic vertebral osteomyelitis [39–43]. In patients with metallic implant devices, evaluation of the spine must take into account another technical difficulty: falsely increased [^{18}F]FDG uptake caused by hypercorrection for tissue attenuation due to the presence of the metallic implant. Therefore, it is very important to evaluate images that have not been corrected for attenuation as well as images that have been corrected, as the latter often show false-positive accumulation of [^{18}F]FDG [45].

A systematic analysis of the literature shows that the sensitivity of all available infection tracers used in the evaluation of spondylodiscitis varies from 63% to 100%, specificity from 36% to 100% and accuracy from 62% to 90%. The presence of [^{18}F]FDG uptake in a vertebral body makes the diagnosis of infection very likely. Nevertheless, interpretation of any abnormal [18F]FDG accumulation must take into consideration the clinical features of the individual patient, because this agent lacks specificity. On the other hand, whole-body acquisition during a single imaging session offers the advantage of detecting unknown sites of infection in the spine and/or in other organs.

Experimental radiopharmaceuticals

111In-biotin scintigraphy

This technique has shown very high sensitivity (90%) and specificity (93%) in the detection of early vertebral infection in a large consecutive series of patients [73]. There is no uptake of radiolabeled biotin by healthy bone tissue, so that uptake of 111In-biotin in the spine is considered to be a pathological finding. In another series of patients in which the added value of SPECT/CT acquisition of 111In-biotin scintigraphy was evaluated [74], this technique consistently showed high diagnostic accuracy, combined with the advantage of distinguishing infection limited to the bone from involvement extending to adjacent soft tissues. When interpreting the SPECT/CT images, it is very important to assess for the presence of tracer accumulation both in images corrected and uncorrected for attenuation, as corrected images can show false-positive uptake of 111In-biotin.

68Ga-citrate PET/CT

68Ga-citrate has been proposed as an infection imaging agent in patients with suspected bone infection, including spondylodiscitis. Its specificity is similar to that of 67Ga-citrate scintigraphy and false-positive results have been reported in patients with spine tumors [77].

Role for therapy follow-up and patient management

Suspicion of spine infection raised on clinical grounds must be confirmed or ruled out with diagnostic imaging, including both radiological and radionuclide procedures. Identifying the true site of infection in the vertebral and/or paravertebral region is crucial for selecting the most appropriate therapeutic strategy according to the extent of infection. In fact, drainage of the abscess is performed and specific antibiotics are given if infection

is limited to the paravertebral soft tissues, while other antibiotics are used when only bone infection is present [78,79]. Although the specific antibiotic is selected on the basis of bacterial resistance testing, different classes of antibiotics are usually used according to the site of infection. It should also be noted that early and correct localization of infection is important for prognostic purposes, since an infection limited to the paravertebral soft tissues has a better outcome than a true bone infection [79,80].

Duration of antibiotic therapy is based on clinical response, normalization of inflammation markers and diagnostic imaging.

The role of nuclear medicine imaging in the follow-up of patients during antibiotic therapy is very important and is based on changes in the degree of uptake of the radiopharmaceutical used for the diagnosis of spine infection, with reduction in the abnormally increased uptake of, for example, [18F]FDG indicating reduction in the infectious process. Accordingly, complete disappearance of pathological uptake of the radiopharmaceutical can support the clinician's decision to discontinue antibiotic therapy.

Conclusion

Nuclear medicine imaging can be considered a valid diagnostic tool in spine infection; it is also complementary to MRI in all cases with equivocal radiological findings, especially in patients with postsurgical spine infection where the diagnostic accuracy of MRI is limited because of the presence of fibrosis and scar tissues. Finally, nuclear medicine imaging is very accurate in the evaluation of treatment response in all patients submitted to antimicrobial therapy.

References

1. Calderone RR, Larsen JM. Overview and classification of spinal infection. *Orthop Clin North Am* 1996; 27:1–8.
2. Mader JT, Calhoun J. Osteomyelitis. In: Mandell GL, Bennett JE, Dolin R (eds). *Principles and Practice of Infectious Diseases*, vol. 1. New York: Churchill Livingstone, 2000, pp. 1182–1196.
3. Carragee EJ. Pyogenic vertebral osteomyelitis. *J Bone Joint Surg Am* 1997;79:874–880.
4. Torda AJ, Gottlieb T, Bradbury R. Pyogenic vertebral osteomyelitis: analysis of 20 cases and review. *Clin Infect Dis* 1995;20:320–328.

5. Honan M, White GW, Eisenberg GM. Spontaneous infectious discitis in adults. *Am J Med* 1996;100: 85–89.

6. Carragee EJ, Kim D, van der Vlugt T, Vittum D. The clinical use of erythrocyte sedimentation rate in pyogenic vertebral osteomyelitis. *Spine* 1997;22:2089–2093.

7. Chen HC, Tzaan WC, Lui TN. Spinal epidural abscesses: a retrospective analysis of clinical manifestations, sources of infection, and outcomes. *Chang Gung Med J* 2004;27:351–358.

8. Perry M. Erythrocyte sedimentation rate and C reactive protein in the assessment of suspected bone infection – are they reliable indices? *J R Coll Surg Edinb* 1996;41:116–118.

9. Sapico FL, Montgomerie JZ. Pyogenic vertebral osteomyelitis: report of nine cases and review of the literature. *Rev Infect Dis* 1979;1:754–776.

10. Lew DP, Waldvogel FA. Current concepts: osteomyelitis. *N Engl J Med* 1997;336:999–1007.

11. Perronne C, Saba J, Behloul Z *et al*. Pyogenic and tuberculous spondylodiskitis (vertebral osteomyelitis) in 80 adult patients. *Clin Infect Dis* 1994;19: 746–750.

12. Wang D. Diagnosis of tuberculous vertebral osteomyelitis (TVO) in a developed country and literature review. *Spinal Cord* 2005;43:531–542.

13. Yoon HJ, Song YG, Park WI, Choi JP, Chang KH, Kim JM. Clinical manifestations and diagnosis of extrapulmonary tuberculosis. *Yonsei Med J* 2004;45: 453–461.

14. Ozuna RM, Delamarter RB. Pyogenic vertebral osteomyelitis and postsurgical disc space infections. *Orthop Clin North Am* 1996;27:87–94

15. Brown EM, Pople IK, de Louvois J *et al*. Spine update: prevention of postoperative infection in patients undergoing spinal surgery. *Spine* 2004;29:938–945.

16. Fang A, Hu SS, Endres N, Brandford DS. Risk factors for infection after spinal surgery. *Spine* 2005;30: 1460–1465.

17. Richards BR, Emara KM. Delayed infections after posterior TSRH spinal instrumentation for idiopatic scoliosis: revisited. *Spine* 2001;26:1990–1996.

18. Hahn F, Zbinden R, Min K. Late implant infections caused by *Propionibacterium acnes* in scoliosis surgery. *Eur Spine J* 2005;14:783–788.

19. Saraph VJ, Krismer M, Wimmer C. Operative treatment of scoliosis with the Kaneda anterior spine system. *Spine* 2005;30:1616–1620.

20. Wimmer C, Gluch H, Franzreb M, Ogon M. Predisposing factors for infection in spine surgery: a survey of 850 spinal procedures. *J Spine Disord* 1998;11: 112–124.

21. Clark CE, Shufflebarger HI. Late-developing infection in instrumental idiopathic scoliosis. *Spine* 1999;24: 1909–1912.

22. Aydinli U, Karaeminogullari O, Tiskaya K. Postoperative deep wound infection in instrumental spinal surgery. *Acta Orthop Belg* 1999;65:182–187.

23. Mader JT Shirtliff ME, Bergquist SC, Calhoun J. Antimicrobial treatment of chronic osteomyelitis. *Clin Orthop Relat Res* 1999;360:47–65.

24. Widmer A. New developments in diagnosis and treatment of infection in orthopedic implants. *Clin Infect Dis* 2001;33:94–106.

25. Mader JT, Wang J, Calhoun JH. Antibiotic therapy for musculoskeletal infections. *J Bone Joint Surg Am* 2001;83-A:1878–1890.

26. Tyrell PN, Cassar-Pullicino VN, Mccall IW. Spinal infection. *Eur Radiol* 1999;9:1066–1077.

27. Chew FS, Kline MJ. Diagnostic yield of CT-guided percutaneous aspiration procedures in suspected spontaneous infectious diskitis. *Radiology* 2001;218: 211–214.

28. Akhtar I, Flowers R, Siddiqi A, Heard K, Baliga M. Fine needle aspiration biopsy of vertebral and paravertebral lesions: retrospective study of 124 cases. *Acta Cytol* 2006 50:364–371.

29. de Lucas EM, González Mandly A, Gutiérrez A. CT-guided fine-needle aspiration in vertebral osteomyelitis: true usefulness of a common practice. *Clin Rheumatol* 2009;28:315–320.

30. Bontoux D, Codello L, Debiais F *et al*. Infectious spondylodiscitis. Analysis of a series of 105 cases. *Rev Rhum Mal Osteoartic* 1992;59:401–407.

31. Longo M, Granata F, Ricciardi K, Gaeta M, Blandino A. Contrast-enhanced MR imaging with fat suppression in adult-onset septic spondylodiscitis. *Eur Radiol* 2003;13:626–637.

32. Struk DW, MunkPI, Lee MT, Ho SGF, Worsley DF. Imaging of soft tissues infections. *Radiol Clin North Am* 2001;39:277–303.

33. Wolansky LJ, Heary RF, Patterson T *et al*. Pseudosparing of the endplate: a potential pitfall in using MR imaging to diagnose infectious spondylitis. *AJR Am J Roentgenol* 1999;172:777–780.

34. Enzmann DR. Infection and inflammation. In: Enzmann DR, DeLaPaz RL, Rubin JB (eds). *Magnetic Resonance of the Spine*. St. Louis: Mosby, 1990, pp. 260–300.

35. Wagner SC, Schweitzer ME, Morrison WB, Przybylski GJ, Parker L. Can imaging findings help differentiate spinal neuropathic arthropathy from disk space infection? Initial experience. *Radiology* 2000;214: 693–699.

36. Kylampaa-Back ML, Suominen RA, Salo SA, Soiva M, Korkala OI, Mokka RE. Postoperative discitis: outcome and late magnetic resonance image evaluation of ten patients. *Ann Chir Gynaecol* 1999;88:61–64.

37. Van Goethem JW, Parizel PM, van den Hauwe L, Van de Kelft E, Verlooy J, DeSchepper AM. The value of

MRI in the diagnosis of postoperative spondylodiscitis. *Neuroradiology* 2000;42:580–585.

38. Grane P, Josephsson A, Seferlis A, Tullberg T. Septic and aseptic postoperative discitis in the lumbar spine: evaluation by MR imaging. *Acta Radiol* 1998;39:108–115.

39. Stumpe KD, Dazzi H, Schaffner A, von Schulthess GK. Infection imaging using whole-body FDG-PET. *Eur J Nucl Med* 2000;27:822–832.

40. Kalicke T, Schmitz A, Risse JH *et al.* Fluorine-18 fluorodeoxyglucose PET in infectious bone diseases: results of histologically confirmed cases. *Eur J Nucl Med* 2000;27:524–528.

41. Zhuang H, Alavi A. 18-Fluorodeoxyglucose positron emission tomographic imaging in the detection and monitoring of infection and inflammation. *Semin Nucl Med* 2002;32:47–59.

42. Schmitz A, Kalicke T, Willkomm P, Grunwald F, Kandyba J, Schmitz O. Use of fluorine-18 fluoro-2-deoxy-D-glucose positron emission tomography in assessing the process of tuberculous spondilitys. *J Spinal Disord* 2000;13:541–544.

43. Gratz S, Dorner J, Fischer U *et al.* ^{18}F-FDG hybrid PET in patients with suspected spondylitis. *Eur J Nucl Med* 2002;29:516–524.

44. Rosen RS, Fayad L, Wahl RL. Increased ^{18}F-FDG uptake in degenerative disease of the spine: characterization with ^{18}F-FDG PET/CT. *J Nucl Med* 2006;47:1274–1280.

45. De Winter F, Gemmel F, Van De Wiele C, Poffijn B, Uyttendaele D, Dierckx R. 18-Fluorine fluorodeoxyglucose positron emission tomography for the diagnosis of infection in the postoperative spine. *Spine* 2003;28:1314–1319.

46. Fuster D, Solà O, Soriano A *et al.* A prospective study comparing whole-body FDG PET/CT to combined planar bone scan with 67Ga SPECT/CT in the diagnosis of spondylodiskitis. *Clin Nucl Med* 2012;37:827–832.

47. Gasbarrini A, Boriani L, Nanni C *et al.* Spinal infection multidisciplinary management project (SIMP): from diagnosis to treatment guideline. *Int J Immunopathol Pharmacol* 2011;24 (1 Suppl 2):95–100.

48. Nanni C, Boriani L, Salvadori C *et al.* FDG PET/CT is useful for the interim evaluation of response to therapy in patients affected by haematogenous spondylodiscitis. *Eur J Nucl Med Mol Imaging* 2012;39:1538–1544.

49. Skanjeti A, Penna D, Douroukas A *et al.* PET in the clinical work-up of patients with spondylodiscitis: a new tool for the clinician? *Q J Nucl Med Mol Imaging* 2012;56:569–576.

50. Zhuang H, Pourdehnad M, Lambright ES *et al.* Dual time point ^{18}F-FDG PET imaging for differentiating malignant from inflammatory processes. *J Nucl Med* 2001;42:1412–1417.

51. Devillers A, Moisan A, Jean S, Arvieux C, Bourguet P. Technetium-99m hexamethyl-propylene amine oxime leucocyte scintigraphy for the diagnosis of bone and joint infections: a retrospective study in 116 patients. *Eur J Nucl Med* 1995;22:302–307.

52. Palestro CJ, Torres MA. Radionuclide imaging in orthopaedic infections. *Semin Nucl Med* 1997;27:334–345.

53. Palestro CJ, Kim CK, Swyer AJ, Vallabhajosula S, Goldsmith SJ. Radionuclide diagnosis of vertebral osteomyelitis: indium-111-leukocyte and technetium-99m methylenediphosphonate bone scintigraphy. *J Nucl Med* 1991;32:1861–1865.

54. Coleman RE, Welch D. Possible pitfalls with clinical imaging of indium-111 leukocytes. *J Nucl Med* 1980;21:122–125.

55. Mok YP, Carney WH, Fernandez-Ulloa M. Skeletal photopenic lesions in In-111 WBC imaging. *J Nucl Med* 1984;25:1322–1326.

56. Fernandex-Ulloa M, Vasavada PJ, Hanslits ML, Volarich DT, Elgazzar AH. Diagnosis of vertebral osteomyelitis: clinical, radiological and scintigraphic features. *Orthopedics* 1985;8:1144–1150.

57. Datz FL, Thorne DA. Cause and significance of cold bone defects on indium-111-labelled leukocyte imaging. *J Nucl Med* 1987;28:820–823.

58. Whalen JL, Brown ML, McLeod R, Fitzgerald RH Jr. Limitations of indium leukocyte imaging for the diagnosis of spine infections. *Spine* 1991;16:193–197.

59. Jacobson AF, Gilles CP, Cerqueira MD. Photopenic defects in marrow containing skeleton on indium-111 leucocyte scintigraphy: prevalence at sites suspected of osteomyelitis and as an incidental finding. *Eur J Nucl Med* 1992;19:858–864.

60. Even-Sapir E, Martin RH. Degenerative disc disease. A cause for diagnostic dilemma on In-111 WBC studies in suspected osteomyelitis. *Clin Nucl Med* 1994;19:388–392.

61. Roelants V, Tang T, Ide C, Laloux P. Cold vertebra on ^{111}In-white blood cell scintigraphy. *Semin Nucl Med* 2002;32:236–237.

62. Gratz S, Dorner J, Oestmann JW *et al.* ^{67}Ga-citrate and ^{99m}Tc-MDP for estimating the severity of vertebral osteomyelitis. *Nucl Med Commun* 2000;21:111–120.

63. Love C, Patel M, Lonner BS, Tomas MB, Palestro CJ. Diagnosing spinal osteomyelitis: a comparison of bone and Ga-67 scintigraphy and magnetic resonance imaging. *Clin Nucl Med* 2000;25:963–977.

64. Dams ET, Oyen WJ, Boerman OC *et al.* ^{99m}Tc-PEG liposomes for the scintigraphic detection of infection and inflammation: clinical evaluation. *J Nucl Med* 2000;41:622–630.

65. Rennen HJ, Boerman OC, Oyen WJ, van der Meer JW, Corstens FH. Specific and rapid scintigraphic

detection of infection with [99mTc]-labelled inter-leukin-8. *J Nucl Med* 2001;42:117–123.

66. Nibbering PH, Welling MM, Paulusma-Annema A, Brouwer CP, Lupetti A, Pauwels EK. [99mTc]-Labelled UBI 29–41 peptide for monitoring the efficacy of anti-bacterial agents in mice infected with *Staphylococcus aureus*. *J Nucl Med* 2004;45:321–326.

67. Welling MM, Visentin R, Feitsma HI, Lupetti A, Pauwels EK, Nibbering PH. Infection detection in mice using [99mTc]-labelled HYNIC and N2S2 chelate conjugated to the antimicrobial peptide UBI 29–41. *Nucl Med Biol* 2004;31:503–509.

68. Sepúlveda-Méndez J, de Murphy CA, Rojas-Bautista JCB, Pedraza-López M. Specificity of [99mTc]-UBI for detecting infection foci in patients with fever in study. *Nucl Med Commun* 2010;31:889–895.

69. Dillmann-Arroyo C, Cantú-Leal R, Campa-Núñez H, López-Cavazos C, Bermúdez-Argüelles M, Mejía-Herrera JC. Application of the ubiquicidin 29–41 scan in the diagnosis of pyogenic vertebral osteo-myelitis. *Acta Ortop Mex* 2011;25:27–31.

70. Sarda L, Cremieux AC, Lebellec Y *et al.* Inability of [99mTc]-ciprofloxacin scintigraphy to discriminate between septic and sterile osteoarticular diseases. *J Nucl Med* 2003;44:920–926.

71. Larikka MJ, Ahonen AK, Niemela O *et al.* Comparison of [99mTc] ciprofloxacin, [99mTc] white blood cell and three-phase bone imaging in the diagnosis of hip prosthesis infections: improved diagnostic accuracy with extended imaging time. *Nucl Med Commun* 2002;23:655–661.

72. De Winter F, Gemmel F, Van Laere K *et al.* [99mTc]-ciprofloxacin planar and tomographic imaging for the diagnosis of infection in the postoperative spine: experience in 48 patients. *Eur J Nucl Med Mol Imaging* 2004;31:233–239.

73. Lazzeri E, Erba P, Perri M *et al.* Scintigraphic imaging of vertebral osteomyelitis with [111In]-Biotin. *Spine* 2008;33:198–204.

74. Lazzeri E, Erba P, Perri M, Doria R, Tascini C, Mariani G. Clinical impact of SPECT/CT with In-Biotin on the management of patients with suspected spine infec-tion. *Clin Nucl Med* 2010;35:12–17.

75. Yao X, Wei D, Soden C Jr, Summers MF, Beckett D. Structure of the carboxyl terminal fragment of the apo-biotin carboxyl carrier subunit of *Escherichia coli* acetyl-coA carboxylase. *Biochemistry* 1997;36:15089–15100.

76. Attwood PV. The structure and the mechanism of action of pyruvate carboxylase. *Int J Biochem Cell Biol* 1995;27:231–249.

77. Nanni C, Errani C, Boriani L *et al.* [68Ga]-citrate PET/CT for evaluating patients with infections of the bone: preliminary results. *J Nucl Med* 2010;51:1932–1936.

78. Livorsi DJ, Daver NG, Atmar RL, Shelburne SA, White AC, Musher DM. Outcomes of treatment for hemato-genous *Staphylococcus aureus* vertebral osteomyelitis in the MRSA era. *J Infect* 2008;57:128–131.

79. Reihsaus E, Waldbaur H, Seeling W. Spinal epidural abscess: a meta-analysis of 915 patients. *Neurosurg Rev* 2000;232:175–204.

80. Priest DH, Peacock JE. Hematogenous vertebral osteomyelitis due to *Staphylococcus aureus* in the adult: clinical features and therapeutic outcomes. *South Med J* 2005;98:854–862.

Clinical cases

Case 1

A 59-year-old male who reported onset of back pain (lumbar-sacral region) 5 months after surgical removal of cutaneous melanoma located in posterior region of neck.

The report of a MR image without contrast stated: "L3–L4: absence of discal pathology. L4–L5: wide ranging disc protrusion, with mild imprint on the anterior profile of the dural sac. L5–S1: focal disc protrusion, median and left paramedian, that results in a mild compression on radicular emergency root of S1. Reduced signal disc."

The patient underwent intradiscal electrothermal therapy of the L5–S1 slipped disc, but symptoms persisted (back pain and partial functional impairment). The report of a repeat MR image without contrast stated: "L5–S1: mild reduction of disc protrusion. Hyperintensity in T2 and STIR of the anterior region of the opposing vertebral bodies, presumably due to the results of thermal ablation," and on further MRI with and without contrast: "L5–S1: sharp increase in the alteration of the signal of the opposing vertebral body surfaces and presence of alteration of the signal in the anterior region of the disc. These findings are suggestive for spondylodiscitis" (Figure 11.1).

However, on ^{111}In-biotin scintigraphy "Scintigraphy with planar and SPECT/CT imaging does not show pathological uptake in the L5–S1 vertebral region. These findings are negative for bacterial spondylodiscitis" (Figure 11.2).

On bone biopsy the final diagnosis was aseptic inflammation.

Teaching point

The differentiation of septic infection from sterile inflammation is crucial to the appropriate choice of therapy for the patient.

Case 2

A 51-year-old male who reported onset of back pain (lumbar-sacral region) 2 months after a surgical procedure for a slipped disc (L4–L5).

The report of a CT image stated: ". . . presence of scarred flogistic tissue in the paravertebral region of L4–L5 with enhancement after contrast medium injection" (Figure 11.3). [^{18}F]FDG-PET/CT was then performed: "Increased uptake of [^{18}F]FDG in the central region of the vertebral body corresponding to L5, suggesting spondylodiscitis" (Figure 11.4).

Teaching point

Functional radionuclide imaging with [^{18}F]FDG-PET is a valid complementary tool to evaluate the presence of spine infection.

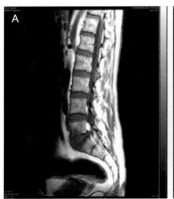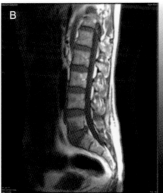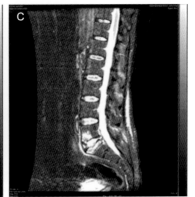

Figure 11.1 (A,B) Sagittal T1-weighted MR image shows decreased signal intensity of the vertebral bodies adjacent to the L4–L5 intervertebral disc. (C) Sagittal T2-weighted MR image shows increased signal intensity in the L4–L5 vertebral bodies and intervertebral disc.

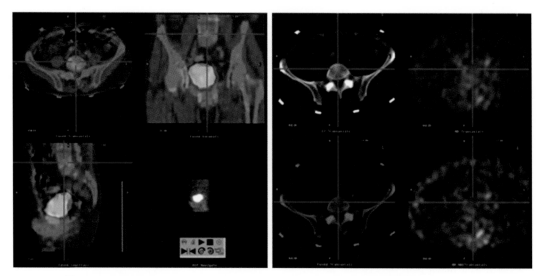

Figure 11.2 ^{111}In-biotin images show no uptake in the L4–L5 vertebral bodies or in the corresponding intervertebral disc.

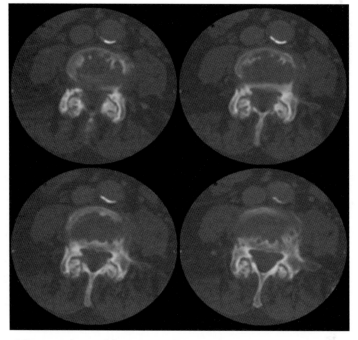

Figure 11.3 Transaxial CT images show endplate erosion of L4–L5, sclerosis near the lytic lesions, hypointensity of the disc and modified intensity in the paraspinal regions.

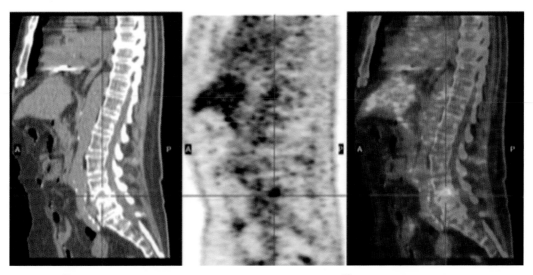

Figure 11.4 [^{18}F]FDG-PET/CT transaxial images show an increased uptake of [^{18}F]FDG in the central region of the vertebral body (L5), suggesting spondylodiscitis.

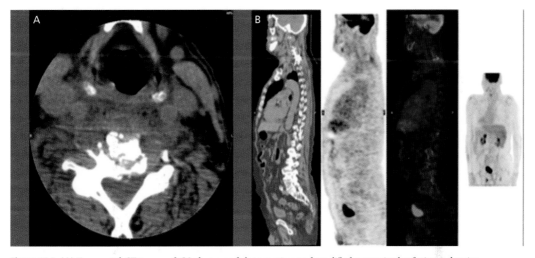

Figure 11.5 (A) Transaxial CT image of C6 shows endplate erosion and modified paraspinal soft tissue density consistent with a spine infection. (B) [^{18}F]FDG-PET/CT sagittal images show increased uptake of [^{18}F]FDG in the cervical spine (C6–C7), suggesting spondylodiscitis.

Case 3

A 75-year-old male who reported onset of cervical back pain and fever.

Both the erythrocyte sedimentation rate (ESR) and C-reactive protein (CRP) level were raised: 48 mm/h and 1.42 mg/dL.

CT imaging suggested the presence of cervical spine infection (Figure 11.5A) and the report on [^{18}F]FDG-PET/CT imaging stated: "Increased uptake of [^{18}F]FDG in the cervical spine (C6–C7), suggesting spondylodiscitis" (Figure 11.5B).

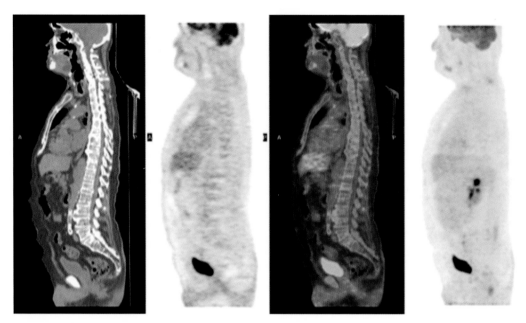

Figure 11.6 [^{18}F]FDG-PET/CT sagittal images show decreased uptake of [^{18}F]FDG in the cervical spine (C6–C7) in comparison to the previous PET/CT (Figure 11.5B), suggesting a good response to antibiotic therapy.

Following a 6-month course of antibiotic treatment, a repeat [^{18}F]FDG-PET/CT scan reported: "Reduced [^{18}F]FDG uptake in the cervical spine, suggesting good response to antibiotic treatment" (Figure 11.6).

Teaching point

Functional radionuclide imaging with [^{18}F]FDG-PET allows the response to treatment to be monitored in patients with infection, especially postsurgical infections.

CHAPTER 12

Nuclear Medicine Imaging of Soft Tissue Infections

Bárbara Morales Klinkert

Fundación López Perez (FALP), Santiago, Chile

Introduction

Soft tissue infections can localize either in superficial skin layers (epidermis, dermis and hypodermis or subcutaneous tissue) or in deeper layers (aponeurotic fascia and muscles). It is common to find localized signs and symptoms, such as regional increased volume, palpable mass, changes in skin temperature, color, hypersensitivity and pain. Soft tissue infections may also include vascular infections and endocarditis, as well as lung and brain infections, but these are beyond the scope of this chapter.

The literature on the usefulness of radionuclide techniques specifically in soft tissue infection of the skin layers is relatively scarce since radiological techniques are more frequently used (see Chapter 5). Some of the commonly used imaging agents in nuclear medicine can accumulate also in areas of sterile inflammation and, therefore, it is mandatory that a radionuclide has high specificity for infection. It is for this reason that the development of an infection-specific imaging agent is an ongoing active area of research [1].

Basic knowledge of the clinical problem

Nuclear medicine images are based on the pathophysiological local changes in acutely inflamed tissues, changes that frequently occur before morphology is altered. The vasodilatation, expansion of the extracellular space and increased concentration of neutrophils are molecular changes in infection that facilitate the accumulation of radiopharmaceuticals such as ^{67}Ga-citrate and the migration of labeled white blood cells (WBCs) into a focus of infection. The abnormal local vascular permeability of inflammation/infection also explains the non-specific accumulation of ^{99m}Tc-methyl diphosphonate (MDP) at inflamed sites during the vascular phase of the bone scan. The local hypermetabolism explains the increased uptake of [^{18}F]fluorodeoxyglucose ([^{18}F]FDG) in PET/CT scans [2].

The diagnosis and precise delineation of infectious foci may be critical in certain clinical states for patient management and therapy follow-up. Radionuclide imaging is often performed as part of a diagnostic work-up. No single test is equally efficacious in all situations, so it is crucial that the type of procedure(s) performed should be optimized for the individual clinical situation of the patient [3,4].

The clinical questions

The critical clinical question to be answered for the referring physician is whether the suspected focus is just inflamed or infected, since the therapeutic approach will be different for the two conditions.

Diagnostic Imaging of Infections and Inflammatory Diseases: A Multidisciplinary Approach, First Edition. Edited by Alberto Signore and Ana María Quintero.

Clinical symptoms and laboratory findings such as WBC count, high C-reactive protein (CRP) and raised erythrocyte sedimentation rate (ESR) are of help, but there is a need to establish a differential diagnosis between infection and inflammation. It is also important to know the precise localization and extent of the focus of infection, and to have an objective quantitative index to use in the follow-up of treatment. Definitive diagnosis is finally provided by percutaneous needle aspiration or biopsy.

Methodological considerations

WBC scintigraphy

[111]In-oxine- and ^{99m}Tc-HMPAO (hexamethylpropylene amine oxime)-labeled WBC scintigraphy are well established and sensitive techniques for soft tissue and bone infection imaging, and are currently the most widely used [4,5], even though the labeling procedure takes about 2–3 hours [6–8].

[111]In-oxine has the advantage of higher stability: its half-life of 72 hours allows delayed imaging, which is particularly valuable for musculoskeletal infection. Disadvantages are the physical characteristics related to photon energies that are not ideal for the gamma-camera.

^{99m}Tc-HMPAO has the advantages of good photon energy for imaging and value in relatively early imaging. Relative disadvantages are the appearance of genitourinary tract activity shortly after injection and colonic activity by 4 hours after injection [9].

WBC uptake depends on intact chemotaxis, the number and type of cells labeled, and the cellular component of a particular inflammatory response. Labeling does not affect the chemotactic response. A leukocyte count of at least 2000/µL is preferred. The technique is especially useful in identifying neutrophil-mediated inflammatory processes, such as bacterial infections [1,3,4].

The reported sensitivity and specificity of radiolabeled WBCs for soft tissue infections ranges from 86% to 90%, with a slightly higher sensitivity for acute infections due to the increased granulocytic response. The accuracy can be enhanced using single-photon emission computed tomography (SPECT)/CT hybrid images that give high anatomical detail and precise localization and extent of the infected focus.

[18F]FDG-PET

FDG is a glucose analog that is transported into cells via glucose transporters. The increased uptake of FDG in inflammation and infection is related to an increased number of glucose transporters.

[18F]FDG-positron emission tomography (PET) is a methodology that has achieved great success in the diagnosis, staging, treatment planning and treatment monitoring of malignant diseases. The introduction of PET/CT technology has enhanced its role in the management of these patients, but the test is not specific for cancer since lesions with inflammatory cells also take up [18F]FDG. [18F]FDG-PET can be used effectively to detect and characterize infectious and inflammatory processes [10–12] and a range of applications have been reported in infection and inflammation [fever of unknown origin (FUO), vasculitis, bacterial endocarditis, sarcoidosis, chronic granulomatous disease and thromboembolic disease] [13,14].

[18F]FDG-PET (now mainly PET/CT) has advantages over other imaging modalities: diagnostic results within 1.5–2 hours, whole-body coverage, optimal spatial resolution (CT), high target-to-background ratio, accurate localization and no reactions to administered radiopharmaceuticals. [18F]FDG-PET has a special role in evaluating cancer patients suspected of infection, especially those with febrile neutropenia. While severe hyperglycemia affects the accuracy of [18F]FDG-PET in the evaluation of malignancies, mild-to-moderate hyperglycemia (250 mg/dL) generally does not appear to affect the technique in the detection of infection and inflammation [10,15].

The standardized uptake value (SUV) can be used as a quantitative and objective index in the follow-up of treatment. Generally, a higher SUV for FDG is expected for malignancies compared with FDG accumulation in infectious or inflammatory disorders, but the index is not sufficiently discriminative. In dual-phase studies, obtaining SUVs at 30 and 90 minutes has also been assessed as a means to differentiate between infection and malignancy, but changes in SUV over time showed considerable overlap in some patients with infection and patients with malignant disease [16].

Common applications of [18F]FDG-PET/CT in soft tissue infections include FUO, HIV–AIDS-related infections and vascular graft infections (see Chapters 14–16). Few publications have reported on its application in infection limited to the skin layers.

Antigranulocyte antibody scintigraphy

[99mTc]-labeled antigranulocyte monoclonal antibody (anti-G mAb) scintigraphy is a simple and well-accepted technique because it does not require isolation of autologous WBCs. The uptake mechanism is based on the migration of the antibody to the focus due to chemotactic behavior and the non-specific uptake of the free antibody due to increased permeability at the focus [3].

Several antibodies have been tested for infection imaging, but their accumulation in sterile inflamed areas is also reported, due to localized hyperemia and increased vascular permeability, thus making the differential diagnosis with infections more difficult. Some authors have also described the possibility that human antimouse antibodies (HAMAs) are induced after repeat administrations and this may limit the use of antibodies in follow-up studies [3,17,18].

Nanocolloids

The main indications for nanocolloids are skeletal and joint infections and inflammation and they have no applications in the evaluation of soft tissue infections [19].

[67Ga]-citrate

Gallium was first shown to accumulate in inflammatory lesions in 1971. It is cheap and available in many countries but has the disadvantage of unfavorable physical characteristics with poor image quality, prolonged acquisition time and a high radiation dose to the patient. Its use is limited to clinical indications such as FUO, chronic osteomyelitis of the spine and lung infections, especially in immunocompromised patients. [67Ga]-citrate has a higher sensitivity for the identification of chronic infections [20].

[99mTc]-ciprofloxacin (Infecton)

[99mTc]-ciprofloxacin (Infecton) is a labeled broad-spectrum antibiotic used in the evaluation of orthopedic, musculoskeletal and postsurgical infections. It is postulated that this labeled quinolone is taken up mainly by viable bacteria and therefore should be a more specific agent for bacterial infection.

It can be distributed as a cold kit to be labeled with [99mTc], which avoids the need to manipulate blood samples, giving very high quality planar and SPECT images.

[99mTc]-MDP bone scintigraphy

Three-phase bone scintigraphy with [99mTc]-MDP has an important role in establishing the differential diagnosis between soft tissue infection (cellulitis) and bone infection (osteomyelitis).

Normal findings and artifacts

WBC scintigraphy

At early images (<1 hour post injection), diffuse uptake in the lungs, vascular structures, kidneys and bladder is considered normal. In delayed images (at 2–4 hours), the normal distribution is symmetric uptake in the reticuloendothelial system (spleen > liver, and skeletal bone marrow) and urinary excretion (kidneys and bladder) (Figure 12.1). In late images (at 24 hours), the distribution is the same, but in 6–8% of cases it is also normal to see colonic uptake secondary to hepatobiliary excretion of [99mTc]-HMPAO. Any other accumulation is considered abnormal.

The manipulation of the WBCs introduces the possibility of cellular damage or clumping that can alter their normal distribution. Unusual localizations of labeled WBCs must be considered, such as at accessory spleens (20–30% autopsy finding) and brain infarcts [21].

Asymmetry must be considered abnormal and suggests increased or decreased uptake. Decreased bone marrow uptake has been described in radiotherapy fields, bone tumors, treated osteomyelitis and disc-space infections after surgery.

[18F]FDG-PET/CT

The normal distribution of FDG includes the brain, myocardium and genitourinary tract. Bone marrow, gastric and bowel activity are variable. Thymic uptake, especially in children, can be prominent. Liver and spleen uptake are generally low-grade and diffuse, although in infection, splenic uptake may be intense.

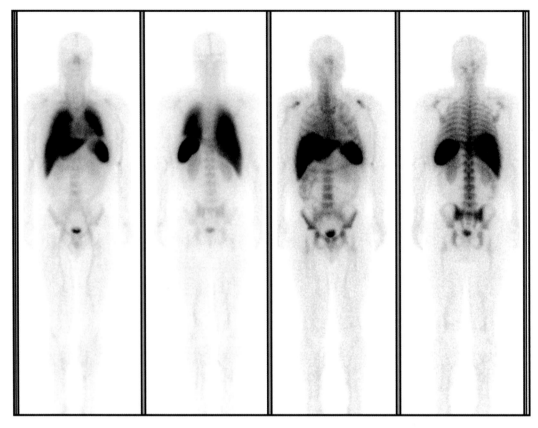

30 minutes **4 hours**

Figure 12.1 Total-body scan acquired 30 minutes and 4 hours after IV administration of 15 mCi of ^{99m}Tc-labeled WBCs. A normal distribution can be appreciated. Lung activity can be seen at the early time point but has disappeared at 4 hours. Spleen uptake is usually higher than liver uptake. Note some bone morrow physiological activity at 4 hours. After 4 hours, intestinal activity appears due to liver excretion of unbound ^{99m}Tc-HMPAO.

Artifacts that can produce focal uptake and are sources of misinterpretation include local inflammatory response to vaccination sites and brown fat uptake due to an inadequate room temperature or to muscular contractions related to patient anxiety or room temperature prior to injection.

^{99m}Tc-ciprofloxacin (Infecton)

Images are usually acquired 2, 4 and 24 hours after IV administration (Figure 12.2) [22]. Additional SPECT/CT images at 4 or 24 hours allow better delineation of soft tissue infection in musculoskeletal applications.

The normal distribution of Infecton is similar to a blood pool image and stable over time, with mild uptake in the heart, great vessels, kidneys and bladder, and faint uptake in whole-body soft tissue. Higher uptake in the first series and in the 4-hour image is considered abnormal. The 20–24-hour image is considered when doubt exists: if the uptake persists, it is considered a positive result; if the uptake reduces, the study is classified as indeterminate.

^{99m}Tc-MDP bone scintigraphy

Normal vascular phases show symmetrical uptake in the great vessels and vascular pool. Normal late phases at 2 or 24 hours post injection show symmetrical uptake in the skeleton according to the osteoblastic activity of the patient. Any soft tissue uptake is considered abnormal (Figure 12.3). If present, artifacts such as contamination of the skin or patient's clothes must be ruled out.

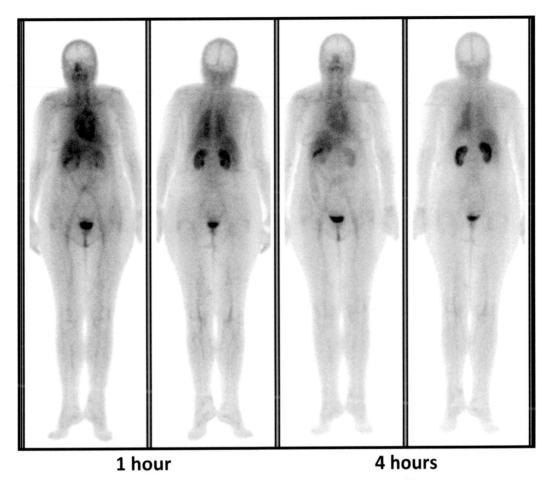

1 hour   **4 hours**

Figure 12.2 Total-body scan acquired 1 and 4 hours after IV administration of 10 mCi of ^{99m}Tc-ciprofloxacin (Infecton). A normal distribution can be appreciated. Note the different biodistribution compared to WBCs in Figure 12.1. This radiopharmaceutical is mainly metabolized by the kidneys and no liver and intestinal activity are seen. No bone marrow activity is also usual.

Pathological findings and significance

The following are crucial in all nuclear medicine techniques to optimize the interpretation of a study: a detailed clinical history of the patient, an optimal technical preparation before the scan and care taken to note the physiological causes of possible artifacts.

Dermatitis

Case reports in the literature have described focal soft tissue uptake of ^{67}Ga-citrate and ^{99m}Tc-labeled WBCs in biopsy-proven erythema nodosum lesions. [^{18}F]FDG uptake has also been shown in these types of skin lesions in patients with the clinical diagnosis

of non-Hodgkin's disease [23–25]. Ultrasound (US) is the first-line imaging technique used in this diagnosis (see Chapter 5) and nuclear medicine procedures have a minimal role, mainly in evaluating moderate-to-severe infections.

Cellulitis

Cellulitis is defined as an acute infection of the skin and subcutaneous tissue. Clinically, it presents as a local defined area of erythema, redness and diffuse swelling of the skin, fever and pain. The most common microorganisms involved are *Staphylococcus aureus* and streptococci, but polymicrobial infection, including with anaerobes, can also be found.

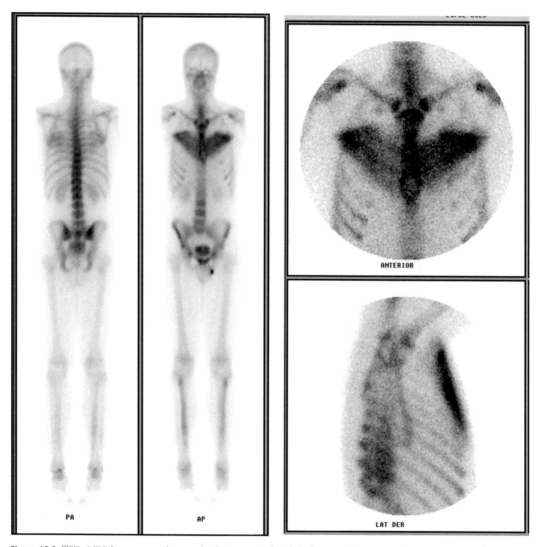

ANTERIOR

LAT DER

PA

AP

Figure 12.3 ^{99m}Tc-MDP bone scan. Abnormal soft tissue uptake of the bone-seeking agent due to recent muscle exercise should be kept in mind in order to avoid misinterpretations.

Early diagnosis and treatment are important to avoid serious complications.

US with color power Doppler can establish the inflammatory element in the subcutaneous tissues, but cannot locate infection unless guided needle samples are taken for laboratory analysis (see Chapter 5). Cellulitis is seen as a poorly defined area of increased CT density or T2 signal intensity within the fat with an amorphous enhancement following contrast infusion (see Chapter 5). Since infections can sometimes mimic the appearance of non-infectious space-occupying lesions radiologically,

nuclear medicine procedures are needed to confirm infection.

Radiolabeled WBCs can detect and delineate the extent of the infectious process and enable prompt treatment, but cannot differentiate cellulitis from abscess formation [26]. The classic finding for cellulitis in a multiphase bone scan is regional or diffusely increased perfusion with either no corresponding increase in bone uptake on static images or only mild diffuse or focally increased uptake due to hyperemia of the adjacent soft tissue infection. In order to confirm the infectious nature of the process, a ^{99m}Tc-HMPAO-labeled WBC scan needs to be performed [26].

Abscesses

Skin layer abscesses are frequently associated with surgical or traumatic wounds. The early diagnosis and precise evaluation of these abscesses as well as deeper abscesses in intensive care unit patients with underlying systemic diseases or occult sepsis is essential if life-threatening complications are to be avoided and appropriate clinical or surgical management provided.

CT scanning has been advocated in the management of abscesses and can show areas of fluid attenuation with peripheral enhancement after intravenous contrast administration; air may occasionally be seen within the abscess [26]. However, the benefits of CT must be weighed against the time necessary to schedule and obtain the scan. ^{99m}Tc-HMPAO-labeled WBCs are sensitive in the detection and confirmation of infectious processes with good quality images. A whole-body image can be obtained, utilizing mobile cameras in the case of very ill patients [27].

Radiolabeled WBCs do not accumulate in normally healing surgical wounds, so the presence of such activity indicates infection. The lateral and oblique views are useful in detecting the existence of a deep skin abscess.

Granulating wounds which heal by secondary intention can appear as areas of intense activity on WBC images even in the absence of infection. Examples include "stomies" (tracheostomies, ileostomies, feeding gastrostomies, etc.) and skin grafts. Vascular access lines, dialysis catheters and even lumbar punctures can all produce false-positive results in the absence of an appropriate clinical history [28,29]. In this case, however, activity at delayed images is lower than that observed at late images.

A ^{99m}Tc-ciprofloxacin scan can also help in the identification of abscesses (Figure 12.4).

Bursitis

Bursitis is the inflammation of the bursa located adjacent to the tendons near the large joints. It is usually a sterile inflammation of the bursal wall as a result of repetitive trauma or mechanical stress. When infection is present, *S. aureus* is the most frequent organism involved. The most commonly affected bursae are those of the olecranon, hip and patella. Treatment of non-infectious bursitis

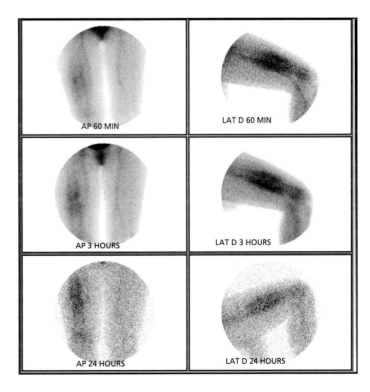

Figure 12.4 ^{99m}Tc-ciprofloxacin scan in an 18-year-old patient with a clinical diagnosis of cellulitis of the right thigh. Planar images show abnormal uptake in the deep soft tissues of the distal portion of the right thigh and in the femur projection, suggesting concomitant osteomyelitis. A deep muscle abscess and a femur osteomyelitis were confirmed.

includes rest, ice and medications for inflammation and pain; infectious bursitis (Figure 12.5) is treated with antibiotics, aspiration and surgery.

Bursitis is usually diagnosed clinically; however, imaging tests such as US and MRI can help to confirm deep localizations (see Chapter 5). The US appearances of infectious and non-infectious bursitis are similar.

Many cases of asymptomatic hip bursitis are an incidental finding on a bone scan and their recognition is important to avoid misinterpretation of an increased trochanteric uptake focus, particularly in patients with malignant diseases, and to aid in the diagnosis and effective management of this treatable condition [30].

A labeled WBC scan may confirm or exclude infection in the presence of non-specific findings on US, MR or bone scan.

Tenosynovitis

Infective tenosynovitis is commonly the result of penetrating trauma, affects the hands and wrists, and is usually caused by *S. aureus* and *S. pyogenes*.

Whenever the possibility of an infective tenosynovitis exists and US or MRI have visualized or delineated a tendon sheath effusion (see Chapter 5), a US-guided aspiration of the tendon fluid will be helpful in differentiating infective from non-infective causes.

Nuclear medicine procedures such as a three-phase bone scan appear to be of value in the differential diagnosis of different localizations and etiologies of tenosynovitis, showing abnormal uptake in vascular and/or late phases [31,32]. Leslie *et al.* described a typical scintigraphic finding in de Quervain tenosynovitis as a focal area of superficial linear hyperemia in the vascular phase and skeletal uptake along the radial aspect of the distal radius in the late phase, corresponding to the anatomical location of the abductor pollicis longus and the extensor pollicis brevis [33,34].

Myositis

Pyomyositis is a suppurative bacterial infection of the muscle. It is relatively uncommon and most commonly affects the larger muscles of the lower limbs. Muscle trauma and hematoma can be precipitating factors and *S. aureus* is the causative organism in most cases. The lack of specific clinical findings means early diagnosis is unlikely.

At an early stage, US reveals diffuse muscle swelling with edema and hyperemia. In late stages and when untreated, abscess formation can be assessed either by US or MRI and percutaneously guided drainage will be needed.

Nathan *et al.* reported the utility of nuclear medicine techniques in pyomyositis, showing the value of fused SPECT/CT imaging with labeled WBCs in differentiating the abnormal soft tissue uptake in muscles from unaffected bone [35]. Abdullah *et al.* showed the same finding when using SPECT/CT with bone scanning agents [36]. The combined use of SPECT/CT labeled WBCs and MRI can provide essential anatomical information to guide drainage procedures.

It is important to consider that scintigraphic techniques using bone-seeking agents lack specificity for infection. Myositis ossificans is a non-infectious process characterized by abnormal heterotopic bone formation involving striated muscle, tendons, ligaments, fasciae and aponeurosis. Whole-body bone imaging may be helpful in determining the full extent of this disease and may do this more accurately and earlier than conventional radiographs. In addition, radiographs tend to underestimate the severity of the disease [37,38]. A case report by Makis *et al.* found that myositis ossificans can mimic an osteoid osteoma on a bone scan [39]. Also, the possibility of abnormal skeletal muscle uptake of bone-seeking agents due to recent muscle exercise should be kept in mind in order to avoid misinterpretations.

Fasciitis

Plantar fasciitis is the most common fasciitis and is characterized by a fusiform thickening of the plantar fascia close to the calcaneal enthesis, with associated fluid collection and increased vascularity. US describes the plantar fascia thickening (threshold value of 4.0 mm) and areas of hypoechogenicity within the proximal plantar fascia. Three-phase radionuclide bone imaging shows the abnormal increased radioisotope uptake within the subcalcaneal region in the vascular phases, indicating the hyperemia of the proximal plantar fascia (Figure 12.6). The plantar uptake in the blood pool images provides prognostic information on the response to localized injection of corticoids into the enthesis [40].

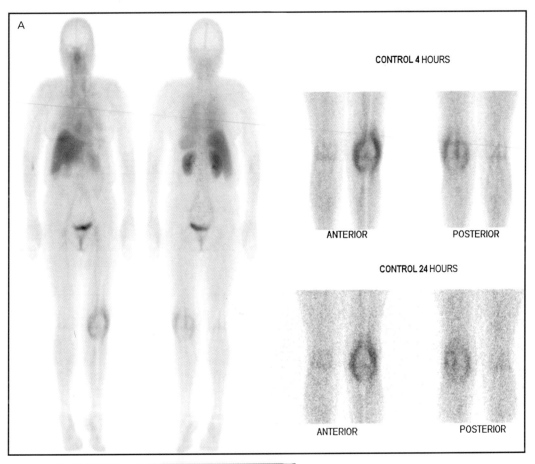

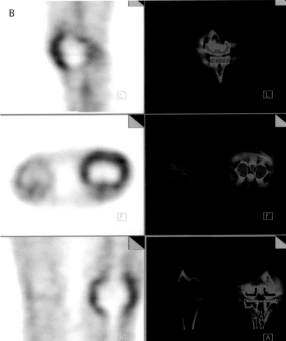

Figure 12.5 ^{99m}Tc-ciprofloxacin scan in a patient with clinically diagnosed bursitis. (A) Planar images show persistent abnormal uptake related to left knee prosthesis-associated inflammation and bursitis. (B) SPECT/CT images clearly show that only soft tissue is involved, excluding an associated osteomyelitis. Biopsy confirmed a *S. aureus* synovial infection.

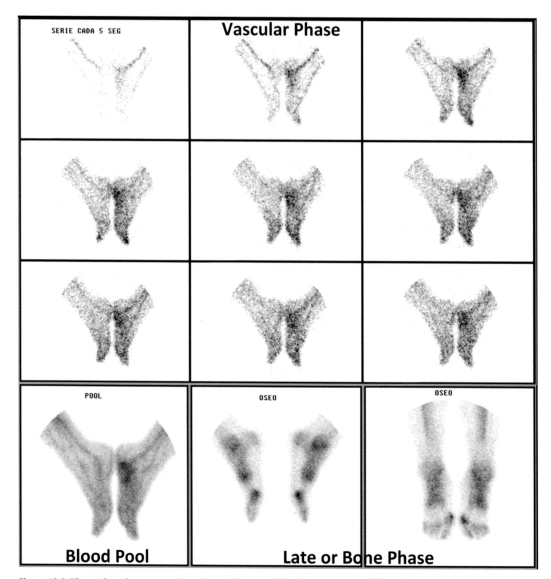

Figure 12.6 Three-phase bone scan of a patient with acute left plantar pain on walking. The vascular and blood pool images show hyperemia of the soft tissue in the plantar of the left foot. No abnormal osteoblastic activity is seen at this level in the late-phase images. This is typical of plantar fasciitis.

The scintigraphic findings are similar to those for tenosynovitis since both pathologies have a similar pathological pathway: tissue changes are thought to proceed from an early reactive phase to progressive degeneration. The tendon appears thickened with focal areas of hypoechogenicity and increased vascularity. Furthermore, the tendon has been found to respond to corticosteroid injection in a similar way to the plantar fascia [41].

Cat scratch disease

The so-called "cat scratch disease" is an infective disease caused by *Bartonella henselae*. It usually appears as a lymphadenopathy that is diagnosed clinically or on US. Bone involvement is rare and is associated with bone pain. In these cases a bone scintigraphy with ^{99m}Tc-MDP may be useful in showing bone involvement. MRI can also show bone disease, but the ^{99m}Tc-MDP scan is generally more sensitive and useful also for therapy follow-up [42].

Implantable device-associated infections

There is an increasing use of implantable medical devices in medical and surgical practice. The most commonly used are intravascular arterial and venous catheters and devices (central venous catheters, pacemakers, portacath, etc.), neurosurgical devices (catheters, reservoirs, stimulators, etc.), respiratory devices, abdominal mesh, urogynecological devices (catheters for dialysis, cosmetic implants, penile implants), dermal fillers, otolaryngological implants, ophthalmological implants and dental implants.

Implantable devices can easily become infected [43] since bacteria tend to adhere to the surface of these devices and this can lead to sepsis or localized infection of the surrounding soft tissues. Bacteria can colonize the surface of the device by adhering to coated proteins (such as fibrin and fibronectin for vascular catheters; and proteins, electrolytes and other organic molecules for urinary catheters). Bacteria can then produce a polysaccharide matrix called a "biofilm" (see Chapter 2) in which the bacteria may grow. In this state, bacteria are difficult to detect and treat. Under unfavorable environmental conditions, microorganisms can detach from the biofilm and become free-floating (planktonic). The presence of planktonic organisms in the bloodstream or urine can lead to sepsis and metastatic infections.

Biofilms, therefore, allow bacterial growth, reduce leukocyte migration and phagocytosis, and reduce antibiotic penetration and treatment of infection (bacteria in biofilms are over 1000 times more resistant to antibiotics than planktonic cells). Radiopharmaceuticals can also only poorly penetrate biofilms and this can make their use in the diagnosis of infection difficult.

From a diagnostic point of view, nuclear medicine is more often indicated than radiological techniques. Although there are limited reports in the literature, any nuclear medicine center will be dealing with these cases on a daily basis. ^{111}In- and

^{99m}Tc-labeled WBCs have the highest diagnostic accuracy; both are better than ^{67}Ga-citrate. More recently, [^{18}F]FDG has been proved useful in some cases of implant-associated infection.

For vascular devices, ^{67}Ga-citrate or radiolabeled WBCs are the most accurate [44–48], although the only other experiences reported have been with [^{18}F]FDG [49–51].

^{111}In- and ^{99m}Tc-labeled WBC scans have been used for neurological infections associated with implants [52,53]. ^{67}Ga-citrate scintigraphy [54] and [^{18}F]FDG have also been used in selected cases [55,56].

Mesh infection can be associated with an enterocutaneous fistula or a superficial incisional surgical site infection [57]. Radiographic imaging (either US, CT or MRI) is useful in the diagnosis of some cases of mesh infection, but as fluid surrounding the mesh can be a normal benign finding [58], radionuclide techniques are usually more accurate in detecting the infection site and extent [59–62].

US, CT and CT/MR peritoneography are particularly helpful for detecting fluid collections in infected peritoneal dialysis catheters, but radiolabeled WBCs (labeled with ^{111}In-oxine [63] or ^{99m}Tc-HMPAO [64]) have also been used to image infected peritoneal dialysis catheter tunnels [65–67]. Imaging with [^{18}F]FDG-PET has also proved to be helpful in diagnosing these tunnel infections [68].

Role for therapy follow-up and patient management

The prompt and appropriate work-up of musculoskeletal soft tissue infections aids early diagnosis and treatment, and decreases the risk of complications resulting from misdiagnosis or delayed diagnosis. US and MRI are the imaging modalities of choice in the evaluation of soft tissue infections [43] (see Chapter 5).

Anatomical techniques such as CT, MRI, US and conventional X-ray rely on the focal changes in density and composition of the affected area to define the lesion, so they can easily detect infection when there is tissue necrosis or abscess formation. MRI is highly sensitive and the fact that ionizing radiation is not used makes it especially valuable in follow-up, but its specificity is low since MRI does not distinguish between infected tissue or effusion and non-specific inflammation. A highly necrotic neo-plasm may also simulate an abscess on MRI [44].

Nuclear medicine techniques, especially labeled WBCs, play an important role in the diagnosis and localization of soft tissue infections in the early phases, in the presence of abnormal landmarks, and in confirming the presence of an infectious process, and have the advantage of providing a whole-body image when searching for occult focus. The high negative predictive value of a normal WBC scan makes this a very useful follow-up technique.

[^{18}F]FDG-PET is known to be useful for determining the effects of therapy in oncological patients, but more recently its use has also been proposed in the evaluation of therapeutic efficacy in infection. Studies in animals have shown that [^{18}F]FDG-PET is accurate in monitoring responses following antibiotic therapy in the setting of soft tissue infection. Other clinical studies have shown that [^{18}F]FDG uptake returned to normal levels after successful antibiotic therapy, even when persistent abnormalities were seen on MRI [10].

Conclusion

Soft tissue infections are, for the most part, accessible to evaluation by US, and this is the first-line investigation for many of them. US-guided aspiration frequently provides sufficient information to determine treatment, thereby helping to minimize long-term morbidity. MRI and CT can be reserved for situations where access is limited or infection is severe and extensive.

In nuclear medicine, several radiopharmaceuticals are available for imaging infection. The value of a labeled WBC scan in different infectious diseases has been well established over the past 20 years, but there is still a need for a more specific agent that can differentiate inflammation and infection.

The role of modern nuclear medicine imaging techniques, such as SPECT/CT and PET/CT, where anatomical and functional information is obtained simultaneously, has contributed to better detection and precise localization of soft tissue infection. The introduction of hybrid techniques is extending the role of nuclear medicine in the diagnosis of infection, not only in the detection and characterization of the focus, but also in the capacity to provide an objective quantitative index to use in the follow-up of treatment.

References

1. Petruzzi N, Shanthly N, Thakur M. Recent trends in soft tissue infection imaging. *Semin Nucl Med* 2009; 39:115–123.
2. Alazraki NP. Radionuclide imaging in the evaluation of infections and inflammatory disease. *Radiol Clin North Am* 1993;31:783–794.
3. Becker W. The contribution of nuclear medicine to the patient with infection. *Eur J Nucl Med* 1995;22: 1195–1211.
4. Peters AM, Danpure HJ, Osman S *et al.* Clinical experience with Tc99m-HMPAO for labeling leucocytes and imaging infection. *Lancet* 1986;2:946–949.
5. Peters AM. The utility of Tc99m-HMPAO leucocytes for imaging infection. *Semin Nucl Med* 1994;24: 110–127.
6. Love C, Palestro CJ. Radionuclide imaging of infection. *J Nucl Med Technol* 2004;32:47–57.
7. Roca M, de Vries EF, Jamar F, Israel O, Signore A. Guidelines for the labelling of leucocytes with In111-oxine. *Eur J Nucl Med Mol Imaging* 2010;37: 835–841.
8. De Vries EF, Roca M, Jamar F, Israel O, Signore A. Guidelines for the labeling of leucocytes with Tc99m-HMPAO. *Eur J Nucl Med Mol Imaging* 2010;37: 842–848.
9. Boerman OC, Rennen H, Oyen WJ, Corstens FH. Radiopharmaceuticals to image infection and inflammation. *Semin Nucl Med* 2001;31:286–295.
10. Kumar R, Basu S, Torigian D, Anand V, Zhuang H, Alavi A. Role of modern imaging techniques for diagnosis of infection in the era of ^{18}F-fluorodeoxyglucose positron emission tomography. *Clin Microbiol Rev* 2008;21:209–224.
11. Basu S, Chryssikos T, Moghadam-Kia S, Zhuang H, Torigian DA, Alavi A. Positron emission tomography as a diagnostic tool in infection: present role and future possibilities. *Semin Nucl Med* 2009;39: 36–51.
12. Glaudemans A, Signore A. FDG-PET/CT in infections: the imaging method of choice? *Eur J Nucl Med Mol Imaging* 2010;37:1986–1991.
13. Love C, Tomas MB, Tronco GG, Palestro CJ. FDG-PET of infection and inflammation. *RadioGraphics* 2005; 25:1357–1368.
14. Bleeker-Rovers CP, de Kleijn EMHA, Corstens FHM *et al.* Clinical value of FDG PET in patients with fever of unknown origin and patients suspected of focal infection or inflammation. *Eur J Nucl Med Mol Imaging* 2004;31:29–37.
15. Zhuang HM, Cortés-Blanco A, Pourdehnad M *et al.* Do high glucose levels have differential effect on FDG uptake in inflammatory and malignant disorders? *Nucl Med Commun* 2001;22:1123–1128.

16. Sahlmann CO, Siefker U, Lehmann K *et al.* Dual time point 2-[^{18}F]fluoro-2′-deoxyglucose positron emission tomography in chronic bacterial osteomyelitis. *Nucl Med Commun* 2004;25:819–823.

17. Thakur ML, Thiagarajan P, White F, Park CH, Maurer PH. Monoclonal antibodies for specific cell labeling: Considerations, preparations and preliminary evaluation. *Int J Rad Appl Instrum B* 1987;14:51–58.

18. Mozley PD, Thakur ML, Alavi A *et al.* Effects of a 99mTc-labeled murine immunoglobulin M antibody to CD15 antigens on human granulocyte membranes in healthy volunteers. *J Nucl Med* 1999;40:2107–2114.

19. Wheeler JG, Slack NF, Duncan A Palmer M, Harvey RF. Tc99m-nanocolloid in inflammatory bowel disease. *Nucl Med Commun* 1990;11:127–133.

20. Vorne M, Soini I, Lantto T, Paakkinen S. Technetium-99m HMPAO-labeled leukocytes in detection of inflammatory lesions: comparison with Gallium-67 citrate. *J Nucl Med* 1989;30:1332–1336.

21. Coleman RE, Welch D. Possible pitfalls with clinical imaging of indium-111 leukocytes: Concise communication. *J Nucl Med* 1980;21:122–125.

22. Amaral H, Morales B, Pruzzo R, Britton KE. Cold–hot mismatch between Tc99m-HMPAO-labeled leukocytes and Tc99m ciprofloxacin in axial skeleton infections: A report of three cases. *Clin Nucl Med* 1999;24:855–858.

23. Winzelberg GG, Rabinowitz J. Whole body Gallium-67 citrate in a patient with sarcoidosis and biopsy proven erythema nodosum. *Clin Nucl Med* 1984;9:418.

24. Cheong KA, Rodgers NG, Kirkwood ID. Erythema nodosum associated with diffuse large B-cell non Hodgkin lymphoma detected by FDG-PET. *Clin Nucl Med* 2003;28:652–654.

25. Peng NJ, Wang JH, Hsieh SP, Jao GH, Tsay DG, Liu RS. Ga-67 and Tc-99m HMPAO labeled WBC imaging in erythema nodosum leprosum reaction of leprosy. *Clin Nucl Med* 1998;23:248–250.

26. Sayit E, Soylev M, Capa G *et al.* The role of technetium-99m-HMPAO-labeled WBC scintigraphy in the diagnosis of orbital cellulitis. *Ann Nucl Med* 2001;15:41–44.

27. Kao CH, Wang SJ. Spread of infectious complications of odontogenic abscess detected by technetium-99m-HMPAO labeled WBC scan of occult sepsis in the intensive care unit. *J Nucl Med* 1992;33:254–255.

28. Datz FL. Abdominal abscess detection: Gallium, ^{111}In-, and ^{99m}Tc-labeled leukocytes, and polyclonal and monoclonal antibodies. *Semin Nucl Med* 1996;26:51–64.

29. Palestro CJ, Love C, Tronco GG, Tomas MB. Role of radionuclide imaging in the diagnosis of postoperative infection. *RadioGraphics* 2000;20:1649–1660; discussion 1660–1663.

30. Allwright SJ, Cooper RA, Nash P. Trochanteric bursitis: bone scan appearance. *Clin Nucl Med* 1988;13:561–564.

31. Kaya M, Tuna H, Tuncbilek N, Cermik TF, Sardogan K. Scintigraphic findings in plant thorn tenosynovitis of finger. *Clin Nucl Med* 2008;33:131–132.

32. Hung GU, Lan Jl, Yang KT, Lin WY, Wang SJ. Scintigraphic findings of *Mycobacterium avium* complex tenosynovitis of the index finger in a patient with systemic lupus erythematosus. *Clin Nucl Med* 2003;28:936–938.

33. Leslie WD. The scintigraphic appearance of de Quervain tenosynovitis. *Clin Nucl Med* 2006;31:602–604.

34. Barber L, Bourke J, Gill G, Graham P. Three phase bone scintigraphy in suppurative tenosynovitis. *Clin Nucl Med* 1995;20:928–929.

35. Nathan J, Crawford JA, Sodee DB, Bakale G. Fused SPECT-CT imaging of the peri-iliopsoas infection using Indium111-labeled leukocytes. *Clin Nucl Med* 2006;31:801–802.

36. Abdullah ZS, Khan MU, Kodali SK, Javaid A. Pyomyositis mimicking osteomyelitis detected by SPEC-CT. *Hell J Nucl Med* 2010;13:277–279.

37. Tyler P, Saifuddin A. The imaging of myositis ossificans. *Semin Musculoskelet Radiol* 2010;14:201–216.

38. Sabatel Hernández G, Moral Ruiz A, Gómez Río M *et al.* Progressive myositis ossificans. Utility of bone scintigraphy. *Rev Esp Med Nucl* 2005;24:195–198.

39. Makis W, Lambert R. Myositis ossificans mimics an osteoid osteoma: a pitfall for Tc-99m MDP planar and SPECT scintigraphy. *Clin Nucl Med* 2010;35:175–177.

40. Frater C, Vu D, Van der Wall H *et al.* Bone scintigraphy predicts outcome of steroid injection for plantar fasciitis. *J Nucl Med* 2006;47:1577–1580.

41. McMillan AM, Landorf KB, Barrett JT, Menz HB, Bird AR. Diagnostic imaging for chronic plantar heel pain: a systematic review and meta-analysis. *J Foot Ankle Res* 2009;2:32.

42. Ismaili-Alaoui N, Vuong V, Marcu-Marin M, Sergent-Alaoui A, Chevallier B, de Labriolle-Vaylet C. Cat-scratch disease and bone scintigraphy. *Clin Nucl Med* 2012;37:772–774.

43. Guggenbichler JP, Assadian O, Boeswald M, Kramer A. Incidence and clinical implication of nosocomial infections associated with implantable biomaterials – catheters, ventilator-associated pneumonia, urinary tract infections. *GMS Krankenhhyg Interdiszip* 2011;6:Doc18.

44. Gutfilen B, Lopes de Souza SA, Martins FP, Cardoso LR, Pinheiro Pessoa MC, Fonseca LM. Use of ^{99m}Tc-mononuclear leukocyte scintigraphy in nosocomial fever. *Acta Radiol* 2006;47:699–704.

45. Lai CH, Chi CY, Chen HP, Lai CJ, Fung CP, Liu CY. Port-A catheter-associated Nocardia bacteremia detected by gallium inflammation scan: a case report and literature review. *Scand J Infect Dis* 2004;36:775–777.

46. Miller JH. Detection of deep venous thrombophlebitis by gallium 67 scintigraphy. *Radiology* 1981;140:183–186.

47. Chiu JS, Tzeng JE, Wang YF. Infection hunter: gallium scintigraphy for hemodialysis access graft infection. *Kidney Int* 2006;69:1290.

48. Sullivan SJ, Quadri SM, Cunha BA. Hickman catheter *Staphylococcus aureus* bacteremia diagnosed by indium-111 scan. *Heart Lung* 1992;21:505–506.

49. Miceli MH, Jones Jackson LB, Walker RC, Talamo G, Barlogie B, Anaissie EJ. Diagnosis of infection of implantable central venous catheters by [^{18}F]fluorodeoxyglucose positron emission tomography. *Nucl Med Commun* 2004; 25:813–818.

50. Bhargava P, Kumar R, Zhuang H, Charron M, Alavi A. Catheter-related focal FDG activity on whole body PET imaging. *Clin Nucl Med* 2004;29:238–242.

51. Mahfouz T, Miceli MH, Saghafifar F *et al.* ^{18}F-fluorodeoxyglucose positron emission tomography contributes to the diagnosis and management of infections in patients with multiple myeloma: a study of 165 infectious episodes. *J Clin Oncol* 2005;23:7857–7863.

52. Medina M, Viglietti AL, Gozzoli L *et al.* Indium-111 labelled white blood cell scintigraphy in cranial and spinal septic lesions. *Eur J Nucl Med* 2000;27:1473–1480.

53. Liberatore M, Drudi FM, Tarantino R *et al.* Tc-99m exametazime-labeled leukocyte scans in the study of infections in skull neurosurgery. *Clin Nucl Med* 2003;28:971–974.

54. Sun SS, Chuang FJ, Chiu KL, Kao CH. Demonstration of ventriculoperitoneal shunt infection on Ga-67 citrate scintigraphy. *Clin Nucl Med* 2002;27:666.

55. Wan DQ, Joseph UA, Barron BJ, Caram P, Nguyen AP. Ventriculoperitoneal shunt catheter and cerebral spinal fluid infection initially detected by FDG PET/CT scan. *Clin Nucl Med* 2009;34:464–465.

56. Rehman T, Chohan M, Yonas H. Diagnosis of ventriculoperitoneal shunt infection using [F-18]-FDG PET: a case report. *J Neurosurg Sci* 2011;55:161–163.

57. Petersen S, Henke G, Freitag M *et al.* Deep prosthesis infection in incisional hernia repair: Predictive factors and clinical outcome. *Eur J Surg* 2001;167:453–457.

58. Sanchez VM, Abi-Haidar YE, Itani KM. Mesh infection in ventral incisional hernia repair: incidence, contributing factors, and treatment. *Surg Infect* 2011;12:205–210.

59. Zuvela M, Antic A, Bajec D *et al.* Diagnosis of mesh infection after abdominal wall hernia surgery – role of radionuclide methods. *Hepatogastroenterology* 2011;58:1455–1460.

60. Lin WY, Chao TH, Wang SJ. Clinical features and gallium scan in the detection of post-surgical infection in the elderly. *Eur J Nucl Med Mol Imaging* 2002;29:371–375.

61. Datz FL. Abdominal abscess detection: gallium, ^{111}In-, and ^{99m}Tc-labeled leukocytes, and polyclonal and monoclonal antibodies. *Semin Nucl Med* 1996;26:51–64.

62. Palestro CJ, Love C, Tronco GG, Tomas MB. Role of radionuclide imaging in the diagnosis of postoperative infection. *RadioGraphics* 2000;20:1649–1660.

63. Kipper SL, Steiner RW, Wilztum KF *et al.* In-111-leukocyte scintigraphy for detection of infection associated with peritoneal dialysis catheters. *Radiology* 1984;151:491–494.

64. Ruiz Solis S, Garcia Vicente A, Rodaco Marina S *et al.* Diagnosis of the infectious complications of continuous ambulatory peritoneal dialysis by ^{99m}Tc-HMPAO labeled leucocytes. *Rev Esp Med Nucl* 2004;23:403–413.

65. Gibel LJ, Hartshorne MF, Tzamaloukas AH. Indium-111 oxine leukocyte scan in the diagnosis of peritoneal catheter tunnel infections. *Perit Dial Int* 1998;18:234–235.

66. Ruiz Solis S, Garcia Vicente A, Rodaco Marina S *et al.* Diagnosis of the infectious complications of continuous ambulatory peritoneal dialysis by ^{99m}Tc-HMPAO labeled leucocytes. *Rev Esp Med Nucl* 2004;23:403–413.

67. Gibel LJ, Quintana BJ, Tzamaloukas AH, Garcia DL. Soft tissue complications of Tenckhoff catheters. *Adv Perit Dial* 1989;5:229–233.

68. Carlos MG, Juliana R, Matilde N *et al.* Hidden clotted vascular access infection diagnosed by fluorodeoxyglucose positron emission tomography. *Nephrology* 2008;13:264–265.

Clinical cases

Case 1

A 37-year-old male with complicated abdominal trauma with retroperitoneal hematoma and a right hip fracture. After hip and abdominal surgery, the patient developed cellulitis of the right thigh. He was given antibiotics.

Laboratory tests showed a CPR of 7 mg/dL, WBC count of 12 000/μL and positive blood cultures for *Acinetobacter baumannii*.

On a plain film there was a right coxofemoral fracture and signs of symphysis disjunction. On US there was a slight increased echogenicity of the subcutaneous tissue of the medial and proximal part of the right thigh. On CT the pubic symphysis disjunction was visualized with a huge hematoma draining to the muscle compartment (internal and external obturator muscle).

^{99m}Tc-ciprofloxacin scintigraphy (Figure 12.7A,B) showed a focus of abnormal increased uptake in the medial part of the right thigh and a larger and intense focus localized under the bladder at the projection site of the pubic symphysis. The line of intense uptake corresponded to a urinary catheter. In the right lateral view (Figure 12.7C), the connection between both foci (skin and pubis) suggests the existence of a cutaneous fistula. A culture from the fistula was positive for *S. aureus*.

Teaching points
• Nuclear medicine techniques have the advantage of being able to obtain a whole-body imaging.
• In this case, not only was a postsurgical abdominal abscess diagnosed, but also two abnormal foci were localized and associated, establishing the diagnosis of a fistula related to the cellulitis process. This prompted surgical drainage of the infected hematoma of the pubis and culture confirmed the diagnosis.

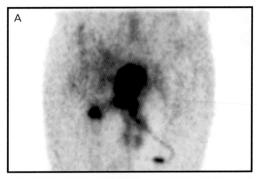

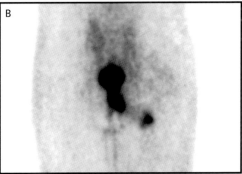

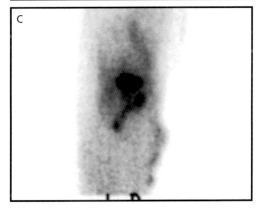

Figure 12.7 (A,B) ^{99m}Tc-ciprofloxacin scintigraphy showing pathological uptake in the medial part of the right thigh and under the bladder behind the pubic symphysis. (C) In the right lateral view, the connection between both foci (skin and pubis) suggests the presence of an infected fistula.

Case 2

Two different patients presented with fever after complicated pancreatitis surgery. US ruled out an intra-abdominal abscess in both cases.

^{99m}Tc-HMPAO-labeled WBC scintigraphy of patient 1 (Figure 12.8A) showed an abnormal linear focus of soft tissue uptake in the middle line of the abdomen in correspondence with the surgical wound and this was more intense at the proximal edge.

^{99m}Tc-HMPAO-labeled WBC scintigraphy of patient 2 (Figure 12.8B,C) showed a linear focus of abnormal soft tissue uptake at the distal edge of the surgical wound. The lateral view (Figure 12.8C)

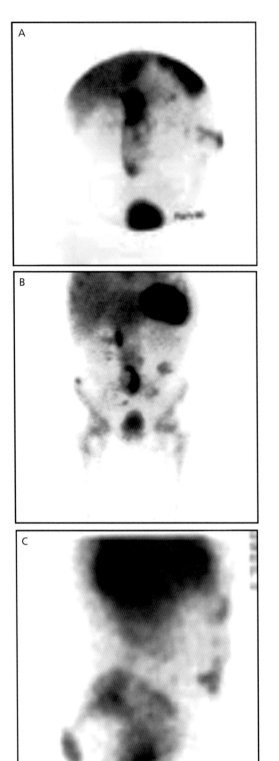

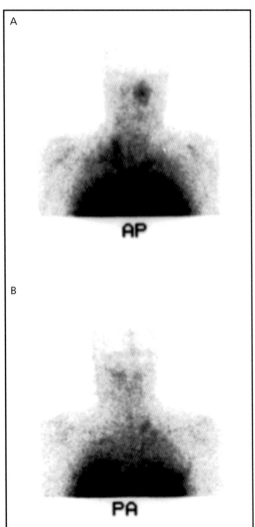

Figure 12.9 (A,B) ^{99m}Tc-HMPAO-labeled WBC scintigraphy showing pathological soft tissue uptake in correspondence with the sternocleidomastoid and pectoralis major muscles.

Figure 12.8 (A) ^{99m}Tc-HMPAO-labeled leukocyte scintigraphy of patient 1 . showing soft tissue uptake in the middle line of the abdomen in correspondence with the infected surgical wound. (B) Anteroposterior and (C) lateral views (lower panel) of ^{99m}Tc-HMPAO-labeled WBC scintigraphy of patient 2 showing linear pathological soft tissue uptake in correspondence with the surgical wound.

confirmed that the focus is superficial in the abdominal wall. Serial wound cultures were positive for *S. aureus*.

In both cases, the images show other small abnormal foci corresponding to the multiple drainage pipes.

Teaching points
• Radiolabeled WBCs do not accumulate in normally healing surgical wounds, so the presence of such activity indicates infection.
• Osteotomies, vascular access lines, dialysis catheters and even lumbar punctures can all produce false-positive results in the absence of an appropriate clinical history.

Case 3
A 31-year-old male who presented with fever and severe dorsal and intercostal pain.

Laboratory tests showed a WBC count of 9500/μL, ESR of 57 mm/h, CRP of 1.5 mg/dL and a cholecystokinin (CCK) of 115 U/mg. Blood cultures were positive for Group A β-hemolytic streptococcus.

Chest CT and X-ray were normal, as were dorsal spine CT and radiographs. US suggested myositis. The right shoulder radiograph was normal.

^{99m}Tc-HMPAO-labeled WBC scintigraphy (Figure 12.9) showed abnormal soft tissue uptake in the right hemithorax corresponding to the sternocleidomastoid and pectoralis major muscles. The focal uptake seen in the anterior projection in the middle of the skull corresponds to active sinusitis.

A guided biopsy confirmed the diagnosis of a non-necrotizing fasciitis with positive cultures for Group A β-hemolytic streptococcus. The patient responded well to antibiotics, without the need for surgery.

Teaching point
US and nuclear medicine are the only imaging techniques that can identify an abnormality at the muscle level.

CHAPTER 13

Nuclear Medicine Imaging of Infections and Inflammatory Diseases of the Abdomen

Josep Martín Comín[1], Alba Rodríguez Gasén[1] and
Christophe Van de Wiele[2]

[1]Hospital Universitari de Bellvitge, L'Hospitalet de Llobregat, Barcelona, Spain
[2]University Hospital Ghent, Ghent, Belgium

Introduction

Although the main imaging modalities in patients with acute abdominal pain are radiological and endoscopic, nuclear medicine can be helpful in many clinical situations [1,2]. Several radionuclide techniques can aid in the diagnosis of these patients and these together with the available radiopharmaceuticals are the focus of this chapter.

Positron emission tomography (PET) and single-photon emission computed tomography (SPECT) are increasingly used to diagnose, characterize and monitor disease activity in the setting of inflammatory diseases of known and unknown etiology. Gallium-67 citrate (^{67}Ga-citrate), white blood cells (WBCs) labeled with technetium-99m (^{99m}Tc) or indium-111 (^{111}In), labeled antigranulocyte monoclonal antibodies (anti-G mAbs) and [^{18}F]fluorodeoxyglucose ([^{18}F]FDG) represent the most widely used radiopharmaceuticals. Several other radiopharmaceuticals are in development for the imaging of inflammation and infection.

Basic knowledge of the clinical problem

There are numerous clinical entities that can cause abdominal infectious–inflammatory diseases. They can present with acute diffused or localized abdominal pain, general discomfort, fever or diarrhea. Nuclear medicine techniques are not useful for differential diagnosis in the acute phase, but rather are a second-line examination to better evaluate disease extent and activity, complications and relapses, and for therapy follow-up.

For accurate image interpretation, the nuclear physician must know both the clinical diagnostic flow-chart and the results of other diagnostic tests [blood tests, endoscopy, computed tomography (CT), magnetic resonance imaging (MRI), ultrasound (US), etc.].

Ulcerative colitis and Crohn's disease are the two main forms of inflammatory bowel disease (IBD). Both are characterized by clinical remissions and relapses that are difficult to predict. The evaluation of disease activity and extent is crucial for prognostic considerations and also for therapy management. Besides, it is as important to establish a differential diagnosis between the two entities, since the therapeutic options are different [3–7]. Contrast-enhanced US and MRI are relevant to this purpose, but endoscopic studies usually provide the definitive diagnosis, although they are limited to the last part of the small bowel and colon, and have to be performed with caution in the acute phases of the diseases.

Diagnostic Imaging of Infections and Inflammatory Diseases: A Multidisciplinary Approach, First Edition. Edited by Alberto Signore and Ana María Quintero.

Both Crohn's disease and ulcerative colitis are believed to result from a combination of immune dysfunction, "dysbiosis" and otherwise normal constituents of the commensal extracellular luminal gut bacteria leaking through an abnormally permeable mucosal layer in genetically predisposed individuals. Alternatively, it has been suggested that both are caused by infection with a facultative intracellular bacterium, *Mycobacterium avium*, subspecies *paratuberculosis* (MAP) [8]. MAP was shown to cause a chronic disease of the intestines in a variety of animals that shares microscopic similarities to Crohn's disease.

Depending on the underlying disease responsible for the abdominal infection, the causative pathogen may differ [9–11]. In diverticulitis, which most commonly affects the sigmoid and descending colon, *Bacteroides* spp., *Peptostreptococcus* spp., Enterobacteriaceae, *Streptococcus viridans* and *Enterococcus* spp. have been isolated. *E. coli* and *B. fragilis* may be grown in cases of acute appendicitis and up to 14 different aerobic and anaerobic bacteria in cases of ruptured appendicitis. The type of pathogen grown in the setting of an abdominal abscess depends upon the location of the abscess; in spleen abscesses, streptococci, staphylococci and *Escherichia coli* are grown, and in pancreatic and pyogenic liver abscesses, *E. coli* and *Klebsiella pneumoniae* are most frequently encountered.

The clinical questions

The clinical questions vary depending on the known or suspected disease.

In appendicitis, approximately 30% of patients may have an unusual clinical presentation and may be misdiagnosed [2], particularly children and the elderly. The time delay to intervention is considered a risk factor for later complications, such as perforation or ulceration. Conventional radiology, CT, US and laparoscopy are the most frequently used diagnostic modalities for appendicitis [12,13], but all have limitations. Radiological techniques using contrast media may miss the diagnosis in up to 20% of cases of gangrenous appendicitis because the appendix may fill with contrast as if there is no disease. US can miss appendices that are atypically localized (up to 10%). In these select difficult cases, nuclear medicine techniques can be helpful as second-line examinations to identify the site of infection.

In cases of IBD, the first question that nuclear medicine must answer concerns the evaluation of disease activity and extent. Other important clinical questions concern the early evaluation of therapy efficacy and the prediction of disease relapse in patients in clinical remission or after surgery. Consensus diagnostic statements and guidelines have recently been jointly prepared by the European Crohn's and Colitis Organization (ECCO), European Society of Gastrointestinal and Abdominal Radiology (ESGAR) and European Association of Nuclear Medicine (EANM). In this consensus paper it emerges that the literature on the role of [18F] FDG-PET imaging in IBD is still very modest compared with that for MRI, CT, endoscopy and WBC scintigraphy [14].

[18F]FDG-PET/CT imaging may have a diagnostic role in the acute phase of IBD, when endoscopic and barium studies may be contraindicated, and in cases of unsuccessful colonoscopy, who are not infrequently children as they may not tolerate such an invasive test. [18F]FDG-PET/CT may also be helpful in differentiating between a flare of IBD versus non-inflammatory processes causing similar symptoms in patients with IBD. Finally, [18F] FDG-PET/CT may be useful in assessing the disease activity of IBD prior to and following therapeutic intervention, as it is a "sensitive method to evaluate the whole intestinal inflammatory burden". The question remains about what the incremental value is of this imaging technique in this setting when compared to other imaging modalities.

In autoimmune pancreatitis (AIP), the main clinical concern is its differentiation from pancreatic carcinoma. [18F]FDG-PET/CT, but not other nuclear medicine techniques, has been shown to have a role in this.

Similarly, in cases of idiopathic retroperitoneal fibrosis (IRF), the clinical question is whether [18F] FDG-PET is a reliable method to evaluate disease activity and whether it can help in differentiating benign from malignant forms of IRF.

Methodological considerations

Inflammation and infection are different processes. Inflammation is a host non-specific immune response that does not require the presence of microorganisms. An acute inflammation (mainly endothelial activation, edema, increased vascular permeability and diapedesis of polymorphonuclear cells into tissues) can be differentiated from a chronic inflammation (little vascular change and diapedesis of mononuclear cells). Acute inflammation occurs after trauma or infection. Chronic inflammation can persist after trauma, ischemia, neoplasm, autoimmunity, graft rejection and degenerative diseases, following infection by some microorganisms such as viruses and fungi. In contrast, the existence of a focus of bacteria may not lead to inflammation in the immunocompromised patient, but still constitutes a site of infection [15]. It has to be considered that all radiopharmaceuticals accumulate to some extent at sites of infection due to the presence of acute inflammation [16–19].

A variety of radiopharmaceuticals have been developed and evaluated to localize and detect areas of inflammation and infection within the body [20] (Table 13.1). Non-specific radiopharmaceuticals are readily available but have important limitations: the accumulation process is slow; in chronic inflam-

mation, vascular permeability tends to normalize and they do not accumulate; and they do not differentiate between sterile inflammation and septic inflammation (infection). In chronic inflammation, WBCs are used to target infections by labeling them *ex vivo* or *in vivo* with labeled anti-G mAbs or labeled peptides [21]. Also, lymphocytes can be targeted using labeled peptides, thus avoiding the need to label them *ex vivo*. Finally, labeled antibiotics, peptides or vitamins can be considered for the direct imaging of the microorganisms responsible for infection.

Labeled white blood cells

^{111}In-oxine, ^{99m}Tc-HMPAO (hexamethylpropylene amine oxime) [22,23] or labeled anti-G mAbs can be used to radiolabel WBCs [22]. For imaging abdominal infections, it is recommended to obtain two sets of images: with ^{99m}Tc-HMPAO, first at 30 minutes and then at 2–3 hours; with ^{111}In-oxine and mAbs, first at 3–4 hours and then at 18–24 hours [24]. It is also recommended to collect time-corrected images (or at least 500 kcounts) in anteroposterior and caudocranial projections, the

Table 13.1 Radiopharmaceuticals used for inflammation/infection imaging based on their physiological mechanism of uptake

Physiological characteristics	Uptake mechanism	Radiopharmaceutical	Type
↑ Blood flow	Non-specific	Ga-citrate	Substrate
↑ Vascular permeability		Polyclonal IgG	Antibodies
↑ Transudation of plasma proteins		Liposomes	Lipids
		Avidin–biotin	Vitamin
↑ Granulocyte infiltration	Granulocytes	Labeled granulocytes	Cells
	Antigen binding	Anti-NCA-95 IgG	Antibodies
		Anti-NCA-90 Fabi	
		Anti-SSEA-1 IgM	
	Specific receptor binding on granulocytes	f-Met-Leu-Phe	Chemotactic peptides
		IL-1	Cytokines
		IL-8	
		PF-4	
		RP517	LTB$_4$ agonists
		DCP11870-11	
↑ Lymphocyte infiltration	Specific receptor binding	IL-2	Cytokines
		IL-12	
↑ Metabolism	Glucose uptake	FDG	Carbohydrate
Presence of microorganisms	Binding to bacteria	Ciprofloxacin	Antibiotic
		Biotin	Vitamin
		UBI 29-41	Peptide

Modified from Rennen *et al.* [20].

latter being of particular interest for the visualization of the rectum. It is good practice to include the lower part of the liver and spleen in the first image (obtained at 30 minutes), as this provides an indirect evaluation of physiological cell biodistribution.

^{67}Ga-citrate

^{67}Ga-citrate has been used for the detection of infection and inflammation since 1971. It has been suggested to form a complex with transferrin and to undergo extravasation at the site of inflammation/infection. Even though its exact mechanism of retention in the infectious lesion has yet to be completely clarified, experimental studies support the hypothesis that ^{67}Ga-citrate is taken up by bacterial siderophores and via transferrin receptors on WBCs [25]. Others have postulated a role for citrate as a substrate for the Krebs' cycle.

Images are usually acquired 48–72 hours after administration due to the high plasma background and low tissue uptake, but its unfavorable imaging characteristics, long physical half-life and low abundance of high-energy gamma radiations mean that high doses of radiation are absorbed and images are of relatively poor image.

^{99m}Tc-besilesomab (Scintimun®)

Besilesomab (BW 250/183) is an antibody directed against the epitope NCA-95 present on the granulocyte surface membrane. It was developed in the 1990s and clinical experience has mainly been in musculoskeletal infections [26]. As it was only recently registered in Europe for osteomyelitis, experience with it is limited.

^{99m}Tc-sulesomab (Leukoscan®)

Sulesomab is a Fab'2 fragment of murine IgG IMMU-MN3, a monoclonal antibody directed against the epitope NCA-90 present on the granulocyte surface membrane. It is registered for the localization and diagnosis of inflammation and infections. However, its biodistribution has limited its clinical application to the study of peripheral bones; there is high uptake in the liver, spleen and urinary and gastrointestinal tracts [27].

^{99m}Tc-fanesolemab

Fanesolemab is an anti-CD15 antibody with very rapid blood clearance. It was initially used for the rapid imaging of acute appendicitis, with excellent results in the USA. Unfortunately, it has been suspended because of safety concerns [28].

^{99m}Tc-infliximab

In active phases of Crohn's disease, increased production and release of tumor necrosis factor alpha (TNFα) by macrophages and monocytes has been described. The use of infliximab, a chimeric human/mouse monoclonal anti-TNFα antibody labeled with ^{99m}Tc, has been proposed by D'Alessandria et al. in patients with IBD for therapy decision-making [29].

Labeled polyclonal human immunoglobulin G

Human immunoglobulin G (HIG) was first labeled with ^{111}In, but because of its poor availability, dosimetry and image quality, this was replaced by ^{99m}Tc. It has been successfully used in the imaging of different inflammatory sites and was able to localize both sepsis and active IBD [30,31]. However, the value of HIG imaging in IBD has been a subject of controversy because of its low sensitivity compared to labeled WBCs [32,33].

Labeled interleukin-2

Interleukin-2 (IL-2) represents the first identified and fully characterized purified human interleukin. It has been labeled with ^{123}I and ^{99m}Tc for SPECT use [34,35] and with ^{18}F for PET use [36]. It binds mainly to activated T-helper-1 lymphocytes. It seems to have an important future role in Crohn's [37,38] and celiac disease [39], particularly in the evaluation of disease extent and activity and in the detection of early relapse.

Labeled antibiotics and antifungals

The first labeled antibiotic to be developed and enter into advanced clinical trials is based on ciprofloxacin, a drug of the fluoroquinolone family, which binds to the DNA gyrase of living bacteria but not to human cells or dead bacteria [40]. Bacterial resistance does not appear to affect binding. Ciprofloxacin has been labeled with ^{99m}Tc (Infecton) and it seems to be pharmacologically stable [41].

The concept of labeled antimicrobial agents has been extended to antifungal drugs. In immunosuppressed patients, fungal infection can pose a real threat to life and its early recognition and treatment are extremely important. This has led to the development of ^{99m}Tc-fluconazole, although results in the preclinical setting need to be confirmed in human trials [42].

Our group has studied the application of labeled cephalosporins (^{99m}Tc-ceftizoxime). Initial results in rats and first clinical experience are promising, but further clinical trials are necessary to prove its utility [43,44].

[^{18}F]Fluorodeoxyglucose

[^{18}F]FDG is known to accumulate at sites of infection and inflammation and in autoimmune diseases. The inflammatory cells produce an excess of glycolytic enzymes and also overexpress glucose transporter isotypes, mainly GLUT-1 and GLUT 3.

In vitro studies of [^{18}F]FDG labeling of human WBCs using mixed/pure preparations of neutrophils and mononuclear cells demonstrated granulocyte uptake of over 78–87% of the activity in mixed preparations, but this was not stable, and the labeling yield ranged from 40% to 80% when pure preparations were used [45]. Despite this limitation, [^{18}F]FDG-labeled WBCs represent a first attempt to develop an infection-specific, positron-emitting radiopharmaceutical.

To date the clinical use of [^{18}F]FDG is limited to pancreatitis and IRF. It is being evaluated in IBD and other abdominal infections.

If a diagnostic quality contrast CT scan is acquired along with the [^{18}F]FDG-PET scan, the dense contrast agent present in the bowel may produce attenuation correction artifacts whereby the bowel appears to have increased activity. Such artifacts may be minimized through the administration of a negative oral contrast agent, e.g. VoLumen (E-Z-EM Inc, Lake Success, NY, USA).

SPECT/CT

Historically planar images have been obtained. With the availability of hybrid gamma-cameras, the possibility of performing SPECT imaging co-registered with CT imaging has improved the capacity of nuclear exams to localize and identify foci of infection/inflammation.

Normal findings and artifacts

The normal distribution of labeled WBCs can differ depending on the isotope used for labeling. If labeled with ^{111}In-oxine, the main tissues where WBCs

accumulate are the spleen and liver (with spleen uptake always higher than liver uptake), with less uptake in the bone marrow and no activity in the gastrointestinal tract and urinary system. If labeled with ^{99m}Tc-HMPAO, the main tissue where there is accumulation is the spleen, followed by the liver and bone marrow, but in this case there is also a variable degree of activity excreted by the liver and kidneys, and present in the gallbladder, bowel and urinary system. Thus, ^{111}In-oxine-labeled WBCs have the better biodistribution for the evaluation of infections in the kidneys, urinary system and gallbladder. ^{111}In-oxine-labeled WBCs also perform better in chronic infections because of the possibility of acquiring good quality late images [20,46].

The normal biodistribution of ^{67}Ga-citrate uptake is the bowel, liver, spleen, bones and urinary system, and therefore it is not an ideal radiopharmaceutical for the imaging of abdominal infections.

[^{18}F]FDG is also physiologically taken up by the bowel, but this uptake varies in distribution and intensity due to several factors, e.g. medications (metformin), fasting and irritable bowel. This may affect the accuracy for imaging IBD patients [47,48]. [^{18}F]FDG uptake in the normal bowel is typically low [standardized uptake value (SUV) of <4], but intense uptake (SUV as high as 10) can occur occasionally, particularly in the right colon. The mechanism of [^{18}F]FDG uptake in the digestive tract is not clearly understood; smooth muscle activity, metabolically active mucosa, swallowed secretions and colonic microbial uptake may be involved.

Gastrointestinal incidentaloma are detected in up to 3% of patients who undergo [^{18}F]FDG-PET/CT imaging [49–51]. Nodular focal and nodular multifocal [^{18}F]FDG uptake is predictive of malignancy and requires further evaluation. Diffuse colonic [^{18}F]FDG uptake is predictive of a normal colonoscopy and a segmental high uptake implies an inflammatory condition.

Pathological findings and significance

Appendicitis

Nuclear medicine techniques have a high accuracy in the diagnosis of appendicitis, but are not used routinely used in clinical practice. Their underutilization is probably due to the emergency requirement for the examination, or the fact that most nuclear medicine departments do not operate a 24-hour service.

Annovazzi *et al.* [2] published a meta-analysis of 24 papers concerning the use of nuclear medicine techniques in the diagnosis of appendicitis. In many of the studies they found a high diagnostic accuracy for ^{99m}Tc-HMPAO- or ^{111}In-oxine-labeled WBCs, ^{99m}Tc-HIG and ^{99m}Tc-anti-G mAb, with the highest sensitivity for the last of these [28], probably due to the severity of the acute inflammation. ^{99m}Tc-anti-G mAb can provide a quick diagnosis within hours. *Ex vivo* labeled WBCs are a valuable option, but are more difficult to organize in an emergency. This highlights the need for the development of faster *in vivo* WBC labeling techniques.

The differential diagnosis in suspected appendicitis includes other acute inflammation, such as ovarian cysts, mesenteric lymphadenitis or bowel intussusceptions; these have a clinical presentation similar to appendicitis and can also show abnormal uptake of these radiopharmaceuticals. The use of SPECT/CT should solve these difficulties.

Published [^{18}F]FDG-PET findings in appendicitis are limited to a number of case reports, but in these it was shown to be able to identify the location of the ongoing infection [52,53].

Inflammatory bowel diseases

The two main forms of IBD, Crohn's disease and ulcerative colitis, differ as to their location and to the nature of the inflammatory changes of the bowel wall identified on microscopy. Crohn's disease most often originates in the terminal ileum but may affect any part of the gastrointestinal tract, from the mouth to the anus (skip lesions). In contrast, ulcerative colitis is restricted to the colon and rectum. At the microscopic level, Crohn's disease affects the whole bowel wall ("transmural lesions"), whereas ulcerative colitis is restricted to the epithelial lining of the gut.

Patients suffering from either Crohn's disease or ulcerative colitis typically present with any of the following symptoms: abdominal pain, vomiting, diarrhea, rectal bleeding, severe internal cramps/muscle spasms in the region of the pelvis, weight loss and various associated complaints or diseases, e.g. arthritis, pyoderma gangrenosum and primary sclerosing cholangitis.

The diagnosis of Crohn's disease and ulcerative colitis depends on direct endoscopic visualization of the colonic and ileal mucosa by wireless capsule endoscopy or double-balloon enteroscopy, and on histological analysis of endoscopically obtained biopsy specimens.

Treatment of IBD is aimed at eliminating symptoms, long-term remission and restoration of quality of life [3–5]. In most cases, this may be achieved through medication. Usually, patients are put on an immunosuppressive treatment, e.g. prednisone, to reduce or eliminate bowel inflammation. Subsequently, patients are switched to a less potent drug to keep the disease in remission, e.g. asacol, a mesalazine. Evaluation of treatment response is through clinical examination [Crohn's disease activity index (CDAI) and ulcerative colitis disease activity index (UCDAI)] and endoscopy. If unsuccessful, a combination of the aforementioned immunosuppression drugs with a mesalazine may be administered. If medication fails to improve symptoms or if precancerous changes in the colon or serious complications occur, surgical intervention, e.g. bowel resection, strictureplasty or a temporary or permanent colostomy or ileostomy, may prove mandatory.

CT and MRI are frequently used to assess the extent of disease not accessible with endoscopy, the extent of any extraintestinal disease and the development of complications [1] (see Chapter 6). However, both techniques require bowel preparation and have a risk of complications, especially when performed in the acute stage of the disease. In contrast to CT, scintigraphic imaging using labeled WBCs is not contraindicated in the acute phase and is well tolerated [2]. Drawbacks of labeled WBC scintigraphy, however, include the hazards associated with withdrawing blood and a limited spatial resolution. When compared to labeled WBCs, [^{18}F]FDG has more favorable kinetics and contrast and a scan can be completed within 2 hours from injection. Furthermore, PET has better spatial resolution and allows for more accurate quantification of tracer uptake. Of interest, contrary to what is seen in malignancy, increased glucose blood levels do not seem to negatively affect [^{18}F]FDG uptake at sites of inflammation. Nevertheless, the role of [^{18}F]FDG-PET in IBD is still being explored and cannot be considered at present as an alternative technique to labeled WBCs for imaging IBD patients.

Therefore, the main nuclear medicine exam currently used in the imaging of IBD is scintigraphy (planar or SPECT or SPECT/CT) with autologous WBCs labeled with ^{111}In-oxine or ^{99m}Tc-HMPAO, each of which has a different aim. ^{99m}Tc-HMPAO-labeled WBCs can be considered the technique of choice in acute phases of disease. The quality of the images is higher and the time to image is shorter. The main drawback, bowel excretion of ^{99m}Tc, depends on the labeling procedure; it is higher if the labeling is performed in saline or phosphate-buffered saline (PBS) and can be overcome by obtaining late images earlier than 2 hours post injection.

Concerning anti-G mAbs, only ^{99m}Tc-besilesomab has been used in this context with excellent results, but it has not been registered in the EU for this purpose (Figures 13.1 and 13.2).

Annovazzi *et al.* [2] published a meta-analysis of 112 studies involving a total of 4388 patients, and in many of which, nuclear medicine techniques were compared to radiological and/or endoscopic techniques. It was observed that labeled WBCs (either with ^{111}In-oxine- or ^{99m}Tc-HMPAO) showed

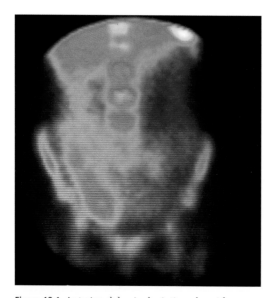

Figure 13.1 Anterior abdominal scintigraphy with ^{99m}Tc-antiG mAb obtained 24 hours post injection in a 35-year-old woman with an ovarian abscess, acute abdominal pain, fever and diarrhea. Note the intense accumulation of labeled antibody in the right iliac fossa. In emergency situations the use of labeled anti-G mAbs is ideal; nevertheless, both 4- and 24-hour images are always required for a correct diagnosis together with SPECT/CT when possible.

a high diagnostic accuracy and could be used with different scopes in the study of IBD. From this meta-analysis it was concluded that alternative nuclear medicine techniques, such as scintigraphy with anti-G mAbs or HIG, because of their lower sensitivity, should only be used when labeled WBCs are not available. Indeed, when compared to ^{99m}Tc-labeled WBCs, in IBD fewer affected segments are detected and the sensitivity and specificity are lower with HIG [33].

For the initial diagnosis of IBD and for differential diagnosis between ulcerative colitis and Crohn's disease, WBC scintigraphy should be considered a second-line imaging technique and used only when radiological and/or endoscopic exams are inconclusive. WBC scintigraphy is highly sensitive for IBD; in the absence of a focal abdominal uptake, the presence of IBD can be excluded (Figure 13.3). Pathological bowel uptake in IBD patients can also be due to an ischemic or infective colitis, or to abdominal bleeding or inflamed tumors. The uptake pattern can be useful for the differential diagnosis between ulcerative colitis and Crohn's disease; if the uptake is in the ileocecal area or in the small bowel, and if there is a patchy distribution of radioactivity, it is more likely that the patient is affected by Crohn's disease. In contrast, when WBC accumulation is focused in the left colon up to the rectum, or diffused throughout the whole colon, it is more likely that the patient has an ulcerative colitis. However, if the scan shows only colon activity, it is not possible to make a differential diagnosis.

Disease extent is usually evaluated by endoscopy, capsule endoscopy or barium studies. WBC scintigraphy, however, usually has a high sensitivity for low-grade acute inflammation in the small bowel and often better shows affected bowel segments than radiological or endoscopic exams, particularly in the jejunum (Figure 13.4). The main drawback of a WBC scan is the lack of anatomical definition, which can be partially resolved by using co-registered SPECT/CT scans with hybrid cameras.

Many other radiopharmaceuticals have been proposed for IBD. D'Alessandria *et al.* studied a population of 10 patients with Crohn's disease with labeled anti-TNFα mAbs and found little presence of TNFα in the affected bowel segments, indicating that caution should be used in the selection of patients for biological therapy with anti-TNFα agents [29].

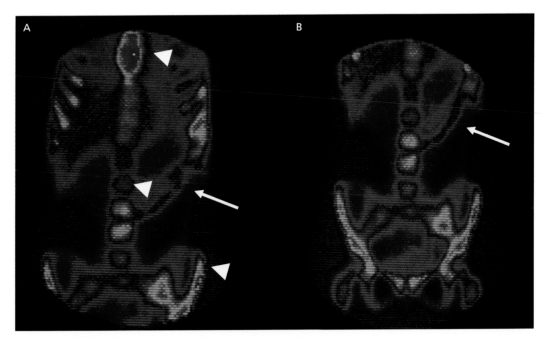

Figure 13.2 Anti-G mAb scan in a 55-year-old man with Crohn's disease. The scan was requested to evaluate the extent of the inflammation. (A) At the 4-hour image there is linear uptake involving the transverse colon (arrow). There is also a high uptake in the bone marrow, spine, sternum and iliac crest (arrowheads), which is typical with radiolabeled anti-G mAbs. (B) At 24 hours the uptake has the same configuration but the bowel-to-background ratio is increased (arrow). Bone marrow uptake is still detectable.

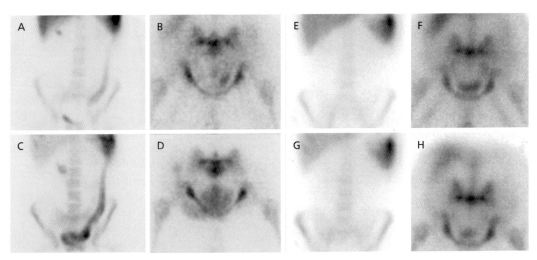

Figure 13.3 ^{99m}Tc-HMPAO-labeled autologous WBC scintigraphy in a 21-year-old man with ulcerative colitis. (A,C,E,G) Anterior abdominal and (B,D,F,H) caudocranial views are shown at 30 minutes (A,B,E,F) and 3 hours (C,D,G,H) after injection of labeled WBCs. The scintigraphy at diagnosis (A–D) clearly shows an inflammatory activity from the left colon to the anus. Note that rectal activity is clearly seen in the caudocranial views (B,D), whereas in the anterior views it is covered by urinary bladder activity (A,C). The patient was treated with 250 mg/day of azathioprine and re-examined 6 months later to evaluate response to treatment (E–H). There is no uptake of labeled WBCs outside of the normal biodistribution pattern, indicating a complete remission.

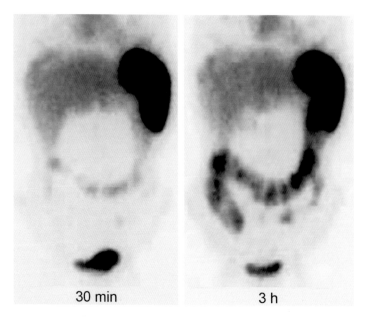

30 min

3 h

Figure 13.4 ^{99m}Tc-HMPAO-labeled autologous WBC scintigraphy in a woman with colonic Crohn's disease. The scan clearly shows that there is no ileal disease. A labeled WBC scan can be used in inflammatory bowel disease in particular to evaluate the extent of disease and its activity, and to monitor the efficacy of therapy, as well as for early prediction of relapse and differential diagnosis of inflamed/fibrotic strictures.

[^{18}F]FDG-PET/CT in the differential diagnosis
Bicik *et al.* prospectively performed [^{18}F]FDG-PET imaging in seven patients with suspected IBD [54]. The imaging results obtained were compared with those for endoscopy and biopsy. In six patients, [^{18}F]FDG uptake proved high in areas of macroscopic disease as well as in areas of biopsy-proven inflammation in the absence of macroscopic disease. Furthermore, [^{18}F]FDG uptake proved higher in patients with a CDAI of greater than 150 or a CAI of greater than 6. Skehan *et al.* performed [^{18}F]FDG-PET imaging in 25 children with suspected IBD; [^{18}F]FDG uptake was identified in five bowel segments [55]. PET results were compared with the gold standard of endoscopy (complete colonoscopy with ileal intubation), radiology or both. The final diagnosis in three children was ulcerative colitis and in 15 children was Crohn's disease. [^{18}F]FDG-PET had a sensitivity and a specificity for identifying inflammation of 71% and 81%, respectively. As complete colonoscopy could only be performed in six of the 19 IBD-positive patients, it was concluded by the authors that [^{18}F]FDG-PET may be a useful adjunct to existing diagnostic modalities in IBD.

Löffler *et al.* retrospectively analyzed the diagnostic potential of [^{18}F]FDG-PET in 23 children (aged 2–16 years; 14 males, nine females) with suspected IBD [56]. Results were compared to endoscopic, his-

tological and abdominal US findings. In all examinations, the presence of inflammation was evaluated in each patient in eight bowel segments (score 1–4). SUVs for [^{18}F]FDG-PET were measured for all segments. Sensitivity, specificity and accuracy were calculated using histology as the standard of reference on a segment-based analysis (pathological if inflammation score ≥ 3 or $SUV_{max}/SUV_{liver} > 1.2$) and for [^{18}F]FDG-PET were 98%, 68% and 83%, respectively; for endoscopy were 90%, 75% and 82%, respectively; and for US were 56%, 92% and 75%, respectively (Figure 13.5). For the small bowel, [^{18}F]FDG-PET was even more reliable (100%, 86% and 90%, respectively).

In a prospective study, Das *et al.* included 17 adult patients with suspected inflammatory diseases of the intestine. First, a low-dose whole-body PET/CT scan [57] was obtained and subsequently, a PET/CT enteroclysis of the abdomen following infusion of 2 L of 0.5% methylcellulose through a nasojejunal catheter. Fourteen patients had abnormal and three had normal PET/CT enteroclysis studies. Twenty-three segments of small intestine and 27 segments of large intestine showed increased [^{18}F]FDG uptake. The detection rate of PET/CT enteroclysis was significantly higher (a total of 50 segments; 23 segments of small intestine and 27 of large intestine) when compared with barium studies (16 segments

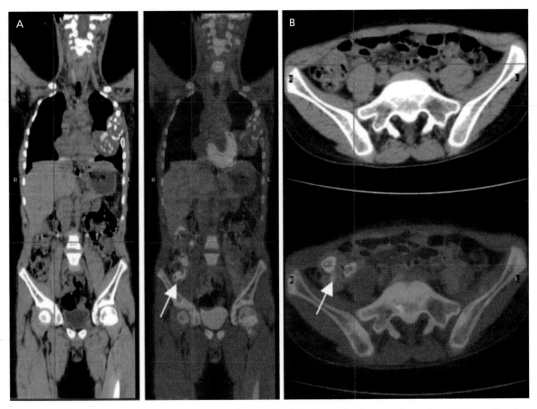

Figure 13.5 [^{18}F]FDG-PET/CT images in a patient with active Crohn's disease in the ascending colon. (A) Coronal and (B) transaxial images showing areas with increased glucose metabolism. An active lymph node is detectable but it is not necessarily an infected site. Arrow indicates activity in the inflamed gut wall, and because the radiopharmaceutical lacks specificity, these areas can be either inflamed or infected.

of small intestine) and colonoscopy (17 segments of large intestine), giving a combined total of 33 segments. In addition PET/CT enteroclysis showed extraluminal [^{18}F]FDG uptake (lymph nodes in two patients, sacroilitis in two patients and mesenteric fat proliferation in five patients).

In summary, [^{18}F]FDG-PET/CT may be useful in IBD when conventional diagnostic studies (radiology and labeled WBC scan) cannot be performed or are inconclusive.

[^{18}F]FDG-PET/CT for assessing and monitoring disease activity

Neurath *et al.* enrolled 59 patients in a prospective study to assess disease activity by [^{18}F]FDG-PET, hydro-MRI and immunoscintigraphy with anti-non-specific cross-reacting antigen 95 anti-G mAb [58]. Colonoscopy could be performed in 28 of the

patients. Twelve patients with irritable bowel syndrome and 20 tumor patients without gut inflammation served as controls. [^{18}F]FDG-PET detected 127 pathological findings (mean SUV$_{max}$ = 4.4) in the terminal/neoterminal ileum (n = 37), small bowel (n = 24) and colon (n = 66) of 54 patients with Crohn's disease, whereas no pathological findings were seen in five patients with Crohn's disease, the control patients with irritable bowel syndrome and the tumor patients without gut inflammation. In contrast, examination with hydro-MRI or anti-G mAbs detected fewer pathological findings in the Crohn's disease patients. Forty-five of the detected foci were accessible to endoscopic verification. The correlation of the foci with endoscopic findings indicated that all three methods had a high specificity (>89%) for detecting inflamed areas in the terminal ileum and colon of patients with Crohn's disease, although hydro-MRI and anti-G mAb scintigraphy proved strikingly less sensitive (40.9% and 66.7%, respectively) versus [18F]FDG-PET (85.4%).

Lemberg et al. assessed the value of PET in identifying active intestinal inflammation compared to conventional endoscopic and radiological studies, including small bowel follow-through and colonoscopy, in a series of 65 children: 55 children with newly diagnosed IBD (n = 37) or symptoms suggestive of recurrent disease (n = 18) and 10 children with recurrent abdominal pain [59]. Thirty-eight patients had Crohn's disease and 17 had ulcerative colitis. PET correctly identified active inflammatory disease in 80% of the children with IBD (81.5% with Crohn's disease; 76.4% with ulcerative colitis) and correctly showed no evidence of inflammation in children with recurrent abdominal pain. [18F]FDG accumulated at sites that corresponded with active disease at colonoscopy and small bowel follow-through in 83.8% and 75.0% of patients, respectively.

Comparable results to those reported above have been obtained by other authors [60–63].

Rubin et al. performed [18F]FDG-PET imaging in 10 patients diagnosed with ulcerative colitis (eight had pancolitis, one extensive colitis and one proctosigmoiditis; median disease duration was 32 years) in a strictly defined remission state [64]. Uptake in each of four colonic segments [rectosigmoid (r–s), descending, transverse and ascending] and distal small bowel were scored on a three-point scale (0 = no uptake or uptake ≥ liver; 1 = uptake somewhat greater than liver; 2 = uptake much greater than liver). While six patients had no increased [18F]FDG uptake, PET demonstrated inflammatory activity in the colon in four patients despite negative endoscopic, histological and symptom assessment: in the r–s region in three patients (one patient with r–s uptake also had ascending colon uptake) and ileal uptake in one patient. The authors concluded that this finding may have important implications for the understanding of ulcerative colitis disease quiescence and that this highly sensitive [18F]FDG-PET imaging modality should be further explored.

In a series by Jacene et al., 17 patients with known Crohn's disease prospectively underwent [18F]FDG-PET/CT before already-planned surgery for obstructive symptoms [65]. Lesions were qualitatively graded on a five-point scale for the presence of increased [18F]FDG uptake consistent with active inflammation. The maximum lean standardized uptake value (SUV_{max}) was determined for lesions that were scored 1 or more. Imaging results were compared with the pathological grading of inflammation and predominant histopathological subtype for each patient's surgical specimen, whether mainly inflammation, fibrosis, or muscle hypertrophy. Thirteen of the 17 patients underwent surgery (median 28 days after PET/CT; range, 2–148 days) and 12 of these 13 had histopathological correlation. Despite the predominant histopathological subtype (inflammation 5; fibrosis 4; muscle hypertrophy 3), acute and chronic inflammation, fibrosis (median 50%; range, 40–90%) and muscle hypertrophy (median 20-fold thickening; range, 9–40-fold thickening) were found in all patients. On PET/CT, 10 of the 12 patients were considered to have active inflammation of the bowel. SUV_{max} was significantly higher in severe than in mild-to-moderate chronic inflammation (8.2 + 2.8 vs. 4.7 + 2.5, p = 0.04). No patient with predominantly fibrosis or muscle hypertrophy (n = 7) had an SUV_{max} greater than 8. The authors concluded that [18F]FDG-PET/CT may be informative for referring gastroenterologists considering medical therapy versus surgery for patients with Crohn's disease who present with obstructive symptoms.

Finally, Spier et al. performed [18F]FDG-PET before and after successful medical therapy in five patients (two with Crohn's disease and three with ulcerative colitis) who presented with moderately active IBD [66]. The mean duration between both scans was 437 days (range, 77–807). Imaging results were related to the clinical activity. Each patient had five bowel segments scored (0–3) on [18F]FDG-PET. All patients showed significant improvement in physician global assessment scores (p = 0.004). The total score of all segments was 32 pre-treatment and 14 post-treatment (p < 0.01). Of 11 pre-treatment active segments, nine (82%) either became inactive or displayed decreased activity, while two showed no change (p < 0.001). Appropriate [18F]FDG-PET determination decreases with successful treatment of inflammation in active IBD and correlates with symptom improvement.

Overall, [^{18}F]FDG-PET bowel activity seems to correlate well with active ongoing inflammation in patients suffering from Crohn's disease and ulcerative colitis, suggesting that it may be a useful non-invasive tool for assessing and monitoring disease activity in patients with IBD (Figure 13.6).

[^{18}F]FDG-PET/CT colonography and PET/CT enterography for assessing disease activity in known IBD

Currently, the extent of involvement and activity of ulcerative colitis is best evaluated by colonoscopy.

Colonoscopy however, carries risk during an acute exacerbation.

Das *et al.* investigated the utility of PET/CT colonography for assessment of extent and activity of ulcerative colitis versus colonoscopy in 15 patients with mild-to-moderately active disease (1-week interval) [67]. A PET activity score based on [^{18}F]FDG uptake and endoscopic mucosal activity was recorded for seven colonic segments of each patient. The PET activity grade of 0, 1, 2 or 3 depended upon the colon segment-to-liver SUV_{max} ratio. The extent of disease was left-sided colitis in five and pancolitis in ten patients. Mean UCDAI was

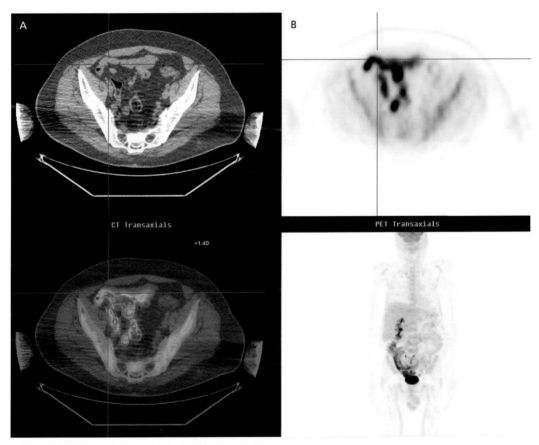

Figure 13.6 [^{18}F]FDG-PET/CT in a patient with clinical relapse of Crohn's disease after therapy: (A) PET/CT fused transaxial slides and (B) maximum intensity projection (MIP). Images show increased uptake of [^{18}F]FDG in the terminal ileum, right colon flexure and ascending colon. [^{18}F]FDG uptake is clearly seen in the gut wall and not in the lumen. This is not always detectable at the level of the ileum and is more frequently observed at the level of the colon. When diagnosis of inflammatory bowel disease has already been made, [^{18}F]FDG can be used to evaluate the efficacy of therapy or, as in this case, the extent of inflammation in clinical relapse.

7.6. The numbers of segments involved as per colonoscopic evaluation and PET/CT colonography were 67 and 66, respectively. There was a fair agreement for extent evaluation between the two modalities (kappa 55.3%, p = 0.02). One patient had grade 0 PET activity, nine had grade 2 and five had grade 3. In six patients, there was a 1:1 correlation between PET activity grade and endoscopic grade. The authors concluded that PET/CT colonography is a novel non-invasive technique for the assessment of extent and activity of disease in patients with ulcerative colitis.

Ahmadi *et al.* studied the role of combined localized PET (lPET) and CT enterography (CTe) in Crohn's disease [68]. Fifty-two lPET/CTe scans were analyzed in this retrospective study; CTe scores and [^{18}F]FDG uptake were quantified. Imaging scores were compared to medical outcome and to C-reactive protein (CRP) levels, erythrocyte sedimentation rate (ESR), the short Inflammatory Bowel Disease Questionnaire and the Harvey-Bradshaw index. The addition of lPET to CTe did not identify additional abnormal segments when compared to CTe alone; 38 (79%) abnormal CTe segments demonstrated increased [^{18}F]FDG uptake (mean SUV$_{max}$: 4.77). Abnormal segments with mucosal enhancement on CTe that did not accumulate [^{18}F]FDG (mean SUV$_{max}$: 1.27) were significantly associated with failure of medical therapy. The authors suggested that a larger trial is warranted to confirm if combined lPET/CTe has an important role in the clinical management of stricturing Crohn's disease.

To conclude, [^{18}F]FDG-PET/CT colonography in ulcerative colitis and PET/CT enterography in Crohn's disease are novel non-invasive techniques for the assessment of disease extent and activity.

Autoimmune pancreatitis

Autoimmune pancreatitis (AIP) is an increasingly recognized type of chronic pancreatitis that is difficult to distinguish from pancreatic carcinoma [69,70]. The most common symptom, present in about 80% of cases of AIP, is obstructive jaundice caused by blocked bile ducts. A cholestatic biochemical profile and serum IgG4 elevation and autoantibodies are usually present. Histopathological examination of the pancreas in AIP shows fibrotic changes with lymphocyte and plasma cell infiltrate.

A capsule-like rim on CT and MRI, which is thought to correspond to an inflammatory process involving peripancreatic tissue, and pancreatic enlargement along with hypointensity on T1-weighted MR images and delayed enhancement on dynamic CT and MR studies are other features of this disorder [71]. Endoscopic retrograde cholangiopancreatography (ERCP) features of AIP include segmental or diffuse irregular narrowing of the main pancreatic duct [72]. Based on these findings, the following diagnostic criteria for AIP have been defined by the Japanese Pancreas Society [73]:

I. Pancreatic imaging studies show diffuse narrowing of the main pancreatic duct with irregular wall (more than one-third of the length of the entire pancreas).

II. Laboratory data demonstrate abnormally elevated levels of serum gamma globulin and/or IgG, or the presence of autoantibodies.

III. Histopathological examination of the pancreas shows fibrotic changes with lymphocyte and plasma cell infiltrate.

For diagnosis, criterion I (pancreatic imaging) must be present with criterion II (laboratory data) and/or III (histopathological findings).

In spite of these criteria, differential diagnosis with pancreatic carcinoma remains difficult and the failure to differentiate AIP from malignancy may lead to unnecessary pancreatic resection. The characteristic mononuclear cell infiltrate of AIP has been found in up to 23% of patients undergoing pancreatic resection for suspected malignancy who are ultimately found to have benign disease. In this subset of patients, a trial of steroid therapy, preferably prednisone, would have prevented a Whipple procedure or complete pancreatectomy for a benign disease, which responds well to medical therapy.

To date, the underlying cause of AIP remains largely unclear but regulatory T cells and a shift of B cells toward IgG4-producing plasma cells are believed to be involved in the development of AIP; histopathological findings of AIP show storiform fibrosis and obliterative phlebitis with diffused infiltration of lymphocytes and IgG4-positive plasma cells [74].

The clinical question in this condition is whether [^{18}F]FDG-PET/CT can help in differentiating AIP from pancreatic carcinoma. To this end, Nakamoto *et al.* performed [^{18}F]FDG-PET in six patients with clinically diagnosed AIP. PET findings were evaluated visually and/or semi-quantitatively using the SUV [75]. In four of the six patients, PET demonstrated intense uptake in the whole pancreas, which appeared swollen on CT, and the accumulation increased with time in three patients. In one patient, intense focal uptake in the pancreatic head was observed and the accumulation decreased over time. In the remaining patient, no abnormal accumulation in the pancreas was observed. Follow-up PET scanning after steroid therapy was performed in three patients and intense [^{18}F]FDG uptake was no longer observed.

Likewise, Nakajo et al. reviewed [^{18}F]FDG-PET/CT findings in six patients with AIP pre- and post-steroid therapy (in five patients) [76]. The initial PET scans were performed 1 and 2 hours after [^{18}F]FDG injection in all six patients. The initial PET scans revealed intense [^{18}F]FDG uptake by AIP in all six patients and pancreas SUV$_{max}$ values increased in four patients and remained stable in two patients. The intense uptake in the pancreas disappeared in five patients during or following steroid therapy and in one patient who showed spontaneous remission of AIP. Of interest, abnormal [^{18}F]FDG uptake by extrapancreatic autoimmune diseases was observed in five of the six patients: sclerosing sialadenitis (n = 5), lymphadenopathy (n = 5), retroperitoneal fibrosis (n = 2), interstitial nephritis (n = 2) and sclerosing cholecystitis (n = 1). Abnormal [^{18}F]FDG uptake disappeared in the salivary glands (n = 4), lymph nodes (n = 4), retroperitoneum (n = 2) and kidneys.

Ozaki et al. compared [^{18}F]FDG-PET findings between 15 patients with AIP and 26 patients with pancreatic cancer [77]. The [^{18}F]FDG-PET findings were evaluated visually or semi-quantitatively using the SUV$_{max}$ and the accumulation pattern of [^{18}F]FDG. [^{18}F]FDG uptake was found in all 15 patients with AIP, whereas it was found in only 19 of the 26 patients (73.1%) with pancreatic cancer. An accumulation pattern characterized by nodular shapes was significantly more frequent in pancreatic cancer, whereas a longitudinal shape indicated AIP. Heterogeneous accumulation was found in almost all cases of AIP, whereas homogeneous accumulation was found in pancreatic cancer. Significantly more cases of pancreatic cancer showed a solitary localization, whereas multiple localization in the pancreas favored the presence of AIP. [^{18}F]FDG

uptake by the hilar lymph node was significantly more frequent in AIP than in pancreatic cancer, and uptake by the lachrymal gland, salivary gland, biliary duct, retroperitoneal space and prostate were seen only in AIP. Comparable results were reported by Lee et al. in a series of 17 patients suffering from AIP and 151 patients suffering from pancreatic cancer [78], by Shigekawa et al. in a series of 18 AIP patients and 20 pancreatic cancer patients [79] and by Kamisawa et al. in a series of 10 AIP patients and 14 pancreatic cancer patients [80].

Matasubayahsi et al. analyzed the usefulness of [^{18}F]FDG-PET in the evaluation of the distribution and activity of systemic lesions of AIP during steroid therapy [81]. In their series, 11 AIP patients had [^{18}F]FDG-PET images evaluated before and 3 months after steroid therapy, and another two cases only before therapy. AIP activity was determined from the level of serum markers, IgG and IgG4, and compared with [^{18}F]FDG-PET findings. In all 13 cases of AIP, a moderate-to-intense [^{18}F]FDG accumulation was recognized in the pancreatic lesion before steroid therapy; 11 (84.6%) showed [^{18}F]FDG accumulation in multiple organs, including the mediastinal and other lymph nodes, salivary gland, biliary tract, prostate and aortic wall. In 11 patients who underwent PET before and after steroid therapy, [^{18}F]FDG accumulation was diminished in almost all systemic lesions, with a mean decrease in SUV$_{max}$ in the pancreatic lesion from 5.12 to 2.69. Similar to the SUV level, serum IgG and IgG4 were decreased in most of the cases after steroid therapy.

In conclusion, [^{18}F]FDG-PET may be useful for detecting AIP and associated extrapancreatic autoimmune lesions and for monitoring disease activity. The presence of diffuse [^{18}F]FDG uptake by the pancreas or concomitant extrapancreatic uptake by the salivary glands can be used to aid in the differentiation of AIP and pancreatic cancer, as can a decrease in [^{18}F]FDG uptake after a short steroid trial.

Idiopathic retroperitoneal fibrosis

Retroperitoneal fibrosis (RPF) is characterized by the development of extensive fibrosis throughout the retroperitoneum, typically centered over the anterior surface of the fourth and fifth lumbar vertebrae [82,83]. This fibrosis leads to entrapment and obstruction of retroperitoneal structures, notably the ureters. Medical treatment frequently leads to residual retroperitoneal masses that may represent active disease or simply consist of inactive fibrotic tissue. Its occasional association with autoimmune diseases and its response to corticosteroids and immunosuppressive therapy suggest that it is probably immunologically mediated. Evidence suggests that RPF is an autoimmune response to an insoluble lipid called ceroid that has leaked through an arterial wall that has been thinned by the presence of atheromatous plaques. Other implicated causes include drugs, abdominal aortic aneurysm, ureteric renal injury, infection, retroperitoneal malignancy, post-irradiation therapy, chemotherapy, hemilaminectomy, hypothyroidism and carcinoid tumor. No genetic predominance is seen in malignant retroperitoneal fibrosis. As no etiological factor is found in up to 70% of patients presenting with RPF, the term idiopathic RFP (IRF) is used.

CT scanning and MRI are the preferred imaging modalities for IRF as they provide superior delineation of the extent of the masses [84,85]. However, CT scans may not be helpful in differentiating benign IRF from malignant IRF. On the other hand, MRI may help in differentiating both conditions, but cannot establish the diagnosis with certainty.

Retrograde pyelography is used in patients with severely impaired renal function. Aortography, venography and lymphangiography may prove of use for assessing the level and extent of occlusion. US can readily demonstrate the degree of obstruction to the ureters and kidneys, and attempts have been made to differentiate benign IRF from malignant IRF by means of color Doppler imaging.

The clinical question is whether [^{18}F]FDG-PET is a reliable means to evaluate disease activity in IRF and whether [^{18}F]FDG-PET/CT can help in differentiating benign from malignant IRF. Vaglio et al. used [^{18}F]FDG-PET imaging to evaluate the metabolic activity of residual masses in a consecutive series of seven IRF patients, all of whom presented with constitutional symptoms and/or pain; six had ureteral involvement [86]. IRF was diagnosed by means of CT, which revealed a peri-aortoiliac mass in all cases. Three patients underwent surgical ureterolysis and two received ureteral stents. Subsequently, five patients received prednisone, one sequential treatment with prednisone and tamoxifen, and one prednisolone plus methotrexate. All of the patients underwent [^{18}F]FDG-PET at varying times after the end of treatment. The presenting signs/symptoms improved in all patients and the levels of acute-phase reactants significantly decreased or normalized. Ureteral obstructive disease resolved in all cases. Post-treatment CT revealed a considerable reduction in the amount of IRF but all of the patients had a residual retroperitoneal mass. [^{18}F]FDG-PET revealed slight aortoiliac [^{18}F]FDG uptake in only one patient; all of the others were negative. No patient relapsed during the follow-up.

Nakajo et al. evaluated the [^{18}F]FDG uptake features in six patients with IRF. [^{18}F]FDG-PET was performed 1 and 2 hours after [^{18}F]FDG injection; uptake was scored using a four-point scale and the intensity uptake quantified (SUV$_{max}$) [87]. On the 1-hour images, intense [^{18}F]FDG uptake was observed in five patients before steroid treatment, but no abnormal uptake was noted in one patient receiving steroid treatment. The SUV$_{max}$ in IRF increased from a mean of 6.0 to 7.6 for all four patients who underwent 1- and 2-hour dual-time point imaging. Abnormal uptake was also noted in the mediastinum and the pancreas in one and two patients, respectively, and the diagnoses of mediastinal fibrosis and AIP were made, respectively. The SUV$_{max}$ was stable or increased in the three lesions of mediastinal fibrosis and AIP. The authors concluded that [^{18}F]FDG-PET may be a reliable means of evaluating disease activity and the extent of IRF, but that dual-time point imaging may not be useful to differentiate malignancy from IRF. Comparable findings were reported by Young et al. in a small series of three IRF patients who underwent [^{18}F]FDG-PET before and after steroid treatment [88].

More recently, Jansen et al. evaluated the value of [^{18}F]FDG-PET in monitoring disease activity and predicting treatment response in a series of 26 patients with IRP who were treated with tamoxifen monotherapy [89]. Patients underwent repeated [^{18}F]FDG-PET (baseline and, if positive, at 3 months) and CT scanning (baseline, 4 and 8 months). Maximal RPF mass thickness in three different view directions was measured on each CT scan; [^{18}F]FDG uptake was semi-quantified using a visual four-point scale. Initial and follow-up [^{18}F]FDG-PET scan results were correlated with clinical, laboratory and CT scan follow-up data. Treatment outcome was the aggregate measure of clinical, laboratory and CT-documented response to tamoxifen. [^{18}F]FDG-PET was positive in 20 patients and these patients had a significantly higher CRP level and larger mass size when compared with patients with a negative [^{18}F]FDG-PET scan result. Visual [^{18}F]FDG-PET score correlated with CRP level and CT-documented mass thickness. The observed [^{18}F]FDG-PET score decrease following treatment correlated with a decrease in ESR but not with CT-documented mass regression. The positive predictive value (PPV) of an initial positive PET scan result was 0.63 and the PPV of a negative follow-up PET scan result in patients with an initial positive [^{18}F]FDG-PET scan result was 0.66. The authors concluded that [^{18}F]FDG-PET is valuable in detecting (recurrent) disease activity, but that short-term follow-up with [^{18}F]FDG-PET cannot be routinely recommended for the therapeutic evaluation of IRF disease in tamoxifen-treated patients.

In summary, [^{18}F]FDG-PET has potential for evaluating disease activity and the extent of IRF (Figure 13.7). Available data suggest FDG-PET may not allow differentiation of benign from malignant IRF.

Other abdominal infections

Intra-abdominal infection (IAI) is an important cause of morbidity and mortality [90–92]. It is the second most commonly identified cause of severe sepsis in the intensive care unit (ICU).

Most IAI results from inflammation and perforation of the gastrointestinal tract, such as appendicitis, peptic ulcer disease and diverticulitis. Diffuse peritonitis may be due to spontaneous perforation, postoperative, post-interventional or post-traumatic causes and mesh-related infections after hernia repair surgery. The lower gastrointestinal tract is most often the location of perforation.

Symptoms of an abdominal infection can vary. Redness, tenderness and swelling of the abdominal region are common, and the area may feel rigid upon palpation. Patients can also experience gastrointestinal distress, along with symptoms of

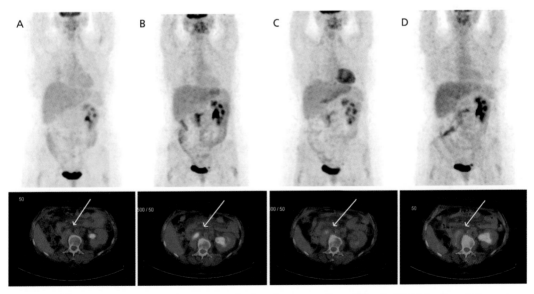

Figure 13.7 [^{18}F]FDG-PET/CT images of a patient with idiopathic retroperitoneal fibrosis. (A) At the time of diagnosis, no significant [^{18}F]FDG uptake was detected. (B) In the control scan after 1 year, the retroperitoneal tissue showed intense [^{18}F]FDG uptake (arrow) and the patient started high-dose steroid therapy. (C) After 10 months of therapy, [^{18}F]FDG uptake was significantly reduced, although it had not ceased completely (arrow) and the therapy was discontinued. (D) After a further year, the lesion showed a new increase in metabolic activity (arrow), indicating a relapse of disease that required new treatment.

organ damage, which can vary from decreased urine output to jaundice. If the infection has progressed, the patient may have an altered level of consciousness, a depressed appetite and a sensation of lethargy and extreme exhaustion. If peritonitis develops, sepsis with acute organ dysfunction may occur, leading to shock, coma and eventually death.

Successful treatment of IAI is based on early and appropriate source recognition, containment and antimicrobial coverage [9–11]. Often the treatment also includes opening up the abdomen for surgical cleaning and debridement; the infected material is removed and the abdominal cavity is flushed with antibacterial cleansers.

Although not a common indication, it has been shown that WBCs labeled with either ^{111}In or ^{99m}Tc can be helpful in selected patients in the diagnosis of acute cholecystitis when other standard radiological exams such as US (the elective imaging tool) cannot give a diagnosis [93,94].

If there is suspicion of abdominal abscess, the diagnostic approaches include US and CT, and nuclear medicine techniques can also be helpful. Radionuclide exams can be useful as a screening test in those patients with fever but without any localizing signs, while CT and US are better at characterizing the nature of infection and its extent.

[67]Ga-citrate has been used for a long time, having good rates of detection of abscesses, but given its drawbacks (time required before obtaining good quality images, false-positives due to colonic activity or malignant tumors, inability to differentiate abscesses from other inflammatory accumulations in adjacent sites). it has now been almost completely abandoned in favor of labeled WBC scintigraphy and, more recently, ^{18}F]FDG-PET.

False-negative results when using ^{67}Ga-citrate can also occur in certain areas of the abdomen, particularly the subphrenic area, because of the normal accumulation of the radionuclide in the liver and spleen. False-negative results have been described also in patients with short duration of symptoms of infection, in neutropenic patients and in patients treated with corticosteroids.

Labeled WBCs, although preferred to ^{67}Ga-citrate, have some limitations. The major problems described have been in the identification of infections near the liver and spleen, and distinguishing between important infections and minor inflammatory processes at surgical incisions or intramuscular injection sites [95]. It has been also reported that ^{111}In-labeled WBCs are unable to detect chronic abscesses or low-grade infections [96].

Mahfouz *et al.* published a study in 248 immunocompromised patients with multiple myeloma in whom a WBC scan could not be performed, to determine the role of ^{18}F]FDG-PET in the diagnosis of occult infections. Results indicated that ^{18}F] FDG-PET could identify cases of colitis, abdominal abscesses and diverticulitis, even in patients with severe immunosuppression [97]. Indeed ^{18}F]FDG can be a useful tool for diagnosing and managing infections even in patients with severe neutropenia or lymphopenia. [18]F]FDG uptake has also been shown to correlate with the degree of human immunodeficiency virus (HIV)-related infection and with the viral load.

Tahara *et al.* reported on two cases of abdominal abscess displaying high uptake of ^{18}F]FDG on PET and suggested that abdominal abscesses should be considered in the differential diagnosis of abdominal masses showing high ^{18}F]FDG uptake in PET studies [98]. In a recent study by Tatli *et al.* of 12 patients, ^{18}F]FDG-PET/CT proved useful in guiding the biopsy of ^{18}F]FDG-avid masses that are either not visible with unenhanced CT or only a portion is ^{18}F]FDG avid [99]. All biopsy procedures yielded diagnostic results; nine were positive for malignancy and three were negative (fibrosis, steatosis and *E. coli* infection).

Bleeker-Rovers *et al.* reported on seven ^{18}F] FDG-PET scans in three patients suffering from autosomal-dominant polycystic kidney disease (ADPKD) [100]. In these patients, ^{18}F]FDG-PET was shown to enable early identification of infection in renal and hepatic cysts, and was useful for monitoring response to treatment (Figure 13.8). In a study by Sallée *et al.*, ^{18}F]FDG-PET proved superior to US, CT and MRI for the identification of infected cysts; among 389 patients suffering from ADPKD, 33 had 41 episodes of cyst infection, including eight definite and 33 likely cases [101].

Role for therapy follow-up and patient management

In IBD patients, labeled WBCs have an important role in therapy follow-up. A specific indication is the

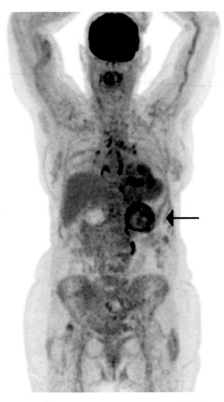

Figure 13.8 [^{18}F]FDG-PET/CT in a patient with a large renal cyst. The uptake of [^{18}F]FDG around the cyst (arrow) is a clear sign of infection of the cyst wall. This was an incidental finding in this patient as the PET scan had been performed for a mediastinal non-Hodgkin lymphoma.

early diagnosis of post-surgical recurrences on pre-anastomotic loops. If quantitative assessment is required, it can be performed in a semi-quantitative way by comparing the activity of WBC uptake with activity in the iliac crest, liver and spleen. The scan should be performed pre-therapy and during therapy. In our experience a normal scan can be detected as early as 48 hours after initiation of steroid therapy.

Signore *et al.* [37] and Annovazzi *et al.* [38] demonstrated that ^{99m}Tc-IL-2 scintigraphy can be a very important step in the non-invasive imaging of patients with Crohn's disease, as well as useful in monitoring the efficacy of therapies in a more objective way.

Further research and clinical trials will allow a better delineation of the clinical role of [^{18}F]

FDG-PET/CT imaging in abdominal infections and particularly in the diagnosis and follow-up of patients with IBD. It certainly holds promise for early evaluation of therapy efficacy as it can visualize the whole inflammatory burden in the bowel with higher sensitivity than labeled WBCs.

Conclusion

Nuclear medicine has an important complementary role to radiology in the diagnosis of abdominal inflammation/infections. The most investigated and accurate technique is the use of ^{111}In-oxine-labeled WBCs.

There are three main areas of development that will condition the future of nuclear medicine imaging in abdominal inflammation/infection: labeled antibiotics, specific peptides such as ^{18}F-IL-2 [36] and [^{18}F]FDG for WBC labeling [45,102].

[^{18}F]FDG-PET/CT imaging is also a promising technique for identifying foci of abdominal infections and for guiding biopsy, but at present its use should be limited to the study of AIP and IRF.

Future availability of hybrid nuclear medicine/MR cameras [103] and new radiopharmaceuticals [104] will open a new important era in the diagnosis and follow-up of this disease.

References

1. Fletcher JG, Fidler JL, Bruining DH, Huprich JE. New concepts in intestinal imaging for inflammatory bowel diseases. *Gastroenterology* 2011;140: 1795–1806.
2. Annovazzi A, Bagni B, Burroni L, D'Alessandria C, Signore A. Nuclear medicine imaging of inflammatory/infective disorders of the abdomen. *Nucl Med Commun* 2005;26:657–664.
3. Triantafillidis JK, Merikas E, Georgopoulos F. Current and emerging drugs for the treatment of inflammatory bowel disease. *Drug Des Dev Ther* 2011;5:185–210.
4. Burger D, Travis S. Conventional medical management of inflammatory bowel disease. *Gastroenterology* 2011;140:1827–1837.
5. Plevy SE, Targan SR. Future therapeutic approaches for inflammatory bowel diseases. *Gastroenterology* 2011;140:1838–1846.
6. Cho JH, Brant SR. Recent insights into the genetics of inflammatory bowel disease. *Gastroenterology* 2011;140:1704–1712.

7. Reenaers C, Louis E, Belaiche J. Current directions of biologic therapies in inflammatory bowel disease. *Ther Adv Gastroenterol* 2010;3:99–106.

8. Thomas Dow C. Cows, Crohn's and more: is *Mycobacterium paratuberculosis* a superantigen? *Med Hypoth* 2008;71:858–861.

9. Mazzei T, Novelli A. Pharmacological rationale for antibiotic treatment of intra-abdominal infections. *J Chemother* 2009;21:19–29.

10. Bodmann KF. Complicated intra-abdominal infections: pathogens, resistance. Recommendations of the Infectliga on antbiotic therapy. *Chirurgie* 2010; 81:38–49.

11. Solomkin JS, Mazuski J. Intra-abdominal sepsis: newer interventional and antimicrobial therapies. *Infect Dis Clin North Am* 2009;23:593–608.

12. Calder JDF, Gajraj H. Recent advances in the diagnosis and treatment of acute appendicitis. *Br J Hosp Med* 1995;54:129–133.

13. Hennelly KE, Bachur R. Appendicitis update. *Curr Opin Pediatr* 2011;23:281–285.

14. Panes J, Bouhnik Y, Reinisch W *et al.* Imaging techniques for assessment of inflammatory bowel disease: Joint ECCO and ESGAR evidence-based consensus guidelines. *J Crohn Colitis* 2013 (published online April 15).

15. Roitt IM. *Essential Immunology*, 9th edn. Oxford: Blackwell Scientific, 1997.

16. Rennen HJ, Boerman OC, Oyen WJ *et al.* Imaging infection/inflammation in the new millenium. *Eur J Nucl Med* 2001;28:241–252.

17. Boerman OC, Rennen H, Oyen WJ *et al.* Radiopharmaceuticals to image infection and inflammation. *Semin Nucl Med* 2001;31:286–295.

18. Petruzzi N, Shanthly N, Thakur M. Recent trends in soft tissue infection imaging. *Semin Nucl Med* 2009; 39:115–123.

19. Martín-Comín J, Benítez Segura A, Roca Engronyat M *et al.* Enfermedad Inflamatoria Intestinal. In: *Medicina Nuclear en la Práctica Clínica*. Madrid: Grupo Aula Médica, 2009, pp. 465–473.

20. Rennen HJJM, Boerman OC, Oyen WJG. Radiomarcadores para el diagnóstico de infecciones y inflamaciones. In: *Diagnóstico de la Inflamación y la Infección en Medicina Nuclear*. Barcelona: J. Martín-Comín & GE Healthcare, 1995, pp. 55–75.

21. Corstens FH, Oyen WJ, Becker WS. Radioimmunoconjugates in the detection of infection and inflammation. *Semin Nucl Med* 1993;23:148–164.

22. de Vries EF, Roca M, Jamar F, Israel O, Signore A. Guidelines for the labelling of leucocytes with (99m) Tc-HMPAO. Inflammation/Infection Taskgroup of the European Association of Nuclear Medicine. *Eur J Nucl Med Mol Imaging* 2010;37:842–848.

23. Roca M, de Vries EF, Jamar F, Israel O, Signore A. Guidelines for the labelling of leucocytes with (111) In-oxine. Inflammation/Infection Taskgroup of the European Association of Nuclear Medicine. *Eur J Nucl Med Mol Imaging* 2010;37:835–841.

24. Martín-Comín J, Prats E. Clinical applications of radiolabelled blood elements in inflammatory bowel disease. *Q J Nucl Med Mol Imaging* 1999;43: 74–82.

25. Tsan MF. Mechanism of gallium-67 accumulation in inflammatory lesions. *J Nucl Med* 1985;26: 88–92.

26. Segarra I, Roca M, Baliellas C *et al.* Granulocyte-specific monoclonal antibody technetium-99m-BW 250/183 and indium-111 oxine labelled leukocyte scintigraphy in inflammatory bowel disease. *Eur J Nucl Med* 1991;18:715–719.

27. Harwood SJ, Valdivia, Hung GL *et al.* Use of sulesomab, a radiolabelled antibody fragment, to detect osteomyelitis in diabetic patients with foot ulcers by leukoscintigraphy. *Clin Infect Dis* 1999;28: 1200–1205.

28. Kipper SL, Rypins EB, Evans DG *et al.* Neutrophil-specific ^{99m}Tc-labeled antiCD15 monoclonal antibody imaging for diagnosis of equivocal appendicitis: clinical evaluation of safety, efficacy and time performance characteristics. *J Nucl Med* 2000;41: 449–455.

29. D'Alessandria C, Malviya G, Viscido A *et al.* Use of ^{99m}Tc labeled anti-TNFα monoclonal antibody in Crohn's disease: *in vitro* and *in vivo* studies. *Q J Nucl Med Mol Imaging* 2007;51:334–342.

30. Fischman AJ, Rubin RH, Khaw BA *et al.* Detection of acute inflammation with ^{111}In-labeled nonspecific polyclonal IgG. *Semin Nucl Med* 1988;18: 335–344.

31. Oyen WJ, Claessens RA, Van der Meer JW *et al.* Indium-111-labeled human nonspecific immunoglobulin G: a new radiopharmaceutical for imaging infectious and inflammatory foci. *Clin Infect Dis* 1992;14:1110–1118.

32. Glaudemans AW, Maccioni F, Mansi L *et al.* Imaging of cell trafficking in Crohn's disease. *J Cell Physiol* 2010;223;562–571.

33. Mairal L, De Lima PA, Martin-Comin J *et al.* Simultaneous administration of ^{111}In-human immunoglobulin and ^{99m}Tc-HMPAO labelled leukocytes in inflammatory bowel disease. *Eur J Nucl Med* 1995; 22:664–670.

34. Signore A, Parman A, Pozzilli P, Andreani D, Beverley PCL. Detection of activated lymphocytes in endocrine pancreas of BB/W rats by injection of ^{123}I-labelled interleukin-2: an early sign of type 1 diabetes. *Lancet* 1987;2:537–540.

35. Chianelli M, Signore A, Fritzberg AR, Mather SJ. The development of Technetium-99m-labelled interleukin-2: a new radiopharmaceutical for the *in vivo* detection of mononuclear cell infiltrates in immune-mediated diseases. *Nucl Med Biol* 1997;24: 579–586.

36. Di Gialleonardo V, Signore A, Glaudemans AWJM, Dierckx RAJO, de Vries EFJ. N-(4-18F-fluorobenzoyl) interleukin-2 for PET imaging of human activated T-lymphocytes. *J Nucl Med* 2012;53:679–686.

37. Signore A, Chianelli M, Annovazzi A *et al.* ^{123}I-Interleukin-2 scintigraphy for the *in vivo* assessment of intestinal mononuclear cell infiltration in Crohn's disease. *J Nucl Med* 2000;41:242–249.

38. Annovazzi A, Biancone L, Caviglia R *et al.* ^{99m}Tc-interleukin-2 and ^{99m}Tc-HMPAO granulocyte scintigraphy in patients with inactive Crohn's disease. *Eur J Nucl Med Mol Imaging* 2003;30:374–382.

39. Signore A, Chianelli M, Annovazzi A *et al.* Imaging of active lymphocytic infiltration in coeliac disease with ^{123}I-interleukin-2 and its response to diet. *Eur J Nucl Med* 2000;27:18–24.

40. Vinjamuri S, Hall AV, Solanski KK *et al.* Comparison of ^{99m}Tc infecton imaging with radiolabelled white-cell imaging in the evaluation of bacterial infection. *Lancet* 1996;347:233–235.

41. Hall AV, Solanski KK, Vonjamuri S *et al.* Evaluation of the efficacy of ^{99m}Tc infecton, a novel agent for detecting sites of infection. *J Clin Pathol* 1998;51: 215–219.

42. Lupetti A, Welling MM, Pauwels EK *et al.* Detection of fungal infections using radiolabelled antifungal agents. *Curr Drug Targets* 2005;6:945–954.

43. Gomes V, Roca M, Martin-Comin J. Marcaje de ceftizoxima con [99m]Tc. *Rev Esp Med Nucl* 2000;19: 479–483.

44. Martín-Comin J, Soroa V, Rabiller G, Galli F, Cuesta L, Roca M. Diagnóstico de la infección ósea con 99mTc-ceftizoxima. *Rev Esp Med Nucl* 2004;23:357.

45. Forstrom LA, Dunn WL, Mullan BP *et al.* ^{18}F-FDG labelling of human leukocytes. *Nucl Med Commun* 2000;21:691–694.

46. Peters AM. The utility of [^{99m}Tc]HMPAO-leukocytes for imaging infection. *Semin Nucl Med* 1994;24: 110–127.

47. de Groot M, Meeuwis AP, Kok PJ, Corstens FH, Oyen WJ. Influence of blood glucose level, age and fasting period on non-pathological FDG uptake in heart and gut. *Eur J Nucl Med Mol Imaging* 2005; 32:98–101.

48. Toriihara A, Yoshida K, Umehara I, Shibuya H. Normal variants of bowel FDG uptake in dual-time-point PET/CT imaging. *Ann Nucl Med* 2011;25: 173–178.

49. Tatlidil R, Jadvar H, Bading JR, Conti PS. Incidental colonic fluorodeoxyglucose uptake: correlation with colonoscopic and histopathologic findings. *Radiology* 2002;224:783–787.

50. Kamel EM, Thumshirn M, Truninger K *et al.* Significance of incidental ^{18}F-FDG accumulations in the gastrointestinal tract in PET/CT: correlation with endoscopic and histopathologic results. *J Nucl Med* 2004;45:1804–1810.

51. Jaruskova M, Belohlavek O. Role of FDG-PET and PET/CT in the diagnosis of prolonged febrile states. *Eur J Nucl Med Mol Imaging* 2006;33:913–918.

52. Ogawa S, Itabashi M, Kameoka S. Significance of FDG-PET in identification of diseases of the appendix – based on experience of two cases falsely positive for FDG accumulation. *Case Rep Gastroenterol* 2009;3:125–130.

53. Koff SG, Sterbis JR, Davison JM, Montilla-Soler JL. A unique presentation of appendicitis: F-18 FDG PET/CT. *Clin Nucl Med* 2006;31:704–706.

54. Bicik I, Bauerfeind P, Breitbach T, von Schulthess GK, Fried M. Inflammatory bowel disease activity measured by positron-emission tomography. *Lancet* 1997;350:262.

55. Skehan SJ, Issenman R, Mernagh J, Nahmias C, Jacobson K. ^{18}F-fluorodeoxyglucose positron tomography in diagnosis of paediatric inflammatory bowel disease. *Lancet* 1999;354:836–837.

56. Löffler M, Weckesser M, Franzius C, Schober O, Zimmer KP. High diagnostic value of ^{18}F-FDG-PET in pediatric patients with chronic inflammatory bowel disease. *Ann N Y Acad Sci* 2006;1072:379–385.

57. Das CJ, Makharia G, Kumar R *et al.* PET-CT enteroclysis: a new technique for evaluation of inflammatory diseases of the intestine. *Eur J Nucl Med Mol Imaging* 2007;34:2106–2114.

58. Neurath MF, Vehling D, Schunk K *et al.* Noninvasive assessment of Crohn's disease activity: a comparison of ^{18}F-fluorodeoxyglucose positron emission tomography, hydromagnetic resonance imaging, and granulocyte scintigraphy with labeled antibodies. *Am J Gastroenterol* 2002;97:1978–1985.

59. Lemberg DA, Issenman RM, Cawdron R *et al.* Positron emission tomography in the investigation of pediatric inflammatory bowel disease. *Inflamm Bowel Dis* 2005;11:733–738.

60. Meisner RS, Spier BJ, Einarsson S *et al.* Pilot study using PET/CT as a novel, noninvasive assessment of disease activity in inflammatory bowel disease. *Inflamm Bowel Dis* 2007;13:993–1000.

61. Louis E, Ancion G, Colard A, Spote V, Belaiche J, Hustinx R. Noninvasive assessment of Crohn's disease intestinal lesions with (18)F-FDG PET/CT. *J Nucl Med* 2007;48:1053–1059.

62. Lapp RT, Spier BJ, Perlman SB, Jaskowiak CJ, Reichelderfer M. Clinical utility of positron emission tomography/computed tomography in inflammatory bowel disease. *Mol Imaging Biol* 2011;13: 573–576.

63. Däbritz J, Jasper N, Loeffler M, Weckesser M, Foell D. Noninvasive assessment of pediatric inflammatory bowel disease with ^{18}F-fluorodeoxyglucose-positron emission tomography and computed tomography. *Eur J Gastroenterol Hepatol* 2011;23:81–89.

64. Rubin DT, Surma BL, Gavzy SJ *et al.* Positron emission tomography (PET) used to image subclinical inflammation associated with ulcerative colitis (UC) in remission. *Inflamm Bowel Dis* 2009;15:750–755.

65. Jacene HA, Ginsburg P, Kwon J *et al.* Prediction of the need for surgical intervention in obstructive Crohn's disease by ^{18}F-FDG PET/CT. *J Nucl Med* 2009;50:1751–1759.

66. Spier BJ, Perlman SB, Jaskowiak CJ, Reichelderfer M. PET/CT in the evaluation of inflammatory bowel disease: studies in patients before and after treatment. *Mol Imaging Biol* 2010;12:85–88.

67. Das CJ, Makharia GK, Kumar R *et al.* PET/CT colonography: a novel non-invasive technique for assessment of extent and activity of ulcerative colitis. *Eur J Nucl Med Mol Imaging* 2010;37:714–721.

68. Ahmadi A, Li Q, Muller K *et al.* Diagnostic value of noninvasive combined fluorine-18 labeled fluoro-2-deoxy-D-glucose positron emission tomography and computed tomography enterography in active Crohn's disease. *Inflamm Bowel Dis* 2010;16: 974–981.

69. Shimosegawa T, Kanno A. Autoimmune pancreatitis in Japan: overview and perspective. *J Gastroenterol* 2009;44:503–517.

70. Buscarini E, Frulloni L, De Lisi S, Falconi M, Testoni PA, Zambelli A. Autoimmune pancreatitis: a challenging diagnostic puzzle for clinicians. *Dig Liver Dis* 2010;42:92–98.

71. Frulloni L, Amodio A, Katsotourchi AM, Vantini I. A practical approach to the diagnosis of autoimmune pancreatitis. *World J Gastroenterol* 2011;17: 2076–2079.

72. Sugumar A, Takahashi N, Chari ST. Distinguishing pancreatic cancer from autoimmune pancreatitis. *Curr Gastroenterol Rep* 2010;12:91–97.

73. Giday SA, Khashab MA, Buscaglia JM *et al.* Autoimmune pancreatitis: Current diagnostic criteria are suboptimal. *J Gastroenterol Hepatol* 2011;26: 970–973.

74. Pezzilli R, Morselli-Labate AM. The concept of autoimmune pancreatitis and its immunological backgrounds. *Expert Rev Clin Immunol* 2010;6: 125–136.

75. Nakamoto Y, Saga T, Ishimori T *et al.* FDG-PET of autoimmune-related pancreatitis: preliminary results. *Eur J Nucl Med* 2000;27:1835–1838.

76. Nakajo M, Jinnouchi S, Fukukura Y, Tanabe H, Tateno R, Nakajo M. The efficacy of whole-body FDG-PET or PET/CT for autoimmune pancreatitis and associated extrapancreatic autoimmune lesions. *Eur J Nucl Med Mol Imaging* 2007;34:2088–2095.

77. Ozaki Y, Oguchi K, Hamano H *et al.* Differentiation of autoimmune pancreatitis from suspected pancreatic cancer by fluorine-18 fluorodeoxyglucose positron emission tomography. *J Gastroenterol* 2008;43: 144–151.

78. Lee TY, Kim MH, Park do H *et al.* Utility of ^{18}F-FDG PET/CT for differentiation of autoimmune pancreatitis with atypical pancreatic imaging findings from pancreatic cancer. *AJR Am J Roentgenol* 2009;193: 343–348.

79. Shigekawa M, Yamao K, Sawaki A *et al.* Is (18) F-fluorodeoxyglucose positron emission tomography meaningful for estimating the efficacy of corticosteroid therapy in patients with autoimmune pancreatitis? *J Hepatobiliary Pancreat Sci* 2010;17: 269–274.

80. Kamisawa T, Takum K, Anjiki H *et al.* FDG-PET/CT findings of autoimmune pancreatitis. *Hepatogastroenterology* 2010;57:447–450.

81. Matsubayashi H, Furukawa H, Maeda A *et al.* Usefulness of positron emission tomography in the evaluation of distribution and activity of systemic lesions associated with autoimmune pancreatitis. *Pancreatology* 2009;9:694–699.

82. Kermani TA, Crowson CS, Achenbach SJ, Luthra HS. Idiopathic retroperitoneal fibrosis: a retrospective review of clinical presentation, treatment, and outcomes. *Mayo Clin Proc* 2011;86:297–303.

83. Vaglio A, Palmisano A, Corradi D, Salvarani C, Buzio C. Retroperitoneal fibrosis: evolving concepts. *Rheum Dis Clin North Am* 2007;33:803–817.

84. Kamper L, Brandt AS, Winkler SB, Ekamp H, Piroth W, Roth S, Haage P. Imaging of retroperitoneal fibrosis. *Med Klin* 2010;105:582–584.

85. Scheel PJ Jr, Feeley N. Retroperitoneal fibrosis: the clinical, laboratory, and radiographic presentation. *Medicine* 2009;88:202–207.

86. Vaglio A, Greco P, Versari A *et al.* Post-treatment residual tissue in idiopathic retroperitoneal fibrosis: active residual disease or silent "scar"? A study using ^{18}F-fluorodeoxyglucose positron emission tomography. *Clin Exp Rheumatol* 2005;23:231–234.

87. Nakajo M, Jinnouchi S, Tanabe H, Tateno R, Nakajo M. ^{18}F-fluorodeoxyglucose positron emission tomography features of idiopathic retroperitoneal fibrosis. *J Comput Assist Tomogr* 2007;31:539–543.

88. Young PM, Peterson JJ, Calamia KT. Hypermetabolic activity in patients with active retroperitoneal fibrosis on F-18 FDG PET: report of three cases. *Ann Nucl Med* 2008;22:87–92.

89. Jansen I, Hendriksz TR, Han SH, Huiskes AW, van Bommel EF. (18)F-fluorodeoxyglucose position emission tomography (FDG-PET) for monitoring disease activity and treatment response in idiopathic retroperitoneal fibrosis. *Eur J Intern Med* 2010;21: 216–221.

90. Nicoletti G, Nicolosi D, Rossolini GM, Stefani S. Intra-abdominal infections: etiology, epidemiology, microbiological diagnosis and antibiotic resistance. *J Chemother* 2009;21:5–11.

91. Menichetti F, Sganga G. Definition and classification of intra-abdominal infections. *J Chemother* 2009;21: 3–4.

92. Mazuski JE, Solomkin JS. Intra-abdominal infections. *Surg Clin North Am* 2009;89:421–437.

93. Lantto E, Järvi K, Laitinen R et al. Scintigraphy with ^{99m}Tc-HMPAO labeled leukocytes in acute cholecystitis. *Acta Radiol* 1991;32:359–362.

94. Fink-Bennett D, Clarke K, Tasi D et al. Indium-111-leukocyte imaging in acute cholecystitis. *J Nucl Med* 1991;32:803–804.

95. Sfakianakis GN, Al-Sheikh W, Heal A et al. Comparisons of scintigraphy with In-111 leukocytes and Ga-67 in the diagnosis of occult sepsis. *J Nucl Med* 1982;23:628.

96. Mc Dougall IR, Naumert JE, Lantieri RL. Evaluation of ^{111}In leukocyte whole body scanning. *AJR Am J Roentgenol* 1979;133:849.

97. Mahfouz T, Miceli MH, Saghafifar S et al. ^{18}F-Fluordeoxyglucose positron emission tomography contributes to the diagnosis and management of infections in patients with multiple myeloma: a study of 165 infectious episodes. *J Clin Oncol* 2005; 23:7857–7863.

98. Tahara T, Ichiya Y, Kuwabara Y et al. High [^{18}F]-fluorodeoxyglucose uptake in abdominal abscesses: a PET study. *J Comput Assist Tomogr* 1989;13: 829–831.

99. Tatli S, Gerbaudo VH, Feeley CM, Shyn PB, Tuncali K, Silverman SG. PET/CT-guided percutaneous biopsy of abdominal masses: initial experience. *J Vasc Interv Radiol* 2011;22:507–514.

100. Bleeker-Rovers CP, de Sévaux RG, van Hamersvelt HW, Corstens FH, Oyen WJ. Diagnosis of renal and hepatic cyst infections by 18-F-fluorodeoxyglucose positron emission tomography in autosomal dominant polycystic kidney disease. *Am J Kidney Dis* 2003;41:E18–21.

101. Sallée M, Rafat C, Zahar JR et al. Cyst infections in patients with autosomal dominant polycystic kidney disease. *Clin J Am Soc Nephrol* 2009;4: 1183–1189.

102. Rini NJ, Palestro CJ. Imaging of infection and inflammation with ^{18}F-FDG-labeled leukocytes. *Q J Nucl Med Mol Imaging* 2006;50:143–146.

103. Glaudemans AW, Quintero AM, Signore A. PET/MRI in infectious and inflammatory diseases: will it be a useful improvement? *Eur J Nucl Med Mol Imaging* 2012;39:745–749.

104. Signore A, Mather SJ, Piaggio G, Malviya G, Dierckx RA. Molecular imaging of inflammation/infection: nuclear medicine and optical imaging agents and methods. *Chem Rev* 2010;110:3112–3145.

Clinical cases

Case 1

A 52-year-old male with ulcerative colitis diagnosed 7 years ago. The patient had two recurrences that were treated with azathioprine and corticosteroids with good response. He was then in maintenance treatment with sulfasalazine.

After a long period of remission, the patient presented with abdominal pain and a 7-day history of diarrhea. Blood tests showed an increased ESR, CRP level and an incipient anemia. A new recurrence was suspected and the referring clinician wanted to know the activity and extent of disease. Therefore, a ^{99m}Tc-HMPAO-labeled WBC scintigraphy was performed (Figure 13.9). The images showed an important inflammatory recurrence in the rectum, sigma, descending colon, half of the transverse colon and also the cecum. After the exam, treatment with azathioprine was administered.

Teaching points
• When a disease has already been diagnosed and a recurrence is suspected, a labeled WBC scan has a great accuracy for the evaluation of disease activity and extent.

• A labeled WBC scan is less accurate for the detection of complications and an MRI should be also performed.
• The combination of these two exams can avoid the need to perform other diagnostic tests, including colonoscopy.

Case 2

A 45-year-old female diagnosed with ulcerative proctitis 2 years ago, with an episode of bloody diarrhea and tenesmus that responded completely to mesalazine treatment.

At consultation, rectal tact and anal inspection were normal. Blood tests showed just a moderate increase in CRP. WBC scintigraphy was performed to evaluate the activity and extent of the disease. Figures 13.10 and 13.11 show the results of the scan and superiority of SPECT/CT images for the detection of mild rectal inflammation. The patient was treated again with mesalazine.

Teaching points
• In IBD, images must always be acquired in anteroposterior and caudocranial views.
• If possible, a SPECT/CT of the abdomen should be acquired for best localization of lesions. This is mandatory for the differential diagnosis of strictures.

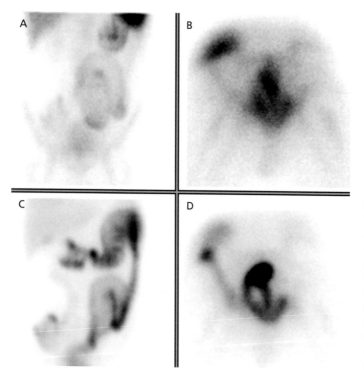

Figure 13.9 ^{99m}Tc-HMPAO-labeled WBC scintigraphy. (A,C) Anteroposterior and (B,D) caudocranial planar views acquired at 30 minutes (A,B) and 3 hours (C,D) after the injection of the labeled cells. An evident pathological accumulation of labeled cells (increasing with time) can be seen in all the planar images, allowing a correct evaluation of disease extent and severity.

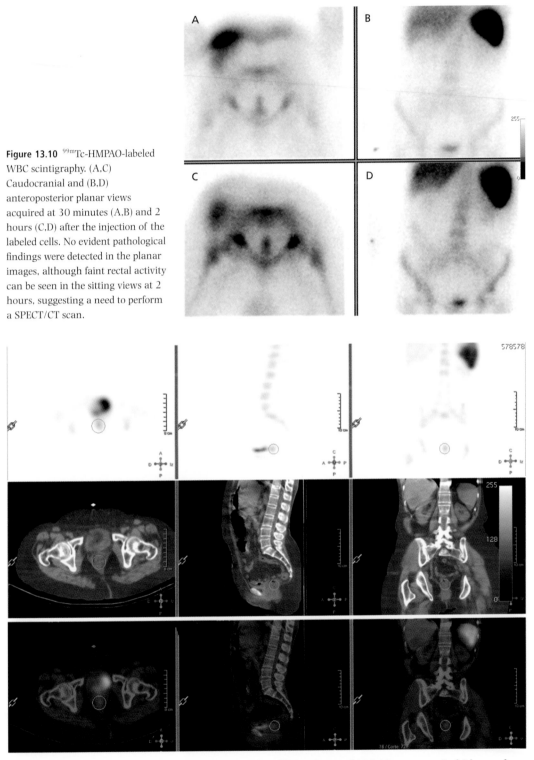

Figure 13.10 ^{99m}Tc-HMPAO-labeled WBC scintigraphy. (A,C) Caudocranial and (B,D) anteroposterior planar views acquired at 30 minutes (A,B) and 2 hours (C,D) after the injection of the labeled cells. No evident pathological findings were detected in the planar images, although faint rectal activity can be seen in the sitting views at 2 hours, suggesting a need to perform a SPECT/CT scan.

Figure 13.11 SPECT/CT processed transaxial (left), sagittal (middle) and coronal (right) images, acquired 3 hours after labeled WBC administration. The blue circle highlights the pathological focus in the rectum that had not been clearly visible in the planar images.

Case 3

A 45-year-old male diagnosed with Crohn's disease 3 years ago and on therapy with azathioprine. One year ago he had presented with an acute episode of colitis and a right colectomy was required.

One week ago, he started to feel discomfort, fever and pain on his right abdominal side. No diarrhea was reported. A blood test demonstrated increased levels of neutrophils and a CT scan was requested. Before CT, a ^{99m}Tc-HMPAO-labeled WBC scintigraphy was performed (Figure 13.12). An abnormal uptake of labeled WBCs was observed in the right side of abdomen at the previous surgery site and this was present on both the 30-minute and 2-hour images. The diagnosis was a postoperative abscess, confirmed later by CT, and treated with antibiotic therapy and CT-guided drainage.

Teaching point

In a patient with a high suspicion of infection, a labeled WBC scan should be performed before the CT scan in order correctly to prepare for the subsequent procedure. In this particular case, the radiologists were already informed about the abscess and thus could immediately organize the CT-guided drainage, avoiding the need to perform the CT scan twice.

Case 4

A 48-year-old female with history of renal polycystic disease of the kidneys. She had a 2-week history of fever, discomfort and dysuria.

A US scan of the abdomen was performed and infection of a renal cyst was suspected. She was therefore referred to nuclear medicine for a scintigraphy with labeled WBCs.

Autologous WBCs were labeled with ^{111}In-oxine and posterior views of the renal area were acquired at 4 and 24 hours post injection. A significant accumulation of labeled WBCs in the left kidney was seen at 4 hours post injection. On the 24-hour image the accumulation in the left kidney was of the same extent but there was increased activity (Figure 13.13).

Teaching point

When the suspicion of infection concerns the kidney, the WBCs must be labeled with ^{111}In-oxine instead of ^{99m}Tc-HMPAO because there is no kidney elimination of the former radiopharmaceutical.

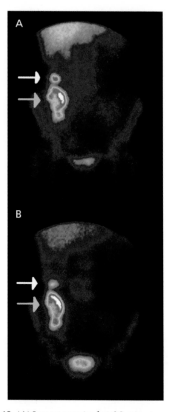

Figure 13.12 (A) Image acquired at 30 minutes post injection of WBCs shows a pathological accumulation of labeled cells on the right side of abdomen. (B) This uptake has increased in the images obtained at 2 hours, thus confirming the infection (yellow arrow). There is a small area in which activity decreases with time (white arrow), which probably corresponds to a sterile inflamed area.

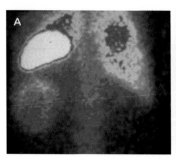
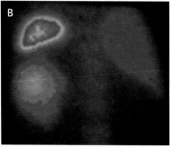

Figure 13.13 Posterior views at (A) 4 and (B) 24 hours post injection of ^{111}In-oxime-labeled WBCs. A significant accumulation of labeled WBCs is seen in both images (but more clearly at 24 hours), confirming the presence of an infected cyst.

CHAPTER 14

Nuclear Medicine Imaging of Vascular Graft Infection: The Added Role of Hybrid Imaging

Ora Israel

Rambam Health Care Campus, Haifa, Israel

Introduction

Vascular grafts replace or bypass occluded or diseased blood vessels of small, medium and large size in order to maintain their patency. Autogenous vascular grafts are vessels taken from another region in the same patient, most commonly the long saphenous vein. Artificial vascular prostheses are produced from biological, synthetic, or biosynthetic materials. Biological implants may be either allografts, e.g. human blood vessels such as removed cadaver vessels, varicose or umbilical veins, or xenografts, which are of animal origin, such as bovine carotid and mammary arteries.

Synthetic grafts are made of either Dacron or polytetrafluoroethylene (PTFE). Dacron grafts are very susceptible to infections since bacteria can adhere to this material. In recent years, Dacron grafts have been coated with collagen, to reduce blood loss, and with antibiotics, to prevent infection. They are inserted mainly in large vessels, such as at aortic and aortoiliac surgery and above-knee bypass. PTFE grafts are most commonly peripheral implants. PTFE is less thrombogenic than Dacron, but is a soft material and therefore prone to kinking around joints. Occlusion of the lumen can occur because of an in-growth healing process. Bleeding at the suture line during and after implantation may cause a seroma, a further site for potential infection.

Autogenous grafts are the mainstay of vascular surgery. Artificial grafts are inserted when autogenous vessels are unavailable or too large to be implanted in small-diameter vessels.

Common complications associated with vascular grafts are occlusion, distal emboli, infection, true and false aneurysms at the site of the anastomosis and erosion into adjacent structures. Infection of biological or prosthetic vascular grafts can have severe outcomes, ranging from loss of a limb to death [1,2].

Basic knowledge of the clinical problem

Vascular graft infection is a rare (incidence ranging from 1% to 6%) but severe complication following reconstructive surgery. Most infections are diagnosed at least 4 months after surgery. The incidence varies with the location of the graft, and is lower in the abdomen and higher for implants below the inguinal region and into the lower extremities. Infection is more common in the inguinal region for aorto-bifemoral and femoro-popliteal bypasses.

Infection is caused either at the time of surgery, during procedures involving the inserted graft

Diagnostic Imaging of Infections and Inflammatory Diseases: A Multidisciplinary Approach, First Edition. Edited by Alberto Signore and Ana María Quintero.

(such as revision or catheterization), or through direct involvement from an adjacent soft tissue focus. Late contamination in cases of bacteremia has also been reported [3]. Once it occurs, vascular graft infection harbors a poor prognosis. It may result in limb loss or even death in over 50% of patients, with an associated morbidity and mortality ranging between 20% and 75% [4–9]. Risk factors for graft contamination include a long preoperative hospital stay or operation time, faulty sterile surgical conditions and emergency procedures. However, infection can also occur despite sterile conditions and meticulous handling of the graft during operation, and even when prophylactic antibiotic treatment is administered. Surgical revision of a graft, especially if performed early (less than a month after the first procedure) is associated with a higher incidence of infection. Postoperative surgical wound infection, mainly groin incisions, skin necrosis, hematomas and seromas can cause graft thrombosis and infection. Remote site infections can lead to graft contamination through hematogenous or lymphatic spread. Infection is more frequently associated with immunosuppressive therapy, diabetes mellitus, cancer and immunological disorders [5,7–12].

Approximately one-third of graft infections are caused by *Staphylococcus aureus*. Additional pathogens are Gram-positive bacteria, such as *Staphylococcus epidermidis*, which are responsible for late, low-grade graft infection and Gram-negative bacteria such as *Pseudomonas* spp., *Klebsiella* spp. and *Escherichia coli*. Polymicrobial infections occur in up to 25% of cases [5,6,11,13,14].

The clinical presentation of vascular graft infection is variable. It may be subtle or stormy depending on the anatomical location and the virulence of the pathogen. Infected abdominal or thoracic grafts have a more indolent course and are therefore more difficult to diagnose. The common presentation includes local pain, redness, a palpable lump and/or secretion in the area of the surgical wound. Infection is suspected in the presence of a draining sinus, a pulsatile mass with signs of local inflammation, or a local superficial process with poor response to antibiotics. Evidence of septic emboli or hypertrophic osteoarthropathy is rare, but when present is strongly suspicious of vascular graft infection. The presence of remote sources of potential contamination, such as infected venous lines, phlebitis,

infected ulcers, osteomyelitis, pneumonia, urinary tract infection or septic emboli, should raise the suspicion of an associated graft infection. Non-specific findings include fever, leukocytosis with left shift and elevated inflammation markers [erythrocyte sedimentation rate (ESR), C-reactive protein (CRP)] [11,13–15].

Once the graft is infected, bacterial eradication is rarely possible. The optimal therapeutic option for an infected vascular graft consists of, as a rule, its surgical removal. At surgery an extra-anatomic bypass is established, the graft is removed, and debridement of the infected and necrotic tissue and reperfusion of the surrounding and distal tissue are performed in staged procedures in a single session. Following surgery, antibiotics are administered for a duration that depends on the type of operation that has been performed and the extent of the infection. If surgery cannot be performed, treatment of the infected graft requires prolonged antibiotic coverage guided by blood cultures.

The clinical questions

In patients with suspected vascular graft infection, accurate and early diagnosis is essential. This will further determine the correct choice of treatment, a decision which is of essential clinical significance. A false-positive diagnosis may lead to unnecessary surgery, while failure to diagnose graft infection is associated with high morbidity [5]. The most challenging clinical question in these patients is to distinguish an infected vascular graft from an infected wound in adjacent soft tissues. This differential diagnosis is the most important factor affecting management of this group of patients.

Methodological considerations

Computed tomography (CT) is the most widely used diagnostic modality in patients with suspected vascular graft infection (see Chapter 7). While diagnostic signs for vascular graft infection on CT include the presence of local perigraft fluid retention and air bubbles, these are present in only about 50% of cases. Signs suggesting an infected prosthesis include thickening of the graft wall, adjacent blurred fat and soft tissue swelling. The sensitivity of CT for detection of infected grafts ranges from 85% to 100%. It decreases in low-grade infections when the incidence of false-negative CT studies is relatively high. The quality of CT studies can be impaired by artifacts caused by metallic clips. False-positive results are caused by postsurgical changes with ectopic air encountered for up to 6 weeks following reconstructive surgery in non-infected cases [3]. The presence of an infected wound, hematoma or lymphocelle in the vicinity of the graft may also mask or mimic an infectious process involving the graft on CT [8,16,17].

The role of magnetic resonance imaging (MRI) in the diagnosis of an infected vascular graft is not clearly defined (see Chapter 7). As for CT, changes in tissue density adjacent to implanted grafts can occur in infection as well as in the presence of hematoma, lymph collection or fibrosis, and are difficult to define precisely. Infection in its early stages is responsible for false-negative studies [8,16]. In a limited number of patients with aortic graft infection, the overall sensitivity of MRI was 68%, associated however with a very high overall specificity of 97% [18].

Occasionally, exploratory surgery is required to confirm the diagnosis of graft infection. Intact grafts are well incorporated into the surrounding tissue, covered at times by fibrotic changes. In contrast, infected grafts are free or poorly incorporated and can be surrounded by turbid fluid, air bubbles or pus.

As morphological abnormalities in patients with an infected vascular graft are often non-specific, the use of a functional and/or metabolic imaging approach has been advocated, with the aim of assessing the clinical significance of anatomical findings or enabling early diagnosis preceding the appearance of structural changes. Nuclear medicine procedures have been used for the diagnosis of infection for more than three decades. The most commonly performed procedures using single-photon emission CT (SPECT) agents are bone scintigraphy (for osteomyelitis), gallium-67 citrate (^{67}Ga-citrate), *in vitro* ^{99m}Tc- or ^{111}In-labeled white blood cell (WBC) scintigraphy, and studies performed with ^{99m}Tc-labeled antigranulocyte monoclonal antibody (anti-G mAb) Fab' fragments. Radiotracers, regardless of whether they are for SPECT or ^{18}F-labeled fluorodeoxyglucose ([^{18}F]FDG) for positron emission tomography (PET), are prima-

rily an expression of function and metabolism at the tissue and cellular level.

Scintigraphic images lack anatomical detail and can only define the gross morphopathology. Integrating metabolic and anatomical information using a single hybrid imaging modality, either SPECT/CT or PET/CT, has significantly improved the diagnostic confidence and test accuracy [19,20]. The wide experience gained from the use of PET/CT as well as SPECT/CT in the assessment of cancer and other disorders has demonstrated that hybrid imaging can confirm the presence of disease and its localization to a specific organ or region of the body. This previously gained experience is now being implemented in the search for the optimal diagnostic modality for infection in general and for vascular graft infection in particular.

Normal and pathological findings and significance

SPECT imaging agents and SPECT/CT

Scintigraphy with ^{67}Ga-citrate and labeled WBCs has been used for the assessment of suspected prosthetic graft infection, particularly in the early stages of disease. ^{67}Ga-citrate studies are of limited value in the assessment of vascular graft infection, with a relatively low reported sensitivity, mainly in abdominal grafts that are obscured by physiological uptake in the liver, spleen and bowel [21].

Labeled WBCs (with either ^{99m}Tc or ^{111}In) is the SPECT agent of choice for detection of infected vascular grafts (Figure 14.1). Their accumulation is determined by a number of mechanisms, including diapedesis, chemotaxis and vascular permeability. Both mixed WBCs and granulocytes can be labeled. When mixed WBCs are labeled, they are characterized by a higher blood pool activity, especially in early images, due to the presence of labeled lymphocytes and residual red blood cells. Damage to the WBCs during the labeling procedure can result in leakage of the radioactivity from the cells and adhesion of labeled WBCs to the vascular endothelium. The overall sensitivity of labeled WBCs for the diagnosis of infected grafts ranges between 53% and 100%. Although not described in detail in the literature, false-negative studies may be related to antibiotic treatment or to the duration of symptoms [22]. The specificity reported in the literature ranges between 50% and 100% as well. False-positive

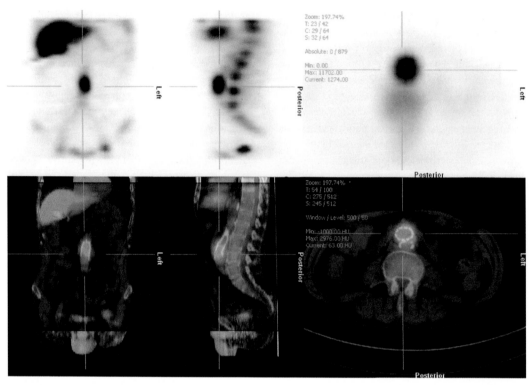

Figure 14.1 SPECT/CT images (SPECT top; fused SPECT/CT, bottom) in a patient with clinical suspicion of an infected aortic graft, 2 hours after IV injection of [99mTc]-HMPAO-labeled WBCs. Coronal (left images), sagittal (middle images) and transaxial sections (right images) show high WBC accumulation within the graft, which is a clear sign of infection.

studies occur in associated conditions such as lymphocelle, hematoma, thrombosis, bleeding and pseudo-aneurysms, as well as due to physiological tracer uptake in recent grafts, less than 1 month after surgery [23].

[111]In-labeled WBC scans have a reported sensitivity ranging between 60% and 100% for the detection of vascular graft infection, depending on its location and time since surgery [18]. A study of 40 patients with suspected infection following abdominal aortic graft insertion compared the performance indices of ^{111}In-labeled WBC scans and MRI. The positive predictive value (PPV) of MRI was higher, 95%, as compared to 80% for ^{111}In-labeled WBCs. The negative predictive value (NPV) of MRI was 80%, which is similar to the 82% for ^{111}In-labeled WBCs, and the authors concluded therefore that MRI should be the primary diagnostic modality in patients with suspected aortic graft infections [18]. A study evaluating the diagnostic value of ^{111}In-labeled WBC scans in 210 patients with sus-

pected infectious processes, involving mainly the musculoskeletal system but including seven patients with suspected graft infection, reported two true positive and five true negative studies for the latter patients, with no cases of erroneous results [24].

In recent years ^{111}In-oxine has been largely replaced by [99mTc]-HMPAO (hexamethylpropylene amine oxime) as the preferred labeling agent in many institutions because of the latter's more favorable physical characteristics, availability, cost and lower radiation burden. SPECT studies performed with [99mTc]-labeled WBCs are of better quality and therefore easier to interpret. Intracellular retention of [99mTc]-HMPAO results from the conversion of a lipophilic into a hydrophilic complex, which further binds to non-diffusible proteins and cell organelles. [99mTc]-labeled WBCs need to be re-injected no later than 1 hour after labeling. The imaging protocol includes scanning at 30 minutes and 2–4 and 24 hours after injection.

[99m]Tc-labeled WBCs have been used successfully for the diagnosis of infected vascular graft with a reported sensitivity and specificity in the range of 82–100% and 75–100%, respectively. Labeled WBC scans have been found to be useful for the detection of vascular graft infection in cases where other imaging modalities showed no characteristic findings. In spite of the high accuracy of WBC scintigraphy, false-positive results have been reported in cases where the infectious process is localized in the vicinity of the graft and therefore can be erroneously interpreted as involving the implant [16,25–28]. False-positive studies can also be caused by cross-labeling of red blood cells and platelets, as well as by increased focal groin uptake of ^{99m}Tc-labeled WBCs due to non-specific perivascular accumulation of granulocytes found early after surgery in non-infected healing wounds or in the healing distal graft anastomosis [29]. Limitations of WBC scintigraphy are related to the time-consuming nature of the technique and the need to handle blood from infected patients [3].

Radiolabeled polyclonal IgG, monoclonal antibodies against granulocyte surface antigens, and leukocyte-avid peptides have the advantages of easy preparation and of availability of easy-to-handle kits. The few published reports that have assessed their role in the diagnosis of graft infection have reported sensitivity and specificity of up to 91% and 100%, respectively [30,31]. A prospective study performed more than 15 years ago evaluated the use of a non-specific protein that accumulates at sites of infection and inflammation, avidin/^{111}In-biotin, for the diagnosis of vascular graft infection. In a study group including 25 patients with 29 grafts, avidin/^{111}In-biotin scintigraphy correctly identified all infected grafts in seven patients, was true negative in 17 patients and false negative in a single infected graft [26]. The main limitations related to the use of these agents are the long imaging time and their slow blood clearance, which can be potentially associated with false-negative studies and thus decreased sensitivity [32].

While the major advantages of nuclear medicine in general, and for assessment of infectious processes in particular, are related to the capability of radiolabeled tracers to define functional or metabolic alterations, a major limitations of these non-invasive tests is the fact that they provide only scarce morphological data. In the absence of precise tomographic landmarks and anatomical details, planar and SPECT procedures are unable to define whether an infectious tracer-avid focus detected on scintigraphy involves a vascular graft. Therefore, both ^{67}Ga-citrate and labeled WBC scans have been used mainly to support a clinically suspected diagnosis of infection, but have not been viewed or used as definitive procedures with respect to impact on patient management.

The ability to integrate functional and morphological information in a single examination with the development of hybrid SPECT/CT imaging devices is of particular value in patients with suspected infection of vascular prostheses [33]. Accurate spatial localization of abnormal foci to a graft or only to the adjacent soft tissues may be impossible unless these highly specific scintigraphic images with low background activity and therefore limited structural information are combined with an anatomical road map (Figure 14.1). Precise alignment of the region of interest during the acquisition of the two components of the SPECT/CT study is crucial to ensure accurate registration and anatomical localization of scintigraphic findings, particularly in the extremities, which are prone to even involuntary patient motion between imaging sequences and which may harbor an infectious process in a structure located very close to several others, as is the case with vascular grafts.

SPECT/CT is a valuable component of labeled WBC imaging in patients with various infectious processes. It contributed significantly to the precise anatomical localization of suspicious foci of increased tracer uptake in a study population of 82 cases, thus enabling the diagnosis of infection and subsequently the precise localization and delineation of its extent in up to half of these patients [33]. This first study assessing the use of SPECT/CT in the evaluation of infection included 24 patients with suspected vascular graft infection scanned with ^{111}In-labeled WBCs. An infected vascular implant was confirmed as the final diagnosis in 10 patients. In one patient, SPECT/CT was false positive misleading with respect to localization of infection involving the vascular graft, which was unconfirmed by further follow-up and clinical outcome. Overall, however, SPECT/CT was more accurate than the combined planar and SPECT study for diagnosis and localization of infection in 63% of patients, providing additional, clinically significant information in 67% of patients with suspected vascular graft infection [33]. A recent study reviewed retrospectively the role of ^{99m}Tc-labeled WBC SPECT/CT in 11 patients with suspected arterial graft infection. Based on clinical outcome, ^{99m}Tc-labeled WBC SPECT/CT studies assessed by visual analysis defined six true positive cases, four true negatives and one false-positive study (in a patient 2 years after insertion of a thoraco-abdominal aortic endograft). Comparing the intensity of ^{99m}Tc-labeled WBC uptake to that of the liver or bone marrow led to slight further improvement in the diagnostic accuracy [34].

[^{18}F]FDG-PET/CT

PET is one of the main non-invasive metabolic imaging modalities. Based on the use of various radiotracers, it provides tomographic imaging data and quantitative parameters of perfusion, cell viability, proliferation and/or metabolic tissue activity. [^{18}F]FDG, at present the most commonly used PET radiopharmaceutical, is an analog of glucose and is taken up by metabolically active cells via glucose transporters and phosphorylated to [^{18}F]2'-FDG-6 phosphate, but not further metabolized. Increased [^{18}F]FDG uptake is related to the metabolic rate of cells involved both in malignant processes and, as repeatedly shown over the last decade, in infectious processes as well. Activated leukocytes, in particular neutrophils, monocytes and macrophages, express high levels of glucose transporters, especially GLUT-1 and -3 [35–38].

[^{18}F]FDG imaging has several advantages over conventional nuclear medicine procedures, mainly labeled WBC scintigraphy. Physiological [^{18}F]FDG background uptake is low, resulting in relatively high target-to-background ratios. Studies are completed within 1–2 hours after tracer administration and there is no need to handle the blood of potentially infected patients.

Increased [^{18}F]FDG uptake may also occur in native vessels. Furthermore, false-positive studies can be due to increased radiotracer activity along implants, grafts and stents, in healing postoperative scars, or in known or unknown malignant disease [39]. These scenarios have to be recognized and differentiated from abnormal [^{18}F]FDG uptake within an infected graft. A pattern of linear [^{18}F]FDG uptake of mild-to-moderate intensity along vascular grafts with no other clinical or laboratory evidence of infection is attributed to a chronic aseptic inflammatory reaction to synthetic grafts, mediated by macrophages, fibroblasts and foreign-body giant cells (Figure 14.2). This occurs more frequently in recently implanted grafts, but has been also described as persisting for years after surgery [46–48]. A focal pattern of intense abnormal [^{18}F] FDG uptake is indicative of the presence of a site of infection (Figure 14.3). The semi-quantitative standardized uptake value (SUV) index has not been validated in infection and therefore it should be used with caution, if at all.

Hyperglycemia has been previously considered as one of the main reasons for false-negative [^{18}F]FDG studies. However, a recent publication has indicated that the false-negative rate in patients assessed for the suspicion of an infectious or inflammatory process is not statistically significantly different between patients with or without diabetes mellitus and with high or normal serum glucose levels at the time of the study [40].

Initial data regarding a potential role of [^{18}F]FDG imaging in the diagnosis of vascular graft infection have been presented as case reports of single patients [41,42]. A single case report has compared the results of CT angiography, [^{18}F]FDG imaging and ^{99m}Tc-labeled WBC imaging in a patient with an aortic graft infection. The only positive test that correctly diagnosed the presence of infection was [^{18}F] FDG-PET [22].

A study that prospectively investigated a heterogenic patient population with suspected bone or soft tissue infection with [^{18}F]FDG and compared this modality with conventional imaging tests; seven patients in this series were assessed for suspected vascular graft infection [43]. Two of these patients were considered as true positives and five as false negatives on [^{18}F]FDG-PET. An additional publication reporting a single-center experience in five patients with suspected prosthetic graft infection demonstrated abnormal [^{18}F]FDG uptake of various intensity in all cases. An infected implant was diagnosed in the three patients with intense tracer uptake [44]. In a study aiming to assess the value of [^{18}F]FDG-PET in 33 patients with suspected aortic graft infection, Fukuchi *et al.* reported that, although the test had a high sensitivity of 91%, the performance of [^{18}F]FDG-PET was hampered by a low specificity of only 64%, as compared to CT

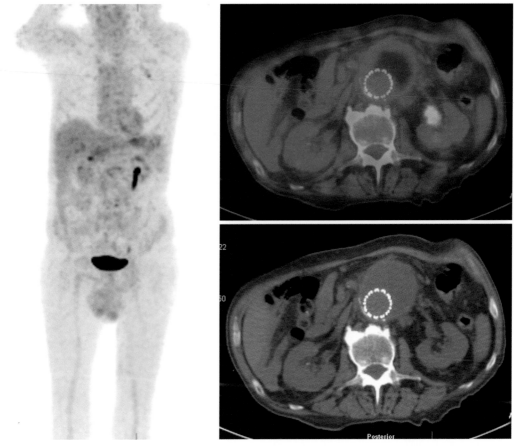

Figure 14.2 [^{18}F]FDG-PET (MIP left; transaxial sections, right) in a patient with an aortic graft. There is a very mild linear uptake of [^{18}F]FDG along the vascular graft (not detectable on the MIP image) with no evidence of infection.

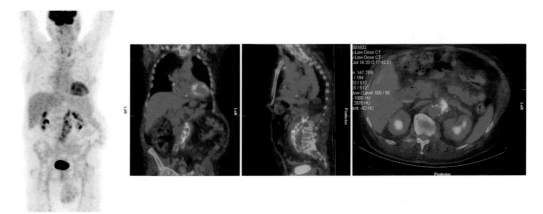

Figure 14.3 [^{18}F]FDG-PET (MIP, coronal, sagittal and transaxial sections, left to right) in a patient with an aortic graft. A focal pattern of intense abnormal [^{18}F]FDG uptake is present and it is indicative of infection.

which had a lower sensitivity of 64% but a specificity of 86% [45].

In spite of its high sensitivity, [^{18}F]FDG-PET is limited in the diagnosis of an infected vascular graft mainly by its lack of ability to precisely define the anatomical localization of increased radiotracer uptake. Correlation of metabolic information provided by [^{18}F]FDG-PET with the anatomical data of CT or MRI is required to accurately localize the site of infection, particularly in cases where the ability to precisely define structures involved by the infectious process can have critical clinical consequences. Visual side-by-side correlation or co-registration of separately performed PET and CT scans of the lower limbs, as would be the case in patients with suspected vascular graft infection, is not accurate enough to localize a focus of increased [^{18}F]FDG uptake to the arterial prosthesis itself or to the surrounding soft tissues. The small size and close proximity of anatomical structures, and the effect of even slight, often involuntary patient motion with positional changes causing misregistration, may lead to inaccurate localization and subsequent false diagnosis [46–48].

Hybrid PET/CT imaging is performed in the same setting on a single device, without changing the patient's position, and allows for correct fusion of the sets of metabolic and anatomical data. Localization of the lesion is facilitated by the concomitant visualization of CT on fused PET/CT images, thus overcoming the limitations of [^{18}F]FDG-PET for the diagnosis of vascular graft infection [46]. On [^{18}F]FDG-PET/CT studies, the presence, intensity and pattern (focal or diffuse) of increased radiotracer activity is defined on the PET component, and the precise localization of the abnormal [^{18}F]FDG foci to the graft or to adjacent soft tissues is determined by using the anatomical map provided by the CT component (Figure 14.2). In patients with a complicated regional anatomy after multiple surgical procedures, PET/CT can also pinpoint the infected implant and differentiate between multiple suspicious findings. In patients with multiple grafts, PET/CT can diagnose or exclude infection involving one or more specific prostheses.

A few case reports provided preliminary evidence suggesting that [^{18}F]FDG-PET/CT can have an incremental value in the assessment of an infected vascular graft [49–51]. In a study aimed at retrospectively assessing the role of [^{18}F]FDG-PET and PET/CT in the diagnosis of patients with fever of unknown origin (FUO), six of seven patients with suspected graft infection had true positive studies, while one case was concluded to be a false positive. Neither true nor false negative studies were found in this limited study group [52]. Keidar et al. prospectively evaluated 39 patients with 69 vascular grafts. The diagnosis of graft infection was confirmed in 15 cases. [^{18}F]FDG-PET/CT was reported as true positive in 14 cases, false negative in one case and false positive in two cases, with a sensitivity, specificity, PPV and NPV of 93%, 91%, 88% and 96%, respectively. Both false-positive results were due to infected hematomas adjacent to the graft and the false-negative study missed involvement of the graft by an infectious soft tissue process located in very close proximity [46]. An additional study assessed 25 patients with clinically suspected vascular prosthetic infection for the incremental value of fused images. The performance of PET/CT was further compared with stand-alone CT. Vascular graft infection was proven in 15 patients by culture. [^{18}F]FDG imaging had a sensitivity of 93%, specificity of 70%, PPV of 82% and NPV of 88% as compared to 56%, 57%, 60% and 58%, respectively, for stand-alone CT [53].

A prospective study assessed the role of [^{18}F]FDG-PET/CT in 76 patients with 96 vascular prosthetic grafts. Evaluated parameters on the PET component included the presence, intensity (graft-to-blood uptake ratio) and pattern (focal or diffuse) of [^{18}F]FDG uptake, and on CT the presence of an anastomotic pseudo-aneurysm and/or of irregular infiltration boundaries. Of all these parameters, only focal [^{18}F]FDG uptake on the PET component and irregular graft boundary on CT were significant predictors of infection (PPV 97%). On the other hand, smooth lesion boundaries with no focal [^{18}F]FDG uptake had a PPV lower than 5%. The overall diagnostic accuracy of [^{18}F]FDG-PET/CT for infection was above 95% in 75% of vascular grafts [54].

Role for therapy follow-up and patient management

The presence of a metabolic response expressed by a decrease or disappearance of abnormal tracer uptake, in particular [^{18}F]FDG, at the site of an infection process may indicate clinical response and guide duration of antimicrobial therapy [55]. There are only scarce and non-structured data regarding the specific use of [^{18}F]FDG imaging in the follow-up of patients with infection and for monitoring response to treatment, and in particular in the follow-up of patients with vascular graft infection, with some evidence suggesting that metabolic response to antimicrobial or anti-inflammatory therapy may indicate further clinical response [35]. While some authors have described a normalization of the [^{18}F]FDG activity after successful treatment of various infectious processes [56], others have shown that [^{18}F]FDG imaging does not effectively identify residual active infection post therapy [57]. Based on current information from meager peer-reviewed literature, [^{18}F]FDG imaging cannot be recommended for monitoring response to treatment in patients with infectious processes and, specifically, in patients with infected vascular grafts. Furthermore, it has been demonstrated that conservative treatment of vascular graft infection consisting of intensive antibiotic therapy is associated with high mortality with a 54% 5-year survival rate, and is considered only in highly compromised patients who cannot tolerate extensive surgery or in those patients with grafts in difficult to access locations that are therefore impossible to excise [1]. This therapeutic option, and thus the need for monitoring response, is limited only to a specific subgroup of patients at high risk for undergoing major surgery [58]. In the majority of patients, removal of the infected graft is the treatment modality of choice for cure and in this clinical setting the need for serial [^{18}F]FDG-PET/CT studies appears to be of less value.

Conclusion

Surgical removal of an infected vascular graft is the most successful treatment option in this group of patients. This justifies the high clinical significance of accurate diagnosis of involvement of the prosthesis by an infectious process. False-positive results may lead to unnecessary major surgery, while false-negative results that fail to diagnose graft infection are related to high morbidity. Combining the anatomical landmarks provided by CT with the presence of functional changes on SPECT or increased metabolism on PET has improved significantly the specificity and diagnostic accuracy of these non-invasive imaging modalities. Specifically, the decrease in the false-positive rate has made precise non-invasive diagnosis of vascular graft infection a reality [59]. Well-controlled studies including large numbers of patients are needed to confirm and further validate the diagnostic performance of SPECT/CT and PET/CT, as well as their role in the management of patients who confront the vascular surgeon with the clinical dilemma of vascular graft infections in general, and their specific challenging scenarios in particular.

References

1. Saleem BR, Meerwaldt R, Tielliu IF, Verhoeven EL, van den Dungen JJ, Zeebregts CJ. Conservative treatment of vascular prosthetic graft infection is associated with high mortality. *Am J Surg* 2010;200:47–52.
2. Stewart AH, Eyers PS, Earnshaw JJ. Prevention of infection in peripheral arterial reconstruction: a systematic review and meta-analysis. *J Vasc Surg* 2007; 46:148–155.
3. Seeger JM. Management of patients with prosthetic vascular graft infection. *Am Surg* 2000;66:166–177.
4. Bandyk DF, Esses GE. Prosthetic graft infection. *Surg Clin North Am* 1994;74:571–590.
5. Bandyk DF. Infection in prosthetic vascular grafts. In: Ratherford RB (ed). *Vascular Surgery*. Philadelphia: WB Saunders, 2005, pp. 875–894.
6. Goldstone J, Moore WS. Infection in vascular prostheses. Clinical manifestations and surgical management. *Am J Surg* 1974;128:225–233.
7. Hallett JW Jr, Marshall DM, Petterson TM *et al.* Graft-related complications after abdominal aortic aneurysm repair: reassurance from a 36-year population-based experience. *J Vasc Surg* 1997;25: 277–284; discussion 285–286.
8. Orton DF, LeVeen RF, Saigh JA *et al.* Aortic prosthetic graft infections: radiologic manifestations and implications for management. *RadioGraphics* 2000;20: 977–993.
9. Vogel TR, Symons R, Flum DR. The incidence and factors associated with graft infection after aortic aneurysm repair. *J Vasc Surg* 2008;47:264–269.
10. Chang JK, Calligaro KD, Ryan S, Runyan D, Dougherty MJ, Stern JJ. Risk factors associated with infection of lower extremity revascularization: analysis of 365 procedures performed at a teaching hospital. *Ann Vasc Surg* 2003;17:91–96.
11. Kolakowski S, Jr. Dougherty MJ, Calligaro KD. Does the timing of reoperation influence the risk of graft infection? *J Vasc Surg* 2007;45:60–64.

12. Szilagyi DE, Smith RF, Elliott JP, Vrandecic MP. Infection in arterial reconstruction with synthetic grafts. *Ann Surg* 1972;176:321–333.

13. Calligaro KD, Veith FJ, Schwartz ML, Savarese RP, DeLaurentis DA. Are gram-negative bacteria a contraindication to selective preservation of infected prosthetic arterial grafts? *J Vasc Surg* 1992;16: 337–345; discussion 345–346.

14. Malone JM, Moore WS, Campagna G, Bean B. Bacteremic infectability of vascular grafts: the influence of pseudointimal integrity and duration of graft function. *Surgery* 1975;78:211–226.

15. Yashar JJ, Weyman AK, Burnard RJ, Yashar J. Survival and limb salvage in patients with infected arterial prostheses. *Am J Surg* 1978;135:499–504.

16. Seabold JE. Imaging of vascular graft infection. In: Murray EP (ed). *Nuclear Medicine in Clinical Diagnosis and Treatment.* Edinburgh: Churchill Livingstone, 1999.

17. Seabold JE, Nepola JV. Imaging techniques for evaluation of postoperative orthopedic infections. *Q J Nucl Med* 1999;43:21–28.

18. Shahidi S, Eskil A, Lundof E, Klaerke A, Jensen BS. Detection of abdominal aortic graft infection: comparison of magnetic resonance imaging and indium-labeled white blood cell scanning. *Ann Vasc Surg* 2007;21:586–592.

19. Bar-Shalom R, Yefremov N, Guralnik L *et al.* Clinical performance of PET/CT in evaluation of cancer: additional value for diagnostic imaging and patient management. *J Nucl Med* 2003;44:1200–1209.

20. Keidar Z, Israel O, Krausz Y. SPECT/CT in tumor imaging: technical aspects and clinical applications. *Semin Nucl Med* 2003;33:205–218.

21. Reyes E, Underwood SR. Nuclear imaging in cardiovascular infection and cardiac transplant rejection. In: Murray EP, Ell PJ (eds). *Nuclear Medicine in Clinical Diagnosis and Treatment.* Edinburgh: Churchill Livingstone, 2004.

22. Gardet E, Addas R, Monteil J, Le Guyader A. Comparison of detection of F-18 fluorodeoxyglucose positron emission tomography and ^{99m}Tc-hexamethylpropylene amine oxime labelled leukocyte scintigraphy for an aortic graft infection. *Interact Cardiovasc Thorac Surg* 2010;10:1423.

23. Palestro CJ, Love C, Bhargava KK. Labeled leukocyte imaging: current status and future directions. *Q J Nucl Med Mol Imaging* 2009;53:105–123.

24. Wanahita A, Villeda C, Kutka N, Ramirez J, Musher D. Diagnostic sensitivity and specificity of the radionuclide (indium)-labeled leukocyte scan. *J Infect* 2007;55:214–219.

25. Liberatore M, Iurilli AP, Ponzo F *et al.* Clinical usefulness of technetium-99m-HMPAO-labeled leukocyte scan in prosthetic vascular graft infection. *J Nucl Med* 1998;39:875–879.

26. Samuel A, Paganelli G, Chiesa R *et al.* Detection of prosthetic vascular graft infection using avidin/indium-111-biotin scintigraphy. *J Nucl Med* 1996;37: 55–61.

27. Williamson MR, Boyd CM, Read RC *et al.* 111 In-labeled leukocytes in the detection of prosthetic vascular graft infections. *AJR Am J Roentgenol* 1986; 147:173–176.

28. Palestro CJ, Torres MA. Radionuclide imaging of nonosseous infection. *Q J Nucl Med* 1999;43:46–60.

29. Chung CJ, Wilson AA, Melton JW, Hartley WS, Allen DM. Uptake of In-111 labeled leukocytes by lymphocele. A cause of false-positive vascular graft infection. *Clin Nucl Med* 1992;17:368–370.

30. LaMuraglia GM, Fischman AJ, Strauss HW *et al.* Utility of the indium 111-labeled human immunoglobulin G scan for the detection of focal vascular graft infection. *J Vasc Surg* 1989;10:20–27; discussion 27–28.

31. Palestro CJ, Weiland FL, Seabold JE *et al.* Localizing infection with a technetium-99m-labeled peptide: initial results. *Nucl Med Commun* 2001;22:695–701.

32. Petruzzi N, Shanthly N, Thakur M. Recent trends in soft-tissue infection imaging. *Semin Nucl Med* 2009; 39:115–123.

33. Bar-Shalom R, Yefremov N, Guralnik L *et al.* SPECT/CT using ^{67}Ga and ^{111}In-labeled leukocyte scintigraphy for diagnosis of infection. *J Nucl Med* 2006; 47:587–594.

34. Lou L, Alibhai KN, Winkelaar GB *et al.* ^{99m}Tc-WBC scintigraphy with SPECT/CT in the evaluation of arterial graft infection. *Nucl Med Commun* 2010; 31:411–416.

35. Vos FJ, Bleeker-Rovers CP, Corstens FH, Kullberg BJ, Oyen WJ. FDG-PET for imaging of non-osseous infection and inflammation. *Q J Nucl Med Mol Imaging* 2006;50:121–130.

36. Bleeker-Rovers CP, Vos FJ, Corstens FH, Oyen WJ. Imaging of infectious diseases using [(18)F]fluorodeoxyglucose PET. *Q J Nucl Med Mol Imaging* 2008; 52:17–29.

37. De Winter F, Vogelaers D, Gemmel F, Dierckx RA. Promising role of 18-F-fluoro-D-deoxyglucose positron emission tomography in clinical infectious diseases. *Eur J Clin Microbiol Infect Dis* 2002;21:247–257.

38. Rennen HJ, Corstens FH, Oyen WJ, Boerman OC. New concepts in infection/inflammation imaging. *Q J Nucl Med* 2001;45:167–173.

39. Wasselius J, Malmstedt J, Kalin B *et al.* High ^{18}F-FDG uptake in synthetic aortic vascular grafts on PET/CT in symptomatic and asymptomatic patients. *J Nucl Med* 2008;49:1601–1605.

40. Rabkin Z, Israel O, Keidar Z. Do hyperglycemia and diabetes affect the incidence of false-negative ^{18}F-FDG PET/CT studies in patients evaluated for infection or inflammation and cancer? A comparative analysis. *J Nucl Med* 2010;51:1015–1020.

41. Tsunekawa T, Ogino H, Minatoya K, Matsuda H, Sasaki H, Fukuchi K. Masked prosthetic graft to sigmoid colon fistula diagnosed by 18-fluorodeoxyglucose positron emission tomography. *Eur J Vasc Endovasc Surg* 2007;33:187–189.

42. Krupnick AS, Lombardi JV, Engels FH *et al*. 18-fluorodeoxyglucose positron emission tomography as a novel imaging tool for the diagnosis of aortoenteric fistula and aortic graft infection – a case report. *Vasc Endovascular Surg* 2003;37:363–366.

43. Stumpe KD, Dazzi H, Schaffner A, von Schulthess GK. Infection imaging using whole-body FDG-PET. *Eur J Nucl Med* 2000;27:822–832.

44. Lauwers P, Van den Broeck S, Carp L, Hendriks J, Van Schil P, Blockx P. The use of positron emission tomography with (18)F-fluorodeoxyglucose for the diagnosis of vascular graft infection. *Angiology* 2007; 58:717–724.

45. Fukuchi K, Ishida Y, Higashi M *et al*. Detection of aortic graft infection by fluorodeoxyglucose positron emission tomography: comparison with computed tomographic findings. *J Vasc Surg* 2005;42:919–925.

46. Keidar Z, Engel A, Hoffman A, Israel O, Nitecki S. Prosthetic vascular graft infection: the role of ^{18}F-FDG PET/CT. *J Nucl Med* 2007;48:1230–1236.

47. Duet M, Laissy JP, Paulmier B *et al*. Inflammatory F-18 fluorodeoxyglucose uptake over arterial bypass prosthesis seen on positron emission tomography can predict acute vascular events. *J Nucl Cardiol* 2006; 13:876–879.

48. Cook GJ, Fogelman I, Maisey MN. Normal physiological and benign pathological variants of 18-fluoro-2-deoxyglucose positron-emission tomography scanning: potential for error in interpretation. *Semin Nucl Med* 1996;26:308–314.

49. Stadler P, Bilohlávek O, Spacek M, Michálek P. Diagnosis of vascular prosthesis infection with FDG-PET/CT. *J Vasc Surg* 2004;40:1246–1247.

50. Keidar Z, Engel A, Nitecki S, Bar Shalom R, Hoffman A, Israel O. PET/CT using 2-deoxy-2-[^{18}F]fluoro-D-glucose for the evaluation of suspected infected vascular graft. *Mol Imaging Biol* 2003;5:23–25.

51. Tegler G, Sörensen J, Björck M, Savitcheva I, Wanhainen A. Detection of aortic graft infection by 18-fluorodeoxyglucose positron emission tomography combined with computed tomography. *J Vasc Surg* 2007;45:828–830.

52. Jaruskova M, Belohlavek O. Role of FDG-PET and PET/CT in the diagnosis of prolonged febrile states. *Eur J Nucl Med Mol Imaging* 2006;33: 913–918.

53. Bruggink JL, Glaudemans AW, Saleem BR. Accuracy of FDG-PET-CT in the diagnostic work-up of vascular prosthetic graft infection. *Eur J Vasc Endovasc Surg* 2010;40:348–354.

54. Spacek M, Belohlavek O, Votrubova J, Sebesta P, Stadler P. Diagnostics of "non-acute" vascular prosthesis infection using ^{18}F-FDG PET/CT: our experience with 96 prostheses. *Eur J Nucl Med Mol Imaging* 2009;36:850–858.

55. Hofmeyr A, Lau WF, Slavin MA. *Mycobacterium tuberculosis* infection in patients with cancer, the role of 18-fluorodeoxyglucose positron emission tomography for diagnosis and monitoring treatment response. *Tuberculosis (Edinb)* 2007;87:459–463.

56. Bleeker-Rovers CP, de Sevaux RG, van Hamersvelt HW, Corstens FH, Oyen WJ. Diagnosis of renal and hepatic cyst infections by 18-F-fluorodeoxyglucose positron emission tomography in autosomal dominant polycystic kidney disease. *Am J Kidney Dis* 2003;41:E18–21.

57. Reuter S, Buck A, Manfras B *et al*. Structured treatment interruption in patients with alveolar echinococcosis. *Hepatology* 2004;39:509–517.

58. Saleem BR, Meerwaldt R, Tielliu IFJ *et al*. Conservative treatment of vascular prosthetic graft infection is associated with high mortality. *Am J Surg* 2010;200: 47–52.

59. Burroni L, D'Alessandria C, Signore A. Diagnosis of vascular prosthesis infection: PET or SPECT? *J Nucl Med* 2007;48:1227–1229.

Clinical cases

Case 1

A 78-year-old woman, who 9 years ago underwent aorto-bifemoral bypass, was referred for [^{18}F]FDG-PET/CT assessment of a solitary lung nodule.

Coronal PET slices demonstrated the presence of diffuse [^{18}F]FDG uptake of mild intensity along the vascular graft. This is consistent with a sterile inflammatory foreign body reaction (Figure 14.4). There was no evidence of vascular graft infection over a follow-up of 48 months.

Teaching point

To evaluate for the presence of an infected vascular graft, the extent, pattern and intensity of [^{18}F]FDG uptake must be taken into consideration.

Case 2

A 65-year-old male who had had synthetic aorto-bifemoral and bilateral femoro-popliteal grafts inserted 6 years prior to the current investigation. Four years later, revision and thrombectomy of the right implant had been necessary.

[^{18}F]FDG-PET/CT was performed for the suspicion of vascular graft infection because of fever and a pus-secreting wound in the right groin (Figure 14.5). On the multislice projection (MIP) PET image (Figure 14.5A) there is an area of intense linear uptake along the right lower limb, from the inguinal region up to the right knee (the area of the lower graft anastomosis). The transaxial PET/CT slice (Figure 14.5B) at the level of the upper thigh demonstrates (arrow) the presence of highly intense focal [^{18}F]FDG uptake involving the right femoro-popliteal graft surrounded by a hypodense mass seen on the CT component (Figure 14.5C), which is consistent with an infectious process involving the implant. The distal tip of both the right and left aorto-bifemoral prostheses is seen in the medial aspect of the thighs on the CT component (arrowheads) with no evidence of increased [^{18}F]FDG uptake or structural abnormalities.

The patient was referred to surgery 2 weeks later. Infection of the right femoro-popliteal graft was confirmed and the implant was removed.

Teaching point

This case highlights the importance of looking at CT images in order to correctly identify the site of [^{18}F]FDG uptake.

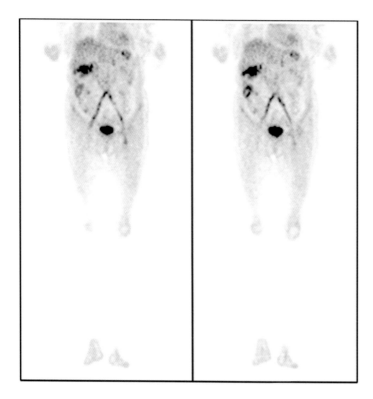

Figure 14.4 Coronal PET images showing diffuse mild [^{18}F]FDG uptake along the aorto-bi-iliac vascular graft, consistent with a sterile inflammatory foreign body reaction.

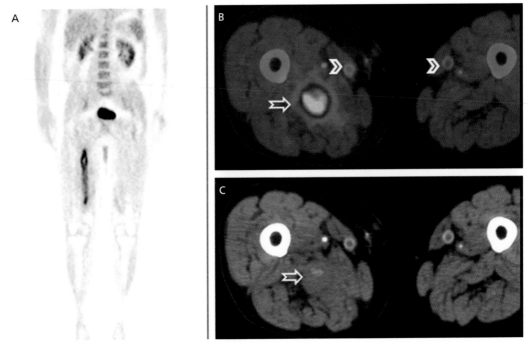

Figure 14.5 FDG-PET/CT. (A) MIP image showing intense linear uptake along the right lower limb. (B) Transaxial PET/CT images localized the pathological [^{18}F]FDG uptake to the femoro-popliteal graft (arrow) surrounded by a hypodense mass seen on the CT (C) consistent with an infection. No [^{18}F]FDG uptake can be seen at the distal tip of both the right and left aorto-bifemoral prostheses (arrowheads).

Case 3

A 53-year-old male patient who had synthetic right ilio-femoral and femoro-popliteal grafts inserted 6 months prior to the current investigation. He was referred with the suspicion of graft infection following complaints of pain in the right limb, fever and a pus-secreting surgical wound at the level of the distal thigh.

A MIP-PET image shows linear, moderately increased [^{18}F]FDG uptake along the right lower limb, with high intensity foci (Figure 14.6A).

PET/CT and CT slices at the level of the inguinal region (Figure 14.6B, left column) show an area of inhomogenous highly intense [^{18}F]FDG uptake in a soft tissue mass surrounding the surgical clips (thin arrows) and the distal portion of the ilio-femoral and proximal tip of the femoro-popliteal implants (open arrow). PET/CT and CT slices at the level of the distal thigh (Figure 14.6B, middle column) show an area of intense [^{18}F]FDG uptake involving the femoro-popliteal graft (open arrow). At the level of the upper calf (Figure 14.6B, right column) an area of high intensity irregular abnormal [^{18}F]FDG uptake in the medial aspect of the soft tissue with postsurgical changes as demonstrated on the CT component (thin arrow) spares the distal tip of the femoro-popliteal graft (arrowhead).

These findings are consistent with an extensive infectious process involving both vascular grafts in the right lower limb and adjacent soft tissues in the inguinal, distal thigh and proximal calf.

Intravenous antibiotic therapy was instituted and the patient was referred for surgical removal of the infected grafts.

Teaching point

This case highlights the importance of looking at CT images in order to correctly identify the site of [^{18}F]FDG uptake.

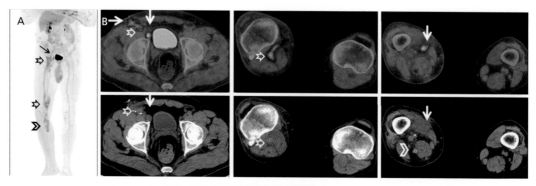

Figure 14.6 (A) MIP-PET image showing a linear, moderately increased [^{18}F]FDG uptake along the right lower limb, with high intensity foci. (B) Coronal PET/CT slices at the level of (right to left) the inguinal region, distal thigh and upper calf, showing areas of highly intense [^{18}F]FDG uptake in soft tissues (thin arrows) and the femoro-popliteal graft (open arrows).

CHAPTER 15

Nuclear Medicine Imaging of Tuberculosis and Human Immunodeficiency Virus

Mike Sathekge[1], Christophe Van de Wiele[2] and Alberto Signore[3]

[1]*University of Pretoria and Steve Biko Academic Hospital, Pretoria, South Africa*
[2]*University Hospital Ghent, Ghent, Belgium*
[3]*"Sapienza" University, Rome, Italy*

Introduction

Acquired immunodeficiency syndrome (AIDS) is a set of symptoms and infections resulting from damage to the human immune system caused by the human immunodeficiency lentivirus-1 (HIV-1) [1]. Globally, it was estimated that in 2007 33.2 million (estimate range, 30.6–36.1 million) people were living with HIV infection or AIDS, an increase from 29.5 million in 2001 [2]. Tuberculosis (TB) is the most serious and most common opportunistic infection, and the most common cause of death in HIV patients [1,2] (Figure 15.1).

Globally, a significant challenge to achieving universal access to HIV prevention, treatment, care and support is the optimization of imaging. In this regard, nuclear medicine with both positron emission tomography (PET) and single-photon emission computed tomography (SPECT) is an integral part of infection imaging. More recent developments rely on PET with [18F]fluorodeoxyglucose ([18F]FDG), a radiopharmaceutical that shows increased (though non-specific) accumulation at sites of abnormally enhanced metabolism (such as tumors or infection). In the case of HIV and TB, gallium-67 (^{67}Ga) imaging offers many practical advantages over indium-111 (^{111}In-oxine)- or technetium-

99m-hexamethylpropylene amine oxime (^{99m}Tc-HMPAO)-labeled white blood cell (WBC; leukocyte) imaging. For example, no cell labeling is required and it can be used in patients with few or no functional white cells. Also, in the case of infection imaging, the highest clinical benefit is achieved by relying on tomographic imaging (SPECT or PET), preferably with hybrid image fusion analysis (SPECT/CT or PET/CT).

Basic knowledge of the clinical problem

HIV primarily infects and kills helper T cells (CD4+ T cells), macrophages and dendritic cells [3]. When CD4+ T-cell numbers decline below a critical level, cell-mediated immunity is lost and the body becomes progressively more susceptible to opportunistic infections as well as malignancies. Initially, as the CD4+ count declines, infections that occur in the general population become more common in HIV-positive patients. For instance, bacterial infections such as *Salmonella*, *Shigella*, *Corynebacterium* and *Mycobacterium tuberculosis* occur with increased frequency when CD4+ counts are 200–500 cells/mm^3 [4]. Only once there is profound impairment of the immune system, with CD4+ counts below

Diagnostic Imaging of Infections and Inflammatory Diseases: A Multidisciplinary Approach, First Edition. Edited by Alberto Signore and Ana María Quintero.

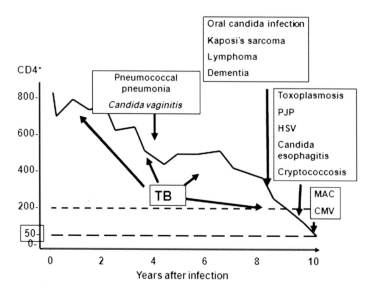

Figure 15.1 Opportunistic diseases in the course of HIV infection. CMV, cytomegalovirus; HSV, herpes simplex virus; MAC, *Mycobacterium avium-intracellulare* complex; PJP, *Pneumococcus jirovecii* pneumonia.

200 cells/mm³, do opportunistic infections that are rarely seen in the general population occur. The presentation of TB is different from that observed in HIV-negative patients, particularly if the CD4+ count is less than 200 cells/mm³: apical predominance is less pronounced, while consolidation, cavitations and hematogenic disseminations are less prevalent [4,5].

Cryptosporidiosis and *Pneumocystis jirovecii* (formerly *P. carinii*) almost always occur when the CD4+ count is less than 200 cells/mm³. *P. jirovecii* is a fungus that causes opportunistic infection, such as pneumonia, in patients with AIDS and other causes of impaired immunity. *P. jirovecii* pneumonia (PJP) continues to be a devastating AIDS-defining illness in HIV-positive patients [6].

Cytomegalovirus (CMV), lymphocytic interstitial pneumonitis (LIP) and atypical mycobacterial infections, such as *Mycobacterium avium–intracellulare* complex (MAC), almost always occur when the CD4+ count is less than 60 cells/mm³ [7]. CMV pneumonia is the third most common finding after pyogenic pneumonia and PJP in patients who are HIV infected. Infections vary from mild to fatal necrotizing CMV pneumonia. Co-infection with pneumocystis is commonly described [8]. The prevalence of CMV pneumonitis is difficult to establish because a positive culture does not distinguish between CMV colonization and invasive infection.

The etiology of LIP is unclear. Typical LIP manifestations are a non-productive cough and mild hypoxemia, together with generalized lymphadenopathy and finger clubbing [6]. LIP may also be associated with painless, bilateral parotid gland enlargement. Although LIP is not confined to HIV-infected children, it is uncommon in HIV-infected adults and rare in HIV-uninfected individuals. Definitive diagnosis of LIP requires lung biopsy.

Malignancies seen in the AIDS setting include HIV-associated lymphoma due to Epstein-Barr virus (EBV), Kaposi's sarcoma (KS) due to KS-associated herpes virus (KSHV) and anogenital cancer due to human papillomavirus (HPV) [9]. While until recently it was assumed that HIV-1 infection plays a passive role in cancer development by impairing the host immune surveillance and increasing the risk of oncogenic virus infection, recent experimental evidence has shown that HIV-1-encoded proteins can directly induce tumor angiogenesis and enhance KSHV transmission to target cells [10]. In addition, clinical evidence suggests that the oncogenicity of HPV is altered by the presence of HIV-1 infection irrespective of the host immune status, and the impact of highly active antiretroviral treatment (HAART) is variable in EBV-related lymphoma and HPV-related cervical cancer, suggesting that additional factors are involved in the pathogenesis of these cancers.

The late stages of severe AIDS render the nervous system susceptible to an array of neurological disorders and at least 40% of HIV-infected patients develop neurological symptoms during the course of their illness. Virtually every component of the nervous system can be afflicted and these neurological disorders cause considerable morbidity and mortality. The neurological problems that occur in HIV-infected individuals may be either primary to the pathogenic processes of HIV infection or secondary to opportunistic infections or neoplasms [11].

The commonest central nervous system (CNS) manifestation of toxoplasma is toxoplasma encephalitis. This presents as focal necrotizing encephalitis with one or more intracerebral mass lesions. Nearly 90% of patients who develop toxoplasma encephalitis have fewer than 200 CD4+ T cells/µL [12,13]. The most common causes of focal brain lesions in patients with AIDS are toxoplasmosis (50%), primary CNS lymphoma (30%) and progressive multifocal leukoencephalopathy (20%) [14].

The most common CNS manifestation of HIV is a chronic neurodegenerative condition characterized by cognitive, central motor and behavioral abnormalities. A variety of names have been given to this syndrome, e.g. AIDS dementia complex, HIV-associated dementia, HIV-associated cognitive motor complex. Recently, HIV-associated neurocognitive disorder (HAND) [15] has become a widely accepted nosology for classifying individuals with varying levels of HIV-associated neurocognitive deficit. HAND is stratified into asymptomatic neurocognitive impairment (ANI), minor neurocognitive disorder (MND) and HIV-associated dementia (HAD). ANI is characterized as a subclinical decline in cognition; MND as a mild decline in cognition in addition to mild impairment in everyday function that affects the more difficult activities of daily living; and HAD by significant decline in cognition along with a significant degree of functional impairment that affects routine activities [16].

The clinical questions

Tuberculosis

In HIV/AIDS and TB infection, early identification and diagnosis of active TB is the key to effective control of the disease [17]. Globally, TB continues to be one of the leading infectious causes of morbidity and mortality, accounting for an estimated 9 million cases and 2 million deaths per year [18].

The effect of the dual HIV and TB epidemics is felt most acutely in developing countries, with recent estimates of dual infection rising rapidly. HIV-infected patients are at a 20-fold increased risk of contracting TB when compared with HIV-non-infected peers [18,19]. Therefore, there is an increasing clinical need for effective imaging for:
• Early identification and diagnosis of TB (key to effective control of the disease);
• Correct identification of extrapulmonary TB and staging of TB (crucially important in order to start anti-TB treatment and coordinate this with antiretroviral treatment for HIV);
• Complement atypical presentation of TB in the HIV-infected patient which is different from that observed in the HIV-negative patient (see above);
• Follow-up of TB patients [in developing countries, multidrug resistant (MDR) and extensively drug resistant (XDR) TB are of serious consequence and thus monitoring of therapy is essential];
• Differentiation between malignancies and TB, which is particularly important for solitary pulmonary nodules (SPNs) (Figure 15.2).

Generalized adenopathy

Available data suggest that HIV binding to resting CD4+ T lymphocytes causes them to home from the blood into lymph nodes, during which process they are induced into apoptosis by secondary signals through the homing receptors [20]. The clinical correlate of this pathophysiological process is peripheral generalized lymphadenopathy with characteristic lymph node morphology that precedes tissue involution and ultimately results in loss of superficial lymph nodes in the later stage of disease [21]. Imaging helps with determining the association between the clinical stage of HIV infection and the pattern of lymphoid tissue activation.

Monitoring the side effects of HAART

A chronic and progressive syndrome of lipodystrophy (peripheral fat loss and/or abdominal obesity) and hyperlipidemia has been reported in up to 60–80% of patients treated with HAART [22, 23]. Hyperinsulinemia, increased C-reactive peptide (CRP) concentration, insulin resistance and impaired glucose tolerance have been frequently observed. In lipodystrophic HIV patients, the available data support the hypothesis that stavudine-related lipodystrophy is associated with increased

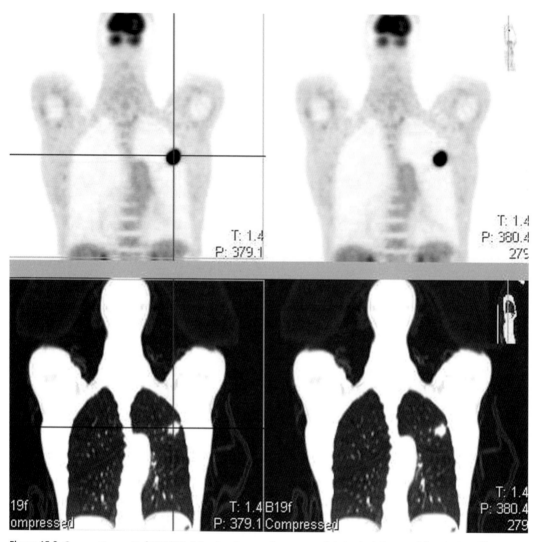

Figure 15.2 Consecutive sagittal PET/CT slides showing a pulmonary nodule in the left upper lobe which is [¹⁸F]FDG avid on double-phase imaging. These features are indistinguishable for malignancy and TB; this patient was proven to have TB.

glucose uptake by adipose tissue as a result of the metabolic stress of adipose tissue in response to HAART. Hence, there is a need for the objective monitoring of the lipodystrophy-inducing effect of newly developed antiretroviral regimens.

Lymphoma

Patients with HIV-1 are at risk for lymphoma, making the differential diagnosis between benign and malignant lymphadenopathy imperative. More specifically, while the implementation of HAART

has resulted in a significant decrease in the incidence of AIDS-defining cancers, the incidence of non-AIDS-defining cancers (NADCs), in particular lung cancer, lymphoma, prostate cancer and skin cancer, has increased, as has the proportion of mortality associated with NADCs in HIV-infected patients [24,25]. The clinical problem is the avoidance of false-positive attribution of [¹⁸F]FDG uptake by lymph nodes to malignant involvement in HIV-positive patients presenting with primary tumors or lymphoma (thus the viral load should be zero).

Brain lymphoma

Primary CNS lymphoma is the second most common mass lesion (after toxoplasmosis) in patients with AIDS, occurring in up to 5% of these patients, although a definite decline in the incidence of HIV-associated CNS lymphoma has occurred in the post-HAART era. This lymphoma is typically of B-cell origin. Almost 100% of affected patients exhibit evidence of EBV in the lymphomatous lesions and the cerebrospinal fluid (CSF) [26]. EBV transformation of chronically activated B cells is probably responsible for lymphoma development. Development of this opportunistic neoplasm is associated with CD4+ lymphocyte counts of less than 100 cells/mm³. The distinction between primary CNS lymphoma and non-malignant lesions due to opportunistic infections, in particular cerebral toxoplasmosis, is important as their treatment is different. Cerebral toxoplasmosis can be effectively treated with medication, whereas primary CNS lymphomas are treated with radiation therapy and corticosteroids. Neither CT nor magnetic resonance imaging (MRI) can reliably distinguish CNS infections such as toxoplasmosis from lymphoma in HIV-1-positive patients.

HIV-associated neurocognitive disorder

Clinically, HAND, formerly AIDS dementia complex, is a subcortical dementia that is characterized by disturbances in cognition, motor performance and behavior. Diagnosis of early HAND is important as many of its symptoms can be caused by other conditions common to people with HIV/AIDS, many of which may be treatable [27]. There is no diagnostic marker or combination of markers for HAND. The diagnosis is made in HIV-positive patients with cognitive impairment after ruling out confounding conditions (CNS opportunistic infections, neurosyphilis, substance abuse, delirium, toxic-metabolic disorders, psychiatric disease, age-related dementias). An essential feature in the diagnosis of HAND is the presence of well-documented cognitive decline and the exclusion of other neurological complications of HIV infection, such as cerebral toxoplasmosis, cryptococcal meningitis, lymphoma and progressive multifocal leukoencephalopathy, conditions that are characterized by focal or heterogeneous [18F]FDG uptake as opposed to the striatal symmetrical hypermetabolism observed in early HAND [28]. Therefore, cerebrospinal fluid (CSF)

examination and imaging studies of the brain are mandatory. CSF analysis should exclude infectious agents other than HIV. CT and MRI changes are only seen with far advanced AIDS dementia when structural changes have occurred. Once the diagnosis of early HAND is established, treatment and management can be optimized.

Pulmonary complications other than tuberculosis

Pulmonary complications are often the initial clinical manifestation of HIV infection. The evaluation of respiratory symptoms in HIV-infected patients can be challenging for a number of reasons. Respiratory symptoms are a frequent complaint among HIV-infected individuals and may be caused by a wide spectrum of illnesses, both HIV-associated and non-HIV-associated conditions. The former include both opportunistic infections and neoplasms. In most situations, there can be considerable variation and overlap in these presentations. Therefore, no constellation of symptoms, physical examination findings, laboratory abnormalities and imaging findings is pathognomonic or specific for a particular disease. Despite a growing knowledge base on PJP, CMV, MAC and Kaposi's sarcoma, their diagnosis continues to be challenging.

The gastrointestinal tract

Most patients with AIDS will have symptoms of gastrointestinal luminal tract disease at some point during their illness. HIV-related disorders may affect all structures from the mouth to the anus. Oral and esophageal lesions, hepatobiliary disorders and diarrhea are the most common [6]. The diagnosis of clinical AIDS is often made by identifying an opportunistic infection or malignant neoplasm of the gastrointestinal tract. Oral and esophageal candidiasis is the most common fungal infection in AIDS patients and dysphagia may be the initial presentation of AIDS [29]. While clinical manifestations of involvement of these organs are protean and usually non-specific, it is important to establish a specific diagnosis promptly in these often critically ill patients. Usually upper gastrointestinal series and endoscopy are adequate diagnostic tools.

Methodological considerations

Patients should be fasted for a minimum of 4 hours before the [18F]FDG-PET/CT whole-body scan. The

[^{18}F]FDG should be administered intravenously using the formula [(body weight/10) + 1)] × 37 MBq. Between injection and scanning (at least 45 minutes), patients must be asked to remain still, covered with a blanket and placed in an environment without auditory stimuli to avoid uptake of the radiotracer at physiological sites excited by these stimuli, which can result in artifacts that have false-positive interpretations. During this activation phase, patients will be instructed to drink 1 L of contrast material (barium diluted in water).

The images should be acquired in a three-dimensional mode using PET/CT. Sixty minutes (or 60 and 120 minutes in dual phase) after injection, the first whole-body scan, with a 3-minute emission scan for each of nine bed positions, should be done from the skull base to the pelvis. Patients must not move while on the scanning table.

Images are usually reconstructed with and without attenuation correction (CT-based) using OSEM (ordered subset expectation maximization) and yield axial, sagittal and coronal slices.

The semi-quantitative analysis of the degree of uptake of the lesions characterized by the FDG-PET/CT scans is commonly based on the standard uptake value (SUV). The SUV represents the activity of the radiotracer in a topographic region of the body image or volume of interest normalized to the weight of the patient and to the quantity of radiotracer administered; hence the formula: SUV = radiotracer activity × weight of the patient/injected dose. This characterizes the relative concentration of the radiotracer in the lesion of interest.

Other radiopharmaceuticals

There is little published work looking at new tracers for PET. This is primarily due to the slow development of non-[^{18}F]FDG tracers. Whilst ^{67}Ga-citrate has been used to identify infection, including TB in HIV-positive patients [30,31], its short half-life precludes the use of this agent as it takes 24 hours to fully bind *in vivo* to the transit proteins, such as lactoferrin and transferrin, that are involved in the targeting of infection. This is clearly not practical with the 68-minute half-life of ^{68}Ga-citrate. It has been suggested that ^{68}Ga-citrate could be complexed to one of the transit proteins but as yet only ^{68}Ga-transferrin has been used to look at the integrity of the alveolar membrane [32]. An alternate approach would be to use [^{18}F]FDG-labeled WBCs for cell labeling. However, there may be two significant problems with this approach: the safety of staff handling HIV-positive blood and the integrity and functioning of labeled WBCs in HIV-positive patients [33].

Normal findings and artifacts

The areas of normal distribution of [^{18}F]FDG include the brain, myocardium and genitourinary tract. Activity in the bone marrow, stomach and bowel is variable. Thymic uptake, especially in children, can also be observed. Hepatic and splenic uptake is generally low grade and diffuse; in the setting of infection, however, splenic uptake can be quite intense. The spleen, an integral part of the body's immune system, performs multiple tasks, including clearance of encapsulated bacteria, production of inflammatory substances (e.g. opsonins) and of immunoglobulin M and immunoglobulin G antibodies, and phagocytosis of infectious agents, in addition to serving as a reservoir of cellular elements, including WBCs [34]. Presumably, the increased splenic activity reflects increased glucose usage by this organ in the setting of infection. It is important to recognize that increased splenic activity does occur in patients with infection and should not automatically be equated with either splenic infection or tumor [34].

Normal variants and artifacts due to physiological causes of uptake include malignant and non-malignant co-morbidity [inflammatory disease (injury, trauma, post treatment) and reactive esophagitis] and thyroid/adrenal morbidity. Artifacts of PET scanning (preparation) occur because of metallic implants, motion, contrast media and detector calibration.

In general, in patients with high [^{18}F]FDG uptake it is difficult to differentiate between a malignancy, HIV infection and TB. Several authors have shown that [^{18}F]FDG uptake continues to increase over time in malignant lesions, whereas in inflammatory lesions uptake decreases or remains stable. However, studies conducted to assess the potential impact of double-phase [^{18}F]FDG-PET versus routine staging in patients suffering from TB confirmed that it is extremely difficult to distinguish TB from malignant involvement [35].

The normal biodistribution of ^{67}Ga-citrate is the liver, spleen, bone, bone marrow, nasopharynx, lacrimal and salivary glands, and gastrointestinal tract, as well as the kidney/bladder in first 24 hours. ^{67}Ga-citrate localization cannot differentiate between tumor and acute inflammation; other diagnostic studies must be added to define the underlying pathology.

Pathological findings and significance

Tuberculosis

Infective sites and activated WBCs of both granulocytic and lymphocytic origin have increased utilization of glucose and it has been known for over 10 years that sites of infection can be localized with [^{18}F]FDG [35,36].

Data on [^{18}F]FDG-PET imaging in patients suffering from tuberculosis (TB) are very limited [37]. In some patients there may be a question whether a site of pulmonary uptake is malignant or benign; in particular whether it is possible to differentiate between TB and tumor. It was thought that though both may have an initially high SUV_{max}, malignant tissues have a greater retention of [^{18}F]FDG between 1 and 2 hours than benign processes such as TB. However, in a prospective series of 31 patients with suspicious pulmonary lesions, low wash-out (i.e. a high retention index for [^{18}F]FDG) was seen in 60% of the benign lesions, including those of 10 patients with TB. This was similar to the high retention index for 62% at the malignant sites of disease; the inference being that late imaging and looking at the wash-out rates or retention index for [^{18}F]FDG is not useful [38] (Figure 15.2).

This finding has been confirmed in a sub-Saharan population. In a group of 30 patients with a high incidence of TB, the SUV_{max} in the benign group was higher than in those with cancer [39], but when using the traditional SUV_{max} cut-off of 2.5, the specificity of [^{18}F]FDG was only 25% for finding cancer. Again, the wash-out of [^{18}F]FDG as measured by change in SUV_{max} was almost identical in the two groups, especially when comparing TB with cancer.

The following are the FDG-PET findings in TB:
• Dual-phase imaging and the use of wash-out rates for [^{18}F]FDG are unlikely to be helpful in differentiating TB from malignancy.
• Pulmonary TB commonly causes an increase in [^{18}F]FDG uptake.

• Lymphadenitis is the commonest extrapulmonary manifestation of TB, but it cannot be distinguished from other causes of abnormal nodal uptake such as HIV and malignancy.
• Uptake is low in tuberculous pleural effusion (Figure 15.3; CT is better than PET in visualizing pleural effusion).
• [^{18}F]FDG-PET detects more sites of extrapulmonary TB than CT, including the joints and bone [40] (Figure 15.3).
• [^{18}F]FDG-PET is essential in monitoring TB treatment (see below).

^{67}Ga-citrate is still used for the detection of pulmonary and extrapulmonary TB, but is limited by being non-specific and incapable of differentiating between TB/infection and inflammation. In mycobacterial lung infections, the commonest ^{67}Ga-citrate scintigraphy pattern is that of patchy or lobar uptake along with hilar and non-hilar nodal uptake (Table 15.1; Figure 15.4). Adding thallium-201 (^{201}Tl) scintigraphy to ^{67}Ga-citrate scintigraphy was shown to increase the specificity for both pulmonary and extrapulmonary TB: a ^{67}Ga-positive/^{201}Tl-negative mismatch pattern in AIDS patients is specific for mycobacterial infections [41]. Extrahilar nodal uptake is more common with atypical mycobacterial infections/MAC, while TB tends to be more commonly limited to hilar uptake [42].

Generalized adenopathy

[^{18}F]FDG-PET data have shown that HIV-1 infection progresses in distinct anatomical steps, with involvement of the upper torso preceding involvement of the lower part of the body, and that the degree of [^{18}F]FDG uptake is related to viral load [43]. The involvement of lymphoid tissue appears to follow a predictable sequence: there is a distinct lymphoid tissue activation in the head and neck during acute disease, a generalized pattern of peripheral lymph node activation in the mid stages and involvement of abdominal lymph nodes during late disease [43,44] (Figure 15.5). [^{18}F]FDG uptake by the lymph nodes of HIV-positive patients was found to be inversely related to CD4 count, thereby supporting the theory of CD4 cell depletion through forced lymph node homing (see above) [45]. Comparison of [^{18}F]FDG uptake in patients who had received HAART and patients who were HAART-naïve revealed different patterns: all the

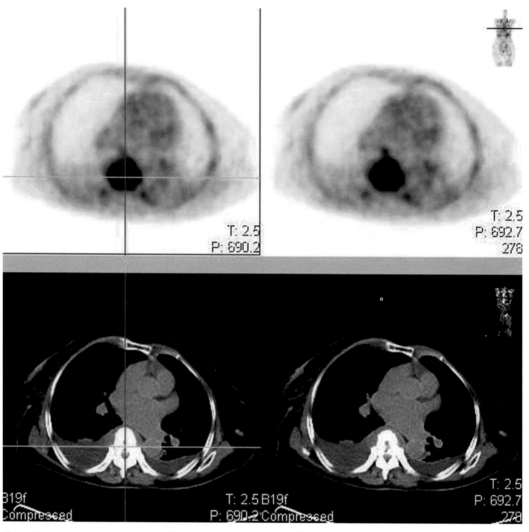

Figure 15.3 Consecutive transaxial PET/CT slides showing intense [^{18}F]FDG in a patient with TB of the spine and low-grade [^{18}F]FDG uptake in a pleural effusion.

Table 15.1 Scintigraphic features in common HIV-associated lesions

Disease	^{67}Ga-citrate lung uptake	^{67}Ga-citrate nodal uptake	^{67}Ga-citrate extrapulmonary uptake	^{201}TlCl uptake	CD4 (cells/mm^3)
TB	Patchy/lobar	Hilar	Various organs (esp. MDR)	Low/none	Variable
MAC	Patchy/lobar	Extrahilar	Various organs	Low/none	<60
PJP	Diffuse, intense	None			<200
CMV	Diffuse, low grade	None	Eye, adrenal, colon, esophagus	None	<50
LIP	Diffuse, low grade	None	Bilateral parotid	None	<50
Kaposi's sarcoma	None	None	None	Focal uptake	<200
Lymphoma	None	Bulky	Spleen	Bulky	<200

CMV, cytomegalovirus; LIP, lymphoid interstitial pneumonia; MAC, *Mycobacterium avium-intracellulare* complex; MDR, multidrug resistant; PJP, *Pneumococcus jirovecii* pneumonia; TB, tuberculosis.

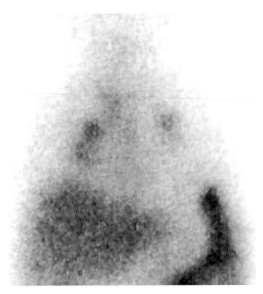

Figure 15.4 ^{67}Ga-citrate anterior planar image of the chest in a patient with HIV showing patchy uptake along with hilar nodal uptake.

HAART-treated patients with either suppressed or high viremia showed a normal pattern, while the HAART-naïve patients with high viremia displayed multiple foci of increased glucose metabolism in the lymph nodes. Together, this finding and the finding of a correlation between the well-established markers of progression to AIDS and positive [^{18}F] FDG-PET in HAART-naïve patients seem to confer prognostic value on [^{18}F]FDG uptake [46].

Lymphoma

Based on studies performed in HIV-positive patients presenting with lymphoma or other malignancy, knowledge of viremia is essential when interpreting [^{18}F]FDG-PET imaging [47]. HIV changes the commonest types of Hodgkin's lymphoma to mixed cellularity and lymphocyte depleted. It is crucial to note that extranodal involvement, such as of the bone marrow, spleen and liver, is common and can easily be seen on PET as it is [^{18}F]FDG avid.

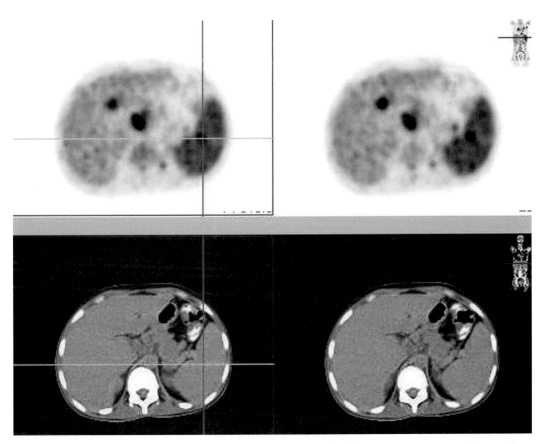

Figure 15.5 Consecutive transaxial PET/CT slides showing nodal and splenic [^{18}F]FDG uptake. It is impossible to make a differential diagnosis between HIV and lymphoma.

Brain lymphoma

The potential of [¹⁸F]FDG-PET to non-invasively differentiate cerebral toxoplasmosis and other infectious diseases from primary CNS lymphoma has been assessed by several authors. Hoffman *et al.* studied individuals with AIDS and CNS lesions with [¹⁸F]FDG-PET [48]. Both qualitative visual inspection of the PET images as well as semi-quantitative analysis indicated that [¹⁸F]FDG-PET was able to accurately differentiate between a lymphoma and a non-malignant etiology for CNS lesions. Similar results were found by other authors [49,50]. Furthermore, O'Doherty *et al.* showed that in 19 patients who were on antitoxoplasmosis treatment, a [¹⁸F]FDG-PET scan was 100% sensitive and specific for identifying primary CNS lymphoma [51]. These studies support the notion that [¹⁸F]FDG-PET may be useful in the management of AIDS patients with CNS lesions since high [¹⁸F]FDG uptake most likely represents a malignant process which should be biopsied for confirmation rather than treated presumptively as infectious.

With regards to general nuclear medicine, ²⁰¹Tl chloride (²⁰¹TlCl) SPECT can localize and characterize brain tumors. Findings in most studies indicate that delayed ²⁰¹TlCl SPECT in extracranial lesions is more specific for lymphoma. This is because an infectious process can sometimes show early uptake of ²⁰¹TlCl, but this then clears relatively quickly compared with uptake by neoplastic lesions in the brain, lungs, mediastinum and abdomen [52–54]. Therefore, in a busy department, early ²⁰¹TlCl SPECT could be dispensed with to save time and only delayed scanning need be performed. Even with delayed ²⁰¹TlCl SPECT, the background ²⁰¹TlCl in the normal brain is still visible (Figure 15.6). Thus, visual inspection (i.e. comparing the ²⁰¹TlCl uptake in the brain to that in the scalp and skull) alone is sufficient to differentiate the normal background from abnormal uptake.

Lee *et al.* further emphasized that sequential ²⁰¹TlCl and ⁶⁷Ga-citrate scanning is highly sensitive and specific in the differentiation of neoplastic from non-neoplastic intracranial mass lesions in patients with AIDS [54]. When the intracranial mass lesions are ²⁰¹TlCl avid, ⁶⁷Ga-citrate SPECT is not necessary, as these lesions have a high probability of being a lymphoma or other neoplasm. Since Kaposi's sarcoma is extremely rare in the CNS, the absence of the ²⁰¹TlCl-positive/⁶⁷Ga-citrate negative pattern is not unexpected [54–56]. In practice, therefore, ⁶⁷Ga-citrate

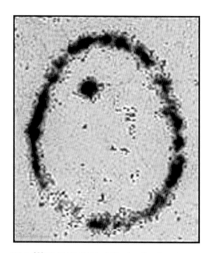

Figure 15.6 ²⁰¹ThCl SPECT of the brain showing an intracranial positive lesion that was proven to be a lymphoma.

Table 15.2 Interpretation of lung scans in HIV-positive patients using ²⁰¹TlCl and ⁶⁷Ga-citrate

	⁶⁷Ga-citrate	*²⁰¹TlCl*
Kaposi's sarcoma	Negative	Positive
Lymphoma	Positive	Positive
Opportunistic infections	Positive	Negative

scanning is probably unnecessary if brain lesions are ²⁰¹TlCl avid. If findings on ²⁰¹TlCl SPECT are negative, ⁶⁷Ga-citrate scanning could be performed to further characterize the lesions and to assist in differentiating infections from infarcts or progressive multifocal leukoencephalopathy (Table 15.2).

HIV-associated neurocognitive disorder

In an early imaging study using [¹⁸F]FDG-PET in patients in the early stage of HAND, Rottenberg *et al.* found relative subcortical hypermetabolism in patients [57]. Disease progression was characterized by reduced glucose uptake in cortical and subcortical gray matter. Van Gorp *et al.* also found a significant relationship between temporal lobe metabolism and the severity of dementia [58]. Finally, during a motor task, von Giesen *et al.* found frontomesial hypometabolism in non-demented HIV-infected subjects [59]. The authors indicated that frontomesial hypometabolism was associated

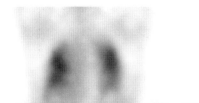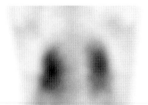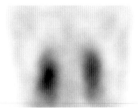

Figure 15.7 ^{67}Ga-citrate SPECT sequential coronal slides of the chest showing diffuse increased bilateral lung uptake in a patient with PJP.

with deteriorating motor performance. Thus, unlike conventional imaging, dementia in AIDS may show early cerebral abnormalities on SPECT and PET scans in the thalamus and basal ganglia [57].

Pneumocystis jirovecii pneumonia

[67]Ga-citrate scintigraphy can detect PJP in asymptomatic patients with normal chest X-rays [60]. Diffuse increased bilateral lung uptake that is more intense than in liver is the commonest pattern (Table 15.1) and has a specificity of 90% for PJP [61] (Figure 15.7). The presence of heterogeneous diffuse lung uptake may have a higher predictive value than homogeneous uptake [62] and when the concurrent chest X-ray is also normal, the specificity approaches 100%.

Cytomegalovirus

[67]Ga-citrate scintigraphy is very useful in CMV. A whole-body ^{67}Ga-citrate scan will demonstrate the following pattern: low-grade lung uptake (Table 15.1) with perihilar prominence [62] associated with eye uptake (due to the frequent presentation of CMV as retinitis; Figure 15.8), adrenal uptake (due to the most frequent pathological findings of CMV as adrenalitis), renal uptake at 48 hours and/or persistent colon uptake with diarrheal symptoms without other pathogens seen in multiple stool specimens [63]. If high-grade pulmonary uptake is seen, superimposed aggressive PCP must be considered.

Lymphocytic interstitial pneumonitis

[67]Ga-citrate scintigraphy appears to have a diagnostic pattern of symmetric parotid uptake (Table 15.1) and low-grade diffuse lung uptake without nodal uptake [64], which can be distinguished from other causes of lung ^{67}Ga-citrate uptake.

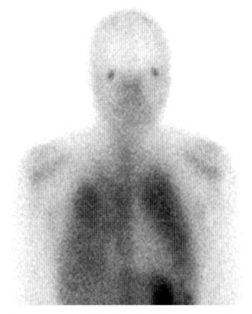

Figure 15.8 Low-grade and diffuse ^{67}Ga-citrate uptake in the lungs associated with lacrimal gland uptake in a patient with CMV.

Kaposi's sarcoma

In the work-up of patients with Kaposi's sarcoma (KS), a negative ^{67}Ga-citrate scan with a positive chest X-ray is often associated with pulmonary KS [61,64]. The absence of accumulation of ^{67}Ga-citrate in KS lesions suggests ^{67}Ga-citrate scanning may be used to differentiate between pulmonary KS and infection in AIDS patients with KS (Table 15.1). Also, the lack of ^{67}Ga-citrate uptake may distinguish KS from lymphoma, which also occurs in AIDS patients and often demonstrates lymph node chain uptake. AIDS-related lymphoma affects the lung less frequently than mycobacterial infection and the neoplasm can be distinguished from infection by its characteristic bulky nodal pattern of

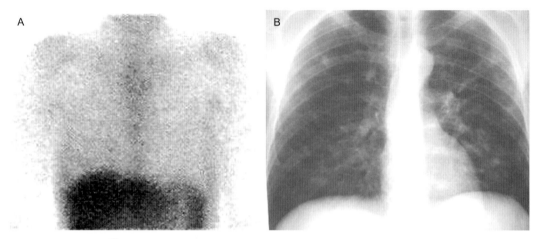

Figure 15.9 A negative ^{67}Ga-citrate scan (A) in a patient with Kaposi's sarcoma, with positive chest radiograph (B) and positive thallium scan (not shown).

uptake. The diagnosis of KS can be confirmed if uptake of ^{201}TlCl is seen in the mass [65]; ^{67}Ga-citrate is less useful (Figure 15.9).

Toxoplasmosis

SPECT imaging with ^{201}TlCl has been shown to localize brain tumors with a good target-to-background ratio, which appears to be related to cell growth rates and blood flow [66,67]. In contrast, ^{201}TlCl does not appear to accumulate in non-neoplastic lesions such as hematomas, radiation necrosis and infectious processes such as toxoplasmosis [67]. Hence, a negative brain ^{201}TlCl SPECT will be consistent with toxoplasmosis for a ring-enhancing lesion on CT or MRI. Thus, a brain ^{201}TlCl SPECT is highly sensitive and specific in patients with AIDS for rapid differential diagnosis of focal brain lesions and increases the likelihood of a diagnostic brain biopsy. Furthermore, Lorberboym *et al.* demonstrated that the sensitivity of brain ^{201}TlCl SPECT is not affected by prior administration of steroids and the retention index of ^{201}TlCl may be a useful measurable variable in distinguishing CNS lymphoma in patients with AIDS from other malignancies or nonmalignant, ^{201}TlCl-avid pathological entities [68].

The gastrointestinal tract

^{67}Ga-citrate uptake in the gastrointestinal track that is equal to or greater than liver uptake, combined with a diffuse colonic uptake that does not change, can be due to CMV infection (when stool cultures are negative), bacterial infections such as salmonellosis or shigellosis, or antibiotic-induced colitis. Multifocal ^{67}Ga-citrate activity is indicative of mycobacterial infection, while bacterial infections such as salmonellosis commonly show diffusely increased activity [63].

In AIDS patients, KS, lymphoma and other tumors can involve the gastrointestinal tract, liver and spleen. An enlarged spleen with reduced uptake of ^{99m}Tc-sulfur colloid on liver–spleen imaging is usually the result of KS in the AIDS patient [69].

Skin lesions

Skin lesions are a common presentation of KS in AIDS patients. Red blood cell (RBC) pooling on ^{99m}Tc-labeled RBC imaging and ^{201}TlCl scintigraphy [13] is useful to distinguish KS from inflammatory skin lesions. Since biopsy is usually diagnostic, nuclear imaging methods can direct diagnosis for KS skin lesions.

Fever of unknown origin

In patients with HIV and fever of unknown origin (FUO), [^{18}F]FDG-PET/CT has emerged as a valuable tool for diagnosis, especially when CT anatomical landmarks are added to PET findings [70].

Role in therapy follow-up and patient management

Tuberculosis

In developing countries, MDR and XDR TB are of serious consequence and thus monitoring of therapy is essential. A major attribute of PET stems from its ability to quantitate [^{18}F]FDG uptake, which allows the infectious or inflammatory processes to be monitored during the early course of the disease. This is especially true in determining the effectiveness of therapy.

It is common for patients with low CD4+ counts and TB co-infection who are treated with antiretroviral treatment to develop immune reconstitution inflammatory syndrome (IRIS) and frequently die because of this condition. Symptoms include new or worsening fever, lymphadenopathy, pulmonary, visceral, CNS or cutaneous disease, which may be severe and life-threatening and must be differentiated from disease progression. Hence, early detection and monitoring of treatment is essential.

The treatment of TB can be problematic, the disease itself may be resistant to standard treatment, and treatment itself is prolonged with regimens in HIV-positive patients being anywhere from 3 to 9 months. Hospitalization for this period of time is not possible so treatment is performed as an outpatient. However, this raises the problem of compliance, especially if the patient starts to feel better. The time course of treatment is empirical and tends to be the maximum needed to treat TB in that clinical situation. However, there can be great variation in the length of the course of treatment required, so an objective method to monitor treatment is required. Using an animal model and TB infection model it has been shown that quantitative [^{18}F]FDG uptake can be used to monitor the effectiveness of treatment [38]. In this study there was a clear correlation between the fall in [^{18}F]FDG uptake in the lungs and successful administration of a bactericidal drug. In contrast, uptake of [^{18}F]FDG increased when an ineffective drug was given and in the control group.

Clinical data remain sparse in extrapulmonary TB; in a recent study [71], SUV$_{max}$ of involved lymph node basins (both early and delayed) and number of involved lymph node basins were significantly higher in non-responders than in responders (respective p values were 0.03, 0.04 and 0.002). Using a cut-off of five or more involved lymph node basins, responders could be separated from non-responders with a sensitivity, specificity and positive and negative predictive value of, respectively, 88%, 81%, 70% and 93%. Using a cut-off of 8.15 for the early SUV$_{max}$ of lymph node basins and of 10 for the late SUV$_{max}$ of lymph node basins, a comparable sensitivity of 88% came at the cost of a lower specificity: 73% and 67%, respectively. In a separate small series, the SUV$_{max}$ in tuberculous lymph nodes returned to normal post-therapy [71].

Aggressive lymphoid proliferations should be differentiated from generalized lymphadenopathy, which does not have a poor outcome, and here again [^{18}F]FDG-PET may play a central role. [^{18}F] FDG-PET scanning could also be indicated for monitoring the efficacy of TB treatment, while [^{18}F]FDG activity may also be a useful tool for evaluating and excluding sites of active disease in the context of targeted screening for latent TB infection before immunosuppressive treatment.

Lipodystrophy

In the clinical setting, [^{18}F]FDG-PET has been shown to allow monitoring of the side effects of HAART, such as lipodystrophy [72]. Because of the low insulin state in these patients, glucose uptake is probably mediated by glucose transporter 1 (GLUT-1) [71]. It is unlikely that increased subcutaneous [^{18}F]FDG uptake is mediated by translocation of the insulin-dependent GLUT-4 transporter, because lipodystrophy is associated with marked insulin resistance. [^{18}F]FDG-PET may become a promising tool to monitor lipodystrophy during the course of HIV treatment. Moreover, in clinical trials, the lipodystrophy-inducing effect of newly developed antiretroviral regimens may be monitored objectively by this approach.

Thymus

The thymus in adults infected with HIV-1 is generally thought to be inactive, both because of age-related involution and viral destruction [73]. The observed increases in the number of CD4+ T cells after HAART have been attributed to thymic reactivation by some authors. The thymic reactivation demonstrates some correlations with visible activity within the thymus, as measured by increased [^{18}F]FDG uptake [74]; however, further studies are needed to validate this process.

Conclusion

PET and SPECT imaging have improved significantly the understanding of the pathogenesis of HIV-1 infection. In addition, [^{18}F]FDG-PET holds great potential in the clinical decision-making of HIV-1 patients presenting with AIDS-related opportunistic infections and malignancies, and for monitoring of side effects of HAART. In this context, the ongoing quest to find better labeling agents may well result in the identification of the ideal PET/CT radiopharmaceutical for imaging infection and inflammation.

References

1. Wainberg M, Jeang K. 25-years of HIV-research. *BMC Med* 2008;31:6–31.
2. UNAIDS/WHO. *AIDS Epidemic Update: December 2007*. Geneva: UNAIDS, 2007. http://data.unaids.org/pub/EPISlides/2007/2007_epiupdate_en.pdf
3. Kelleher H, Zaunders J. Decimated or missing in action: CD4+ T cells as targets and effectors in the pathogenesis of primary HIV infection. *Curr HIV/AIDS Rep* 2006;3:5–12.
4. Haramati LB, Jenny-Avital ER, Alterman D. Thoracic manifestations of immune restoration syndromes in AIDS. *J Thoracic Imaging* 2007;22:213–220.
5. Lacombe C, Lewin M, Monnier-Chollet L et al. Imaging of thoracic pathology in patients with AIDS. *J Radiol* 2007;88:1145–1154.
6. George R, Andronikou S, Theron S et al. Pulmonary infections in HIV-positive children. *Pediatr Radiol* 2009;39:545–554.
7. Cohen PT, Sande M, Volberding P. Clinical spectrum of HIV disease. In: *The AIDS Knowledge Base: A Textbook of HIV*. Boston: Little Brown, 1994.
8. Graham SM. Non-tuberculosis opportunistic infections and other lung diseases in HIV-infected infants and children. *Int J Tuberc Lung Dis* 2005;9:592–602.
9. Cadogan M, Dalgleish A. HIV induced AIDS and related cancers: chronic immune activation and future therapeutic strategies. *Adv Cancer Res* 2008;101:349–395.
10. Aoki Y, Tosato G. Neoplastic conditions in the context of HIV-1 infection. *Curr HIV Res* 2004;2:343–349.
11. Simpson DM, Tagliati M. Neurologic manifestations of HIV infection. *Ann Intern Med* 1994;121:769–785.
12. Mill J. *Pneumocystis carinii* and *Toxoplasma gondii* infections in patients with AIDS. *Rev Infect Dis* 1986;8:1001–1101.
13. Levy RM, Bredesen DE, Rosenblum ML. Neurological complications of the acquired immunodeficiency syndrome (AIDS): experience of UCSF and review of the literature. *J Neurol* 1985;62:775–798.
14. Ciricillo SF, Rosenblum ML. Use of CT and MR imaging to distinguish intracranial lesions and to define the need for biopsy in AIDS patients. *J Neurosurg* 1990;73:720–724.
15. Antinori A, Arendt G, Becker JT et al. Updated research nosology for HIV-associated neurocognitive disorders. *Neurology* 2007;69:1789–1799.
16. Woods SP, Moore DJ, Weber E et al. Cognitive neuropsychology of HIV-associated neurocognitive disorders. *Neuropsychol Rev* 2009;19:152–168.
17. Zou W, Foussat A, Houhou S. Acute upregulation of CCR-5 expression by CD4+ T lymphocytes in HIV-infected patients treated with interleukin-2. *AIDS* 1999;13:455–463.
18. World Health Organization. *Global Tuberculosis Control Report. Surveillance Planning Financing*. Geneva: WHO, 2009.
19. UNAIDS. *Report on the Global AIDS Epidemic*. Geneva: UNAIDS, 2008.
20. Cloyd M, Chen J, Wang I. How does HIV cause AIDS? The homing theory. *Mol Med Today* 2000;6:108–111.
21. Lederman M, Margolis L. The lymph node in HIV pathogenesis. *Semin Immunol* 2008;20:187–195.
22. Carr A. Diagnosis, prediction and natural course of HIV-1 protease inhibitor-associated lipodystrophy, hyperlipidemaemia, and diabetes mellitus: a cohort study. *Lancet* 1999;353:2093–2099.
23. Behrens G, Stoll M, Schmidt R. Lipodysystrophy syndrome in HIV infection: what is it, what causes it and how can it be managed? *Drug Saf* 2000;23:57–76.
24. Bedimo R. Non-AIDS-defining malignancies among HIV-infected patients in the highly active antiretroviral therapy era. *Curr HIV/AIDS Rep* 2008;5:140–149.
25. Crum-Cianflone N, Hullsiek K, Marconi V et al. Trends in the incidence of cancers among HIV-infected persons and the impact of antiretroviral therapy: a 20-year cohort study. *AIDS* 2009;23:41–50.
26. Lee VW, Antonacci V, Tilak S, Fuller JD, Cooley TP. Intracranial mass lesions: sequential thallium and gallium scintigraphy in patients with AIDS. *Radiology* 1999;211:507–512.
27. Price R, Spudich S. Antiretroviral therapy and central nervous system HIV type-1 infection. *J Infect Dis* 2008;197:S294–S306.
28. Simpson DM, Tagliati M. Neurologic manifestations of HIV infection. *Ann Intern Med* 1994;121:769–785.
29. Klein RS, Harris CA, Shell CB et al. Oral candidiasis in high risk patients as the initial manifestation of the acquired immunodeficiency syndrome. *N Engl J Med* 1987;311:354–358.
30. Buscombe JR, Oyen WJ, Corstens FH, Ell PJ, Miller RF. Localization of infection in HIV antibody positive patients with fever. Comparison of the efficacy of Ga-67 citrate and radiolabeled human IgG. *Clin Nucl Med* 1995;20:334–339

31. Buscombe JR, Buttery P, Ell PJ, Miller RF. Patterns of Ga-67 citrate accumulation in human immunodeficiency virus positive patients with and without Mycobacterium avium intracellulare infection. *Clin Radiol* 1995;50:483–488

32. Schuster DP, Markham J, Welch MJ. Positron emission tomography measurements of pulmonary vascular permeability with Ga-68 transferrin or C-11 methylalbumin. *Crit Care Med* 1998;26:518–525.

33. Prvulovich EM, Miller RF, Costa DC *et al*. Immunoscintigraphy with a ^{99Tm}-labelled anti-granulocyte monoclonal antibody in patients with human immunodeficiency virus infection and AIDS. *Nucl Med Commun* 1995;16:838–845

34. Love C, Tomas MB, Tronco GG, Palestro CJ. FDG PET of infection and inflammation. *RadioGraphics* 2005; 25:1357–1368.

35. Sathekge MM, Maes A, Pottel H, Stoltz A, van de Wiele C. Dual time-point FDG PET-CT for differentiating benign from malignant solitary pulmonary nodules in a TB endemic area. *S Afr Med J* 2010; 100:598–601.

36. Jeong YJ, Lee KS. Pulmonary tuberculosis: up-to-date imaging and management. *AJR Am J Roentgenol* 2008;191:834–844.

37. Glaudemans AW, Signore A. FDG-PET/CT in infections: the imaging method of choice? *Eur J Nucl Med Mol Imaging* 2010;37:1986–1991.

38. Sathekge M, Buscombe JR. Can positron emission tomography work in the African tuberculosis epidemic? *Nucl Med Commun* 2011;32:241–244.

39. Lan XL, Zhang YX, Wu ZJ, Jia Q, Wei H, Goa ZR. The value of dual time point ^{18}F FDG PET imaging for the differentiation between malignant and benign lesions. *Clin Radiol* 2008;63:756–764.

40. Sathekge M, Maes A, Kgomo M, Stoltz A, Pottel H, Wiele C. Impact of FDG PET on the management of TBC treatment. A pilot study. *Nuklearmedizin* 2010; 49:35–40.

41. Tatsch K, Knesewitsch P, Kirsch CM *et al*. The place of 67Ga scintigraphy in the primary diagnosis and follow-up evaluation of opportunistic pneumonia in patients with AIDS. *Nuklearmedizin* 1988;27:219–225.

42. Abdel-Dayem HM, Naddaf S, Aziz M *et al*. Sites of tuberculous involvement in patients with AIDS. Autopsy findings and evaluation of gallium imaging. *Clin Nucl Med* 1997;22:310–314.

43. Sathekge M, Goethals I, Maes A, Wiele C. Positron emission tomography in patients suffering from HIV-1 infection. *Eur J Nucl Med Mol Imaging* 2009;36: 1176–1184.

44. Scharko A, Perlman S, Pyzalski R, Graziano F, Sosman J, Pauza C. Whole-body positron emission tomography in patients with HIV-1 infection. *Lancet* 2003;20: 959–961.

45. Sathekge M, Maes A, Kgomo M, Wiele C. Fluorodeoxyglucose uptake by lymph nodes of HIV patients is inversely related to CD4 cell count. *Nucl Med Commun* 2010;31:137–140.

46. Lucignani G, Orunesu E, Cesari M *et al*. FDG-PET imaging in HIV-infected subjects: relation with therapy and immunovirological variables. *Eur J Nucl Med Mol Imaging* 2009;36:640–647.

47. Sathekge M, Maes A, Kgomo M, Pottel H, Stolz A, Van De Wiele C. FDG uptake in lymph-nodes of HIV+ and tuberculosis patients: implications for cancer staging. *Q J Nucl Med Mol Imaging* 2010;54:698–703.

48. Hoffman JM, Waskin HA, Schifter T *et al*. FDG-PET in differentiating lymphoma from nonmalignant central nervous system lesions in patients with AIDS. *J Nucl Med* 1993;34:567–575.

49. Villringer K, Jager H, Dichgans M *et al*. Differential diagnosis of CNS lesions in AIDS patients by FDG-PET. *J Comput Assist Tomogr* 1995;19:532–536.

50. Heald A, Hoffman JM, Bartlett J, Waskin H. Differentiation of central nervous system lesions in AIDS patients using positron emission tomography (PET). *Int J STD AIDS* 1996;7:337–346.

51. O'Doherty M, Barrington S, Campbell M, Lowe J, Bradbeer C. PET scanning and the human immunodeficiency virus-positive patient. *J Nucl Med* 1997;38: 1575–1583.

52. Lee VW. The importance of a delayed scan in thallium imaging for tumors (letter). *J Nucl Med* 1992;33: 463–465.

53. Lee VW. Delayed thallium scan for the diagnosis of AIDS-related pulmonary Kaposi sarcoma and other complications (letter). *Clin Nucl Med* 1995;20: 568–570.

54. Lee VW, Cooley TP, Fuller J, Ward RJ, Farber HW. Pulmonary mycobacterial infections in AIDS: characteristic pattern of thallium and gallium findings. *Radiology* 1994;193:389–392.

55. Waxman AD, Eller D, Ashook G *et al*. Comparison of gallium-67 citrate and thallium-201 scintigraphy in peripheral and intrathoracic lymphoma. *J Nucl Med* 1996;37:46–50.

56. Abdel-Dayem HM, Bag R, DiFabrizio L *et al*. Evaluation of sequential thallium and gallium scans of the chest in AIDS patients. *J Nucl Med* 1996;37:1662–1667.

57. Rottenberg DA, Moeller JR, Stotler SC *et al*. The metabolic pathology of the AIDS dementia complex. *Ann Neurol* 1987;22:700–706.

58. Van Gorp W, Mandelkern M, Gee M *et al*. Cerebral metabolic dysfunction in AIDS: findings in a sample with and without dementia. *J Neuropsychiatry Clin Neurosci* 1992;4:280–287.

59. von Giesen H, Antke C, Hefter H, Wenserski F, Seitz R, Arendt G. Potential time course of human immunodeficiency virus type 1-associated minor motor deficits:

electrophysiologic and positron emission tomography findings. *Arch Neurol* 2000;57:1601–1607.

60. Bitran J, Beckerman C, Weinstein R *et al.* Patterns of gallium-67 scintigraphy in patients with acquired immunodeficiency syndrome and AIDS related complex. *J Nucl Med* 1987;28:1103–1106.

61. Woolfenden JM, Carrasquillo JA, Larson SM *et al.* Acquired immunodeficiency syndrome Ga-67 citrate imaging. *Radiology* 1987;162:383–387.

62. Kramer EL, Sanger JH, Garay SM *et al.* Diagnostic implications of Ga-67 chest scan patterns in human immunodeficiency virus-seropositive patients. *Radiology* 1989;170:671–679.

63. Ganz WI, Serafini AN. Role of nuclear medicine and AIDS: overview and perspective for the future. *Q J Nucl Med* 1995;39:169–186.

64. Zuckier LS, Ongseng F, Goldfarb GR. Lymphocytic interstitial pneumonitis: a cause of pulmonary galliurn-67 uptake in a child with acquired immunodeficiency syndrome. *J Nucl Med* 1988;29:707–711.

65. Lee VW, Rosen MP, Baum A *et al.* AIDS-related Kaposi sarcoma: finding in thallium 201 scintigraphy. *AJR Am J Roentgenol* 1988;151:1233–1235.

66. Lorberboym M, Baram J, Feibel M, Hercbergs A, Lieberman L. A prospective evaluation of ^{201}Tl single-photon emission computerized tomography for brain tumor burden. *Int J Radiat Oncol Biol Phys* 1995;32:249–254.

67. Black KL, Hawkins RA, Kim KT, Becker DP, Lerner C, Marciano D. Use of ^{201}Tl SPECT to quantitate malig-nancy grade of gliomas. *J Neurosurg* 1989;71: 342–346.

68. Lorberboym M, Estok L, Machac J *et al.* Rapid differential diagnosis of cerebral toxoplasmosis and primary central nervous system lymphoma by thallium-201 SPECT. *J Nucl Med* 1996;37:1150–1154.

69. Ganz WI, Heiba H, Ganz SS *et al.* Use of liver spleen scintigraphy to detect immune status and Kaposi sarcoma in AIDS patients. *Radiology* 1987; 165(P):97.

70. Castaigne C, Tondeur M, Wit S, Hildebrand M, Clumeck N, Dusart M. Clinical value of FDG-PET/CT for the diagnosis of human immunodeficiency virus-associated fever of unknown origin: a retrospective study. *Nucl Med Commun* 2009;30:41–47.

71. Sathekge M, Maes A, Kgomo M, Stolz A, Van De Wiele C. Use of ^{18}F-FDG PET to predict response to first-line tuberculostatics in HIV-associated tuberculosis. *J Nucl Med* 2011;52:1–6.

72. Sathekge M, Goethals I, Maes A, Wiele C. Positron emission tomography in patients suffering from HIV-1 infection. *Eur J Nucl Med Mol Imaging* 2009;36: 1176–1184.

73. Tsong Fang H, Colantonio A, Uittenbogaart C. The role of the thymus in HIV infection: a 10 year perspective. *AIDS* 2008;22:171–174.

74. Hardy G, Worrell S, Hayes P *et al.* Evidence of thymic reconstitution after highly active antiretroviral therapy in HIV-1 infection. *HIV Med* 2004;5:67–73.

Clinical cases

Case 1

A 31-year-old male presented with intermittent high-grade fever and chills. Considering his HIV-positive status in a TB-endemic country, a diagnosis of TB was considered. Sputum examination confirmed the presence of tuberculous bacilli. The patient was started on antitubercular treatment (ATT).

The complete hemachrome was unremarkable. CRP and ESR were raised at 8.7 mg/dL and 72 mm/h respectively. Blood and urine cultures were negative. Viral load was not detectable. Chest X-ray showed left upper lobe disease with soft puffy infiltrates and cavitation.

The pre-therapy scan demonstrated intense [^{18}F]FDG uptake in the upper zone of the left lung with mediastinal and hilar lymph node uptake (Figure 15.10). The right lung was morphologically normal with no abnormal [^{18}F]FDG uptake. Physiological [^{18}F]FDG uptake was noted in the brain, myocardium, liver, bone marrow, bowel and urinary tract. A repeat study after 12 weeks of therapy showed faint [^{18}F]FDG uptake in the mediastinal lymph node and lung (Figure 15.10). There was an approximately 80% reduction in the [^{18}F]FDG uptake in these sites, indicating good ongoing metabolic response to ATT, which corresponded to the clinical re-evaluation. This enabled the patient to continue with his ATT and rule out MDR TB.

Teaching point

[^{18}F]FDG-PET can be used to monitor ATT response and thus enable early detection of drug resistance in TB. This will allow for the initiation of an appropriate treatment, which may significantly affect patient survival.

Case 2

A 27-year-old HIV-positive male developed fevers and night sweats. The patient was admitted to hospital and it was thought that his symptoms may have been due to TB. He underwent lymph node biopsy, which was negative for TB and malignancy.

The viral load was 176 262 copies/mL and the CD4 count was 232 cells/µL.

Intense [^{18}F]FDG uptake was seen in multiple cervical lymph nodes, including axillary and mediastinal lymph nodes. As expected, [^{18}F]FDG uptake was also seen in the collecting system and the bladder (Figure 15.11).

Teaching point

[^{18}F]FDG-PET data have shown that HIV-1 infection progresses in distinct anatomical steps, with distinct lymphoid tissue activation in the head and neck during acute disease, a generalized pattern of peripheral lymph node activation at the mid stages and involvement of abdominal lymph nodes during late disease, suggesting that lymphoid tissues are engaged in a predictable sequence.

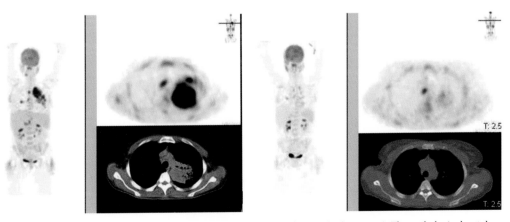

Figure 15.10 [^{18}F]FDG-PET/CT performed before (left images) and after therapy (right images). The pathological uptake in the left lung and mediastinum before therapy almost completely disappeared after therapy.

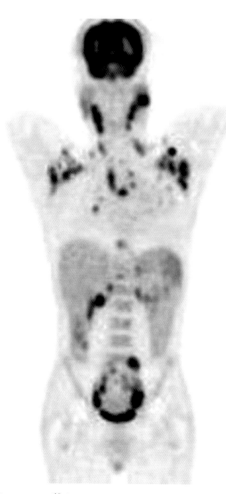

Case 3

A 31-year-old HIV-positive female on HAART (stavudine, lamivudine and efavirenz) with clinical evidence from physicians' and patient's reports of fat wasting from the face, buttocks, limbs and upper trunk, accumulation of fat in the abdomen or over the dorsocervical spine and no history of anabolic steroids, glucocorticoids or immunomodulators within 3 months of assessment.

The viral load was less than 50 copies/mL and the CD4 count was 442 cells/μL. The fasting cholesterol was 0.83 mmol/dL and triglyceride was 0.32 mmol/dL, and fasting CRP was 0.45 mmol/dL.

A coronal image of the patient under HAART showed increased $[^{18}F]$FDG uptake in subcutaneous fat (Figure 15.12).

Teaching points
• Apoptosis is an energy-dependent phenomenon that is accompanied by increased $[^{18}F]$FDG utilization.
• Accordingly, the increase in the mean SUV of the subcutaneous fat of patients suffering from HIV-related lipodystrophy under HAART therapy may theoretically reflect ongoing apoptosis and may allow quantitative non-invasive monitoring of lipoatrophy.

Figure 15.11 $[^{18}F]$FDG MIP image showing pathological uptake in multiple cervical, axillary and mediastinal lymph nodes.

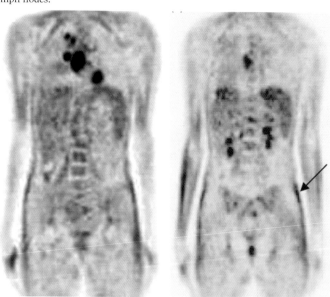

Figure 15.12 Sequential coronal section of an $[^{18}F]$FDG-PET scan in a patient under HAART with lipodystrophy. Images show increased $[^{18}F]$FDG uptake in the lungs, mediastinum and subcutaneous fat (arrow).

CHAPTER 16

Nuclear Medicine Imaging of Fever of Unknown Origin

François-Xavier Hanin and François Jamar

Université Catholique de Louvain, Brussels, Belgium

Introduction

Fever (or pyrexia) of unknown origin (FUO) has for the last 50 years been a major topic of interest for internists. A definite diagnosis for the fever may be difficult to find and in some patients, may never be found. The definition of the clinical situation has evolved over the years in parallel with developments in diagnostic medicine. The progress in medical imaging (but also microbiology, serology, molecular biology) has promoted functional imaging as a complementary modality to, or perhaps even a substitute for, morphological imaging. One of the advantages of functional imaging using radioactive tracers is that a specific function can be observed, although the drawback is that, if this very function is not involved (e.g. neutrophil migration in abscesses), the goal cannot be reached and the patient remains at the start level. Nuclear medicine has therefore tried to develop methods that combine sufficient sensitivity and specificity to circumvent the clinical problem. White blood cells (WBCs) and non-specific human immunoglobulins (HIGs) labeled with either ^{111}In or ^{99m}Tc, ^{67}Ga-citrate and [^{18}F]fluorodeoxyglucose ([^{18}F]FDG) were developed for this purpose and their use is reviewed in this chapter.

Basic knowledge of the clinical problem

FUO has been recognized for decades as an extremely difficult challenge. It encompasses a number of clinical situations and diagnoses that cannot be classified as a purely nosological entity. However, final diagnoses in such patients can be as benign as drug-related fever or an autoimmune disorder, or as severe as low-grade septicemia or cancer. Petersdorf and Beeson in the early 1960s proposed a definition of FUO: recurrent fever over 38.3 °C, lasting for 2–3 weeks and undiagnosed after 1 week of inhospital investigation [1]. Owing to the evolution of diagnostic medicine and management habits, this definition was modified to no diagnosis after appropriate inpatient (3 days) or outpatient (2 weeks) evaluation [2]. The effect of this change was to eliminate the benign pyrexia syndromes and other benign causes of fever. Following the HIV infection epidemics, the criteria were further changed and Durack and Street proposed the following classification: classic FUO (in non-immunocompromised patients), neutropenic FUO, nosocomial FUO and FUO associated with HIV infection [3]. This classification does not include specific entities for non-HIV-related immunocompromised patients or postoperative fever.

Diagnostic Imaging of Infections and Inflammatory Diseases: A Multidisciplinary Approach, First Edition. Edited by Alberto Signore and Ana María Quintero.
© 2014 John Wiley & Sons, Inc. Published 2014 by John Wiley & Sons, Inc.

Diagnosis in FUO patients is challenging because fever may be a very atypical expression of the underlying disease. Over 200 diagnoses are to be considered and these typically are divided into four groups: infection, neoplasia, non-infectious inflammatory disorders (e.g. granulomatous diseases, arthritis, vasculitis and others) and no final diagnosis [4]. The first three categories account for approximately 50% of patients, with no final diagnosis found in the remaining 50% of cases [5]. It is noteworthy that the spectrum of FUO changed between the 1960s and 1990s with fewer cases of infection and malignancy in the latter decade and more inflammatory fever and undiagnosed cases [6]. Interestingly, patients with no final diagnosis have a good prognosis [1,2,7–9]. Other series report more cancers and infection as the cause of fever in up to 50%. The distribution of causes obviously depends on the local epidemiology, e.g. the high prevalence of tuberculosis (TB) in some populations [10–12], but also on changing epidemiology with time: fever related to HIV infection for instance was unknown in the initial reports on FUO and has been excluded from later publications on true FUO, as it was by then considered to be a separate entity. Further, it must be kept in mind that some patients present with rare manifestations of common diseases, a feature that was recognized a long time ago by Petersdorf and Beeson [1].

It is therefore important to establish diagnostic criteria that allow for a rapid but also reasonable approach to an acceptable diagnosis, i.e. a diagnosis that can be substantiated by sufficient clinical evidence, even in the absence of formal proof. Such criteria were established for true FUO patients by a multicenter effort of Dutch internists who developed a comprehensive algorithm including potential diagnostic clues (PDCs) [5,8]. PDCs are defined as all localizing signs, symptoms or abnormalities pointing towards a specific diagnosis. They must be collected along with a systematic review of the medical history, current symptoms, clinical examination and obligatory diagnostic tests, including standard laboratory tests, serology, blood and urine microbiology, tuberculin test, chest X-ray and abdominal ultrasound (US) or computed tomography (CT) scan. PDCs can be misleading but they often help to limit the number of possible diagnoses. In patients without PDCs, fundoscopy and cryoglobulins are found useful in the early phase of the work-up; in patients older than 55 years, temporal

artery biopsy is useful in a later phase, as are abdominal and chest CT and bone marrow biopsy, although Mourad et al. argued against the latter procedure because of its low yield (<2%) [6]. Although CT and MRI are commonly used in FUO patients, no systematic research has been prospectively undertaken in these patients.

Besides true FUO as described above, a number of clinical presentations may be associated with elevated inflammatory markers, leukocyte counts and/or fever. In some patients with fever and a previous medical history such as diabetes mellitus or recent surgery, there is a strong suspicion that fever is related to infection, although evidence is lacking. These patients are sometimes included in FUO series but should rather be classified as having *occult infection* [13].

Finally, it is unclear from the literature on nuclear medicine studies, especially retrospective studies, whether strict FUO criteria were applied to all patients, as illustrated by the statement by Hilson *et al.* that "The PUO had been present for several days to several weeks, and routine investigations including blood . . . had not determined its origin" [14]. This must be kept in mind when comparing studies. Sarcoidosis is a good example of the need for this, since some patients will present with true FUO whereas others may have fever and other features suggesting a granulomatous disorder (e.g. cutaneous or eye involvement).

A comprehensive meta-analysis was published by Mourad *et al.* on the diagnostic value of several tests in the work-up of FUO [6]. This analysis together with recent reports of diagnostic algorithms may help the reader to better understand the diagnostic strategy applied in this condition [5,15]. These data will not be discussed further as this chapter focuses on nuclear medicine techniques in FUO and related disorders.

The clinical questions

The use of functional imaging in FUO is directed to obtaining a rapid diagnosis or clues toward it. It is anticipated that when the diagnostic scope is wide, the sensitivity and specificity will not be as high as it might be when a very precise question is being asked, such as infection of orthopedic hardware. The questions raised in the following sections can be summarized as:

• What can nuclear medicine offer in FUO?

• Can nuclear medicine provide an *all-purpose radiotracer* that will help most patients or do more specific techniques need to be recommended?

• Is nuclear medicine able to help in assessing the effect of treatment and detecting potential treatment failure?

Methodological considerations

Several tracers have been proposed for the diagnosis of FUO. The most widely used are ^{67}Ga-citrate, ^{111}In-labeled WBCs, ^{99m}Tc-labeled antigranulocyte monoclonal antibodies (anti-G mAbs), ^{111}In- and ^{99m}Tc-labeled human non-specific immunoglobulins (HIGs) and, more recently, [^{18}F]FDG. Table 16.1 summarizes the characteristics of each tracer. It is clear that radiolabeled immunoglobulins and ^{67}Ga-citrate are not the optimal choice. The effective doses necessitate reducing the injected activities for labeled WBCs. [^{18}F]FDG and labeled mAbs have a better dosimetric profile (but note that the dose from concomitant CT must also be considered). Hybrid imaging combining a nuclear scan with a CT scan can be used with all tracers but has not been reported for labeled immunoglobulins. Nevertheless, in most cases, whole-body imaging is required to optimize the probability of finding a clue to diagnosis. None of the methods described has specific contraindications, but careful identification of possible pregnancy is necessary in all female patients. When using radiolabeled monoclonal antibodies, the risk of human antimouse antibodies (HAMAs) should be kept in mind in patients previously exposed to similar (non-human) antibodies. It is essential to fully explore the clinical records of the patient, not only for reporting but also for adapting the imaging protocol to the individual situation: for instance, in a patient with a previous history of a total knee prosthesis and FUO, the [^{18}F]FDG-PET scan must include the knees in the field of view.

Normal findings and artifacts

Because the search for the cause of FUO implies whole-body scanning, extensive knowledge of the normal biodistribution of the tracers is necessary for appropriate reporting. The uptake in normal organs and potential artifacts are described in Table 16.2. In a clinical setting where every organ can be involved, it must be kept in mind that sites of normal uptake may in turn become sites of abnormal uptake because of increased/decreased activity or unexpected asymmetry. In addition, every abnormal uptake may not indicate the cause of FUO and may potentially be misleading. For instance, the serendipitous finding of a small tumor in a patient with an inflammatory disorder can be regarded as a true positive finding in that it discloses something that actually exists and can be confirmed, or as a false positive in that it points towards a pathology that does not explain the patient's symptoms. This is especially true with [^{18}F]FDG-PET.

Pathological findings and significance

Findings in FUO

^{67}Ga-citrate

This tracer is highly non-specific but for many years was almost the only tracer to be considered in FUO. ^{67}Ga-citrate binds to several extracellular and intracellular targets, such as transferrin and lactoferrin (in neutrophils). By its very non-specific nature, ^{67}Ga-citrate proved useful in infection (e.g. spondylodiscitis and liver abscesses), inflammation [e.g. sarcoidosis (Figure 16.1) and rheumatoid arthritis] and cancer (e.g. lymphoma and hepatoma). Its poor physical properties are a major drawback, but the major problem is a very complex biodistribution with a slow blood clearance, necessitating delayed acquisitions of up to 3 days post injection. ^{67}Ga-citrate also suffers from a very high effective dose, i.e. 22 mSv for a standard activity of 220 MBq [16].

Limited prospective experience was gained in FUO using ^{67}Ga-citrate. Results were rather disappointing even if initial reports in the 1970s were enthusiastic [14,17]. Two large retrospective studies and two prospective comparisons with [^{18}F]FDG are available [18–21]. Knockaert *et al.* reported in 1994 a large series of 145 patients in whom 46 turned out not to have a final diagnosis [18]. The ^{67}Ga-citrate scan was abnormal in 82 patients but useful only in 42 (29% of the recruited patients). US and CT scanning were only useful in 6% and 14%, respectively. Interestingly, only one-third of patients with normal scanning ended up with a final diagnosis. Habib *et al.* were less fortunate by ending with 41 abnormal scans amongst 102 patients, but only 21 of these were considered useful and only two decisive with regards to the

Table 16.1 General characteristics of radiopharmaceuticals used in fever of unknown origin

	^{67}Ga-citrate	^{111}In-labeled WBC	^{111}Tc-WBC	^{99m}Tc-mAb	^{111}In-HIG	^{99m}Tc-HIG	[^{18}F]FDG
Emission	Gamma	Gamma	Gamma	Gamma	Gamma	Gamma	Positron
Energy (keV)	93–300*	173 and 245	140	140	173 and 245	140	511 (γ)
Half-life (hours)	78	67	6	6	67	6	1.83
Availability	Unrestricted	Specialized	Specialized	Unrestricted°	Limited**	Limited**	Specialized°
Preparation	No	In vitro	In vitro	Cold kit	In-house	In-house	No
Imaging time (minutes)	60–90	60–90	60–90	45–60	60–90	60	15–30
Time to diagnosis	3 days	1 day	4–24 hours	4–24 hours	1–2 days	4–24 hours	3 hours
Biodistribution	Complex	Simple	Complex	Simple	Complex	Complex	Complex
Image quality	Poor	Good	Good	Good	Fair	Good	High

*Higher energy peak of 394 keV is usually not used for imaging.
**Labeled HIG is not available commercially and should be prepared locally.
°Availability or use depends on marketing authorization in each country.

Table 16.2 Normal distribution of radiopharmaceuticals used in fever of unknown origin at usual imaging time

	^{67}Ga-citrate	^{111}In-labeled WBC	^{99m}Tc-labeled WBC	^{99m}Tc-mAb	^{111}In-HIG	^{99m}Tc-HIG	$[^{18}F]$FDG
Blood vessels	Up to 48 hours	None after 6 hours	None after 6 hours	None after 6 hours	Up to 48 hours	Up to 24 hours	None after 90 minutes
Kidney	+/++	−	+	(+)	+/++	++	++
Liver	++	+	+	+	++	+	+
Spleen	(+)	++	++	++	+	+	(+)
Bone marrow	(+)	++	++	++	+	−	−
Bowel	+/+++	−	After 3–4 hours	−	(+)	−	+/++
Urine (bladder)	+	−	+	+	+	++	++
Salivary glands	+	−	−	−	−	−	−
Bone	+	−	−	−	−	−	−
Artifacts	None	Swallowed WBCs in bowel	Non-specific bowel activity	−	−	Thyroid, stomach	Brown fat, muscle, brain, myocardium

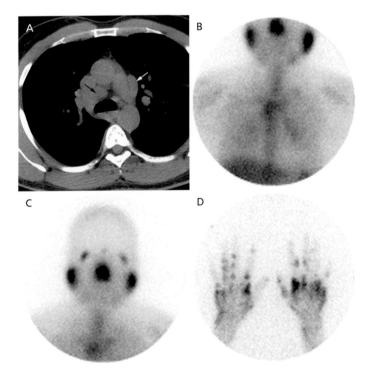

Figure 16.1 Patient with sarcoidosis imaged with ^{67}Ga-citrate. (A) CT scanning shows abnormal lymph nodes in the mediastinum (arrows). (B) These are positive on the ^{67}Ga-citrate scan, more intensely on the left side. (C) The scan also discloses the so-called *Panda sign*, i.e. increased uptake in the lachrymal and salivary glands and (D) intense joint uptake related to sarcoidosis arthritis.

general work-up [19]. Meller *et al.* studied 20 patients prospectively with ^{67}Ga-citrate compared to $[^{18}F]$FDG coincidence imaging and found a diagnosis in 18 patients. $[^{18}F]$FDG appeared superior but ^{67}Ga-citrate, in spite of a lower sensitivity (45% vs. 86% for $[^{18}F]$FDG), displayed an excellent specificity (100% vs. 84% for $[^{18}F]$FDG) [20]. The study by

Blockmans *et al.* in 58 patients again showed a better performance for $[^{18}F]$FDG (using a full-ring scanner) than for ^{67}Ga-citrate [21]. The comparison performed in 40 patients showed that $[^{18}F]$FDG was helpful in 35% of the patients as compared to 25% for ^{67}Ga-citrate, and both methods were non-contributory in 42% of the patients.

Radiolabeled HIG

Since infection or acute inflammation is established as the cause of fever in only a minority of patients [2], ^{111}In-HIG was thought preferable to labeled WBC scanning in suspected cases of infections that are not associated with a neutrophilic infiltrate, such as viral, mycobacterial, fungal and parasitic infections [22]. However, in most studies using ^{111}In-HIG, only pyretic patients with a high likelihood of infection or inflammation were included, which influences the results. In a retrospective analysis of 24 immuno-competent patients with FUO, ^{111}In-HIG proved useful in 10 of 16 patients, whereas in the other patients with normal studies, no infection could be demonstrated. Proven inflammatory processes were missed in only one patient with endocarditis and infection of a renal cyst [23]. In this setting, ^{111}In-HIG has an accuracy that approaches that of ^{111}In-labeled WBCs [24–26]. If localizing symptoms are present, CT may be the preferred technique, whereas [^{18}F]FDG-PET scanning has recently emerged in FUO [27]. ^{99m}Tc-HIG appeared slightly more useful in immunocompromised patients [28].

[111]In-labeled WBCs

Radiolabeling of WBCs (essentially neutrophils) was developed in the 1970s as a specific tracer for infection imaging. Labeling must be *in vitro*, which is a demanding procedure that necessitates both expertise and adequate infrastructure. Neverthe-less, the labeling method is now well standardized and provides high yields and purity [29]. Labeled WBCs have proved very useful in a number of clini-cal indications due to the high specificity of target-ing. Anything other than liver, spleen and bone marrow uptake must be considered abnormal.

In FUO, labeled WBC scanning has not proved very successful because the technique precisely targets neutrophil infiltrates in tissues (diapedesis), mainly as a consequence of the presence of bacte-ria. It was therefore anticipated that ^{111}In-labeled WBCs would perform poorly as an aid to the diag-nosis of FUO. Although it has been effective in iden-tifying patients with infections, these represent only approximately 25% of the patients, and it has failed to diagnose any of the other causes of FUO to any significant extent. Schmidt *et al.* reported that ^{111}In-labeled WBCs were useful in only 22% of 32 patients with fever [30]. Six had infection and one non-Hodgkin's lymphoma. None of the patients with a negative scan developed infection. In a retro-spective study of 28 patients, 11% of whom had pyogenic infection, Davies *et al.* [31] showed a very high negative predictive value (90%) but a disap-pointing positive predictive value of 38% for ^{111}In-labeled WBCs, confirming not only that this scanning performs poorly in FUO but also, when a low prevalence of infection is expected, that the spe-cificity may not be as high as expected, possibly because readers try to give a diagnostic clue in par-ticular situations where this is not appropriate. MacSweeney *et al.* [32] reported slightly better results in a retrospective study of 25 patients, with an overall accuracy of 91% in postoperative fever versus only 52% in spontaneous FUO, which led to the previously described concept of *occult infec-tion* [13] (Figure 16.2). Surprisingly, Tudor *et al.* reported an average distribution of the causes of FUO in 58 patients (33% infection, 41% non-infectious or malignant and 26% no diagnosis) and a very low sensitivity for infection (20%), albeit a high specificity (100%), performances that were similar to US [33]. They also showed that all positive scans were found within 4 weeks of the onset of

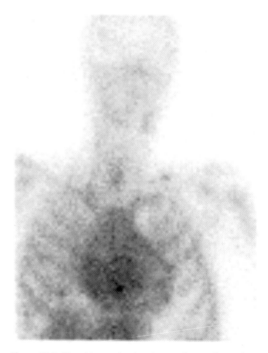

Figure 16.2 Heart transplant patient at 2 months with fever and inflammatory reaction. The ^{111}In-labeled WBC scan discloses intense pericardial activity, corresponding to acute infectious pericarditis. Autopsy performed 2 days later confirmed infection with *Staphylococcus aureus* and *Aspergillus fumigatus*.

symptoms. Data published more recently by Seshadri *et al.* on 54 patients [34] were disappointing as well, with negative and positive predictive values of 56% and 83%, respectively, in postoperative fever (37%) and of 94% and only 20%, respectively, in spontaneous FUO (including two-thirds without a final diagnosis). Kjaer *et al.* reported good results especially in patients with raised C-reactive protein (CRP), regardless of the neutrophil counts [35]. They also found that ^{111}In-labeled WBCs were superior to [18F]FDG, with a sensitivity of 71% and a specificity of 92% in a series of 19 patients, including 37% without a diagnosis and considered true negatives, whereas [18F]FDG showed a high rate of false-positive cases that were not confirmed. Although, [99mTc]-hexamethylpropylene amine oxime (HMPAO)-labeled WBCs are widely used and efficiently labeled [36] (Figure 16.3), no specific report of their use in FUO is available.

[99m]Tc-antigranulocyte monoclonal antibodies

Several antibodies directed against neutrophil membrane receptors have been produced and labeled with [99m]Tc. Such mAbs have the advantage of being available as a ready-to-use kit, avoiding the need for *in vitro* cell separation and labeling. Their biodistribution is hampered by a relatively slow blood clearance, slow penetration in tissues due to their large size and relatively high liver, marrow and spleen uptake. Further, they may induce immunization against murine antibodies (HAMAs), which may preclude their further use in follow-up. BW 250/183, an antibody directed against the nonspecific cross-reacting antigen 95, is commercially available and has been widely used in infections (Figure 16.4). In a retrospective study of 34 patients with FUO [37], the positive and negative predictive values for infection were only 88% and 52%, respectively, in a series where 59% of the patients had infection and only 11% no final diagnosis. In the infection patients, remarkably, the diagnostic performance was poor for endocarditis. Meller *et al.*, in a study of 51 patients, showed that the method was helpful in 27% overall and in only 12 of 18 patients with infection [38]. BW 250/183's use in FUO should be restricted to patients with diagnostic clues pointing towards possible pyogenic infection, e.g. postoperative fever.

[18F]FDG

During the last decade, [18F]FDG has been studied as a potential all-purpose tracer in patients with FUO. [18F]FDG is a positron-emitting labeled analog of glucose that is taken up avidly in many tumor tissues as a consequence of increased expression of membrane glucose transporters (GLUTs) and intracellular hexokinase. Further studies have shown that cells involved in infection and inflammation, especially neutrophils and the monocyte/macrophage family, but also fibroblasts, also express high levels of GLUTs, especially GLUT-1 and -3, leading to the accurate positive diagnosis of inflammatory processes using [18F]FDG imaging. From limited experimental studies, although no single cell has been found to specifically take up the radiolabeled tracer, the technique appears to be able to identify inflammatory and infectious diseases from the glycolytic activity of the cells responsible for the response to the infectious process and to the inflammatory reaction.

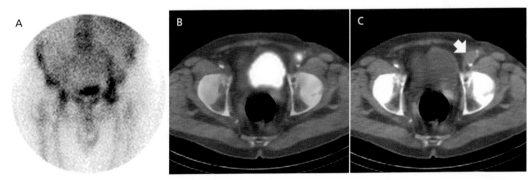

Figure 16.3 ^{99m}Tc-HMPAO-labeled WBC scintigraphy in a patient with an iliofemoral arterial bypass placed 2 months previously and persistent fever. (A) The planar image at 20 hours clearly shows abnormal uptake in the groin. (B) The SPECT/CT fusion image confirms that the labeled WBC uptake corresponds to intraprosthetic uptake. (C) This is anatomically delineated by the CT scan (arrow).

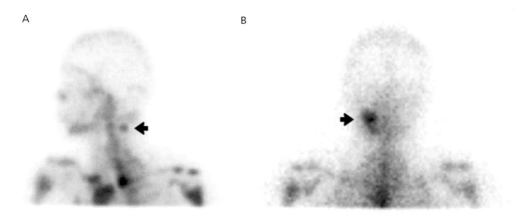

Figure 16.4 (A) Six-hour and (B) 20-hour images obtained after injection of [99mTc]-antigranulocyte antibody (BW 250/183). The early image shows discrete uptake in the middle cervical spine (arrow), whereas the delayed image shows wider uptake with reduced background, corresponding to a *Staphylococcus aureus* cervical abscess secondary to local steroid infiltration.

[18F]FDG-PET using modern scanners is usually coupled to a CT scanner. PET/CT is a rapid technique that allows diagnosis in a few hours after injection. Image quality is high and, with the coupling to the high-resolution morphological imaging of CT, provides high detection accuracy (Figures 16.5 and 16.6).

The biodistribution of [18F]FDG is complex and numerous normal variants of uptake have been described, which should lead to caution when interpreting whole-body scanning. In particular, physiological uptake in the brain, myocardium, skeletal muscle, liver, bowel, bone marrow, brown fat and urinary tract must be considered. Uptake by previously known or occult malignancy should always be considered (see Clinical case 1 below; Figures 16.8 and 16.9). Interestingly, the more recent PET scanners allow rapid imaging with relatively low injected activities, resulting in effective doses in the range of 3.5–7.0 mSv per scan (1.9×10^{-2} mSv/MBq) [39]. It should be noted that if a CT scan is added, the exposure to X-rays must be added to the effective dose.

Numerous reports have described the diagnostic performances of [18F]FDG-PET or PET/CT in FUO. As opposed to oncology studies, the interpretation of the data cannot always be expressed using the classical sensitivity and specificity parameters. These studies, as expected, contained a variable proportion of patients without a final diagnosis, for which sensitivity and specificity are not appropriate

parameters. Therefore, negative and positive predictive values are often calculated.

Table 16.3 presents a summary of studies selected on the basis of the number of recruited patients and a clear presentation of inclusion criteria [20,21,35,40–49]. All studies followed the Durack and Street's criteria [3], sometimes with minor deviations (e.g. temperature >38 °C instead of 38.3 °C, or variations in the duration of in- or outpatient work-up before referral to nuclear medicine). All but two of these studies are single-center and six of the 14 are prospective. One study did not exclude HIV-infected patients (seven of 81 patients), but was included in this presentation since results were very comparable to the average of the other studies [49]. Half of the total 583 patients were imaged using a PET scanner or PET/CT scanner. On average, 35% of the patients ended up with no final diagnosis (8–53%), with PET disclosing abnormal findings in two-thirds of the patients (43–92%). On average, [18F]FDG-PET was helpful in 46% of the patients (16–90%), the percentage being clearly higher when using combined PET/CT (57%) than with PET alone (36%). The wide range of results is certainly related to the different recruitment schedules. Two studies compared [18F]FDG-PET and [67Ga]-citrate scintigraphy and showed that the diagnostic yield of [18F]FDG-PET was higher. Only one study compared [18F]FDG-PET and [111In]-labeled WBC scanning, and showed a better sensitivity and specificity for the latter, mainly related to non-

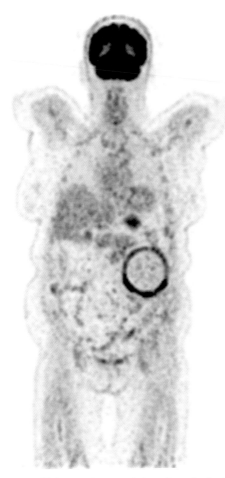

specific [18F]FDG findings considered to be false positives. This study had an intrinsic bias in that patients recruited for [18F]FDG-PET had initially been referred for 111In-labeled WBC scanning. The proportion of patients with infection or inflammation was however in the usual range for such studies, namely 37% (seven of 19 patients).

According to a recent meta-analysis [50], nine studies (four with CT) met the criteria for classic FUO. A final diagnosis was obtained in 242 of the total of 388 patients (62%) and [18F]FDG-PET was positive in 240 patients (62%) and considered helpful in 177 (46%). The statistical analysis of the five [18F]FDG-PET studies without CT gave a pooled sensitivity of 83% (95% CI: 73–90%) and a pooled specificity of 58% (95% CI: 49–66%). This was improved in the four studies that added CT scanning: 98% (95% CI: 94–100%) and 86% (95% CI: 75–93%), respectively. Interestingly, the benefit with CT was mainly related to the reduction in false-positive cases, rather than to the improved anatomical accuracy. Overall, [18F]FDG-PET seemed to perform particularly well in cases of neoplasia (23 cases) and was slightly, but not significantly, less sensitive in infection and non-infectious inflammation (see Clinical case 2 below; Figure 16.10).

In the only prospective multicenter study published so far [42], an analysis of 70 patients with a very rigorous diagnostic algorithm, a final diagnosis was obtained in 35, giving [18F]FDG-PET a positive and negative predictive value of 70% and 92%, respectively, and it was useful in 33% of the entire population. Interestingly, this study demonstrated

Figure 16.5 [18F]FDG-PET coronal view of a patient with fever and raised CRP. A large cystic-shaped image is visible in the left flank, but this cannot be anatomically defined from the PET image.

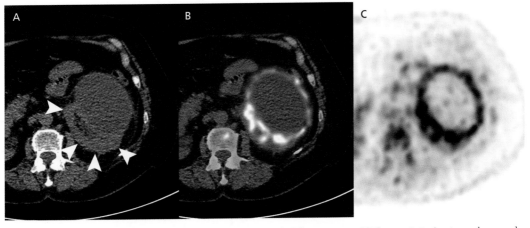

Figure 16.6 Transverse [18F]FDG-PET, fusion and CT slices clearly delineate normal kidney activity (cortex, calyces and pelvis; arrowheads in A), whereas the remaining activity corresponds to an infected benign renal cyst (B and C).

Table 16.3 Summary of studies using FDG-PET or PET/CT in fever of unknown origin

Study	Design (number of patients)	Method	Patients without diagnosis (%)	Abnormal PET findings (%)	PET helpful (%)	Direct comparison
Meller et al. 2000 [20]	Prospective (20)	Dual-head coincidence	2 (10)	13 (65)	11 (55)	$>^{67}$Ga
Blockmans et al. 2001 [21]	Prospective (58)	PET full ring	20 (36)	46 (79)	24 (41)	$>^{67}$Ga
Lorenzen et al. 2001 [40]	Retrospective (16)	PET full ring	3 (18)	12 (75)	11 (69)	
Bleeker-Rovers et al. 2004 [41]	Retrospective (35)	PET full ring	16 (46)	15 (43)	13 (37)	
Kjaer et al. 2004 [35]	Prospective (19)	PET full ring	7 (37)	10 (53)	3 (16)	$<^{111}$In-labeled WBC
Buysschaert et al. 2004 [42]	Prospective (74)	PET full ring	35 (47)	53 (72)	19 (26)	
Bleeker-Rovers et al. 2007 [15]	Prospective multicenter (70)	PET full ring	37 (53)	33 (47)	23 (33)	
Keidar et al. 2008 [43]	Prospective (48)	PET/CT	19 (40)	27 (56)	22 (46)	
Federici et al. 2008 [44]	Retrospective (10)	PET/CT	3 (30)	5 (50)	5 (50)	
Balink et al. 2009 [45]	Retrospective (68)	PET/CT	24 (35)	41 (60)	38 (56)	
Ferda et al. 2009 [46]	Retrospective (48)	PET/CT	4 (8)	44 (92)	43 (90)	
Kei et al. 2010 [47]	Retrospective (12)	PET/CT	5 (42)	7 (58)	5 (42)	
Palosi et al. 2011 [48]	Retrospective (24)	PET/CT	7 (29)	13 (54)	11 (46)	
Kubota et al. 2011 [49]	Retrospective multicenter (81)	PET/CT or PET + CT	22 (27)	52 (64)	42 (52)	
Average (all studies)	583		204 (35)	371 (64)	270 (46)	
Average (PET/CT only)	291		84 (29)	189 (65)	166 (57)	

that [^{18}F]FDG-PET was of limited value in patients in whom fever persisted but erythrocyte sedimentation rate (ESR) and CRP were normal. This was confirmed in another study in which the FUO in six patients with normal ESR, CRP and WBC counts who were true negatives on [^{18}F]FDG-PET/CT, subsequently resolved without further treatment [45]. A Japanese multicenter study, however, showed no correlation between the diagnostic relevance of [^{18}F]FDG-PET and CRP, ESR and WBC counts, suggesting that these parameters are not predictive of the diagnostic performance of PET [49]. It must however be noted that in this study, HIV-infected patients were not excluded from the retrospective analysis, which may have marginally influenced the results.

One study was not included in Table 16.2 [51]: this study retrospectively analyzed the results obtained in 69 children with a mean age of 8.1 years (range: 0.2–18.1 years) in whom a final diagnosis was found in 37 (54%). [^{18}F]FDG-PET or PET/CT was useful to the diagnosis in 45% of the 77 scans; remarkably, 63 (82%) of the scans were abnormal with a different distribution from that in adults, *viz* only 10 (14%) and four (6%) cases of infection and neoplasm, respectively. These data are most encouraging and should prompt prospective studies in the field, provided appropriate inclusion criteria are defined to target a non-oncological pediatric population.

Although the number of evaluable studies remains limited, there is now evidence that [^{18}F]FDG-PET/CT should be considered a first-line diagnostic tool in patients with FUO in whom conventional diagnostic procedures have not been successful. This has not been studied prospectively in FUO, but excellent results in the very difficult setting of prolonged fever in the intensive care unit have been reported by Simons *et al.* [52] and should encourage the development of a protocol for [^{18}F]FDG-PET/CT scanning at a very early stage of the work-up of FUO. This may turn out to be highly cost-effective as it may reduce the number of procedures that need to be performed and hence the hospitalization costs. The additional value of combining the whole-body [^{18}F]FDG-PET study with a whole-body CT study with iodinated contrast injection remains to be prospectively evaluated, although data reported by Ferda *et al.* [46] and Balink *et al.* [45] in a retrospective setting are already convincing.

A few methodological points should be made regarding performing and interpreting [^{18}F]FDG-PET/CT in FUO. First, hyperglycemia does not seem to preclude an accurate diagnosis, as may be the case in many cancers [27,53]. Second, steroid therapy should be avoided prior to scanning, especially in elderly patients, since it may cause false negatives in (giant cell) arteritis (GCA) [54] as it efficiently controls the inflammatory process (see Clinical case 3 below; Figure 16.11). Third, although used by some authors, semi-quantitative indices and standard uptake values (SUVs) are not recommended and interpretation should rather rely on visual analysis of combined functional and morphological images; however, it is worth noting that the respective contribution of PET and CT in PET/CT studies has not been studied as such. Finally and most importantly, it must be kept in mind that there is no infallible way of differentiating infection and neoplasia in discrete foci of abnormal uptake. This drawback is inherent to the strategic choice (i.e. lack of specificity) and in FUO is by far outweighed by the high sensitivity!

Atypical FUO and related disorders

Sarcoidosis

[^{18}F]FDG-PET has emerged as a very valuable tool in evaluating sarcoidosis. The whole-body tomographic capability together with the physical properties of [^{18}F]FDG-PET as compared with ^{67}Ga-citrate scintigraphy explains why the latter has been almost completely abandoned in this indication [55]. The method is well suited for whole-body evaluation of this very polymorphic disorder (see Clinical Case 2 below; Figure 16.10). It is useful for the diagnosis and staging of the disease at a number of anatomical sites [56,57] and seems to be helpful for assessing the effect of treatment, especially with steroids [58]. It is, however, essential to keep in mind that [^{18}F]FDG-PET/CT will not substitute for pathology: in particular, the differential diagnosis with lymphoma is impossible with certainty and, therefore, a pathological diagnosis will be required in patients with enlarged lymph nodes. [^{18}F]FDG-PET/CT may, however, help to identify the correct and easiest node to biopsy.

Vasculitis

In inflammatory or immune conditions, [^{18}F]FDG-PET has proved very promising for assessing large-vessel arteritides, such as GCA and Takayasu's disease. This has been observed in dedicated studies and in subsets of studies in patients with FUO [27]. The sensitivity (77–92%) and specificity (89–100%) were found to be high in untreated patients with GCA and inflammatory markers (see Clinical case 3 below; Figure 16.11). A lower sensitivity was observed under immunosuppressive therapy (e.g. steroids). It must be noted that [^{18}F]FDG-PET does not allow reliable diagnosis and monitoring of localized temporal arteritis [59].

HIV-related infection(s) (see also Chapter 15)
During the first years of the HIV infection epidemic, ^{67}Ga-citrate and later ^{99m}Tc-HIG (which is no longer available) were used and were found to be helpful [28]. Over recent years, [^{18}F]FDG-PET has emerged as the method of choice.

In AIDS, there is a typical and well-defined anatomical sequence to the appearance of [^{18}F]FDG-avid lymph nodes, starting with those in the upper part of the torso and then involving the lower part of the body [60]. In addition, the degree of uptake is related to viral load [61] and this increases in the event of treatment withdrawal [62]. This pattern has been hypothesized to be related to a forced homing of CD4+ lymphocytes in lymph nodes [61]. Furthermore, a correlation between the markers of AIDS progression (such as the percentage of CD8+/CD38+/RO+ T cells) and [^{18}F]FDG uptake in non-treated patients indicates that prognostic information could be gathered from [^{18}F]FDG-PET. [^{18}F]FDG uptake has been shown to be strongly associated with response to antiretroviral treatment [63]. In addition, ^{18}F-FDG-PET can play a role in the management of infectious and oncological complications of AIDS, such as opportunistic infections, lymphoma, Kaposi's sarcoma and AIDS-related dementia complex [60,64]. Nevertheless, the involvement of lymph nodes related to viral load may complicate the interpretation of results [65]. Therefore, biological data and treatment and personal history of the patient are mandatory for correct interpretation.

Tuberculosis (see also Chapter 15)
[^{18}F]FDG-PET has not been widely used in tuberculosis (TB). An interesting pilot study [66] developed a dual-time point method to better characterize TB involvement in HIV-negative patients. It is, however,

essential to keep in mind that [^{18}F]FDG-PET/CT will not substitute for pathology: in particular, the differential diagnosis with lymphoma or sarcoidosis is impossible with certainty with [^{18}F]FDG-PET/CT and a pathological diagnosis will be required in patients with enlarged lymph nodes. [^{18}F]FDG-PET/CT may, however, help to identify the correct and easiest node to biopsy. Other granulomatous diseases such as sarcoidosis, coccidioidomycosis, histoplasmosis and cystomycosis can be misleading [67].

Role in therapy follow-up and patient management

The impact of nuclear medicine techniques, especially [^{18}F]FDG-PET and labeled WBC scanning, on patient management is illustrated in Table 16.3. So far, there is very little evidence, if any, that [^{18}F]FDG-PET may have a prominent role in assessing response to treatment in FUO patients. An example is given in Figure 16.7, which is of a patient with previously treated septicemia and residual inflammatory signs, but persistent low-grade mastoiditis. In sarcoidosis, [^{18}F]FDG-PET can be useful for monitoring therapy response during and after steroid therapy, as reported in a series of 20 patients by Braun *et al.* [68]. The quantitative relationship between [^{18}F]FDG uptake and inflammatory remnants allows SUV to be used to evaluate the response during steroid therapy or after completion of treatment. In vasculitis, such as GCA, [^{18}F]FDG-PET has proved useful in assessing the extent of the disease and in monitoring the disease activity during therapy. The well-established relationship between viral load and [^{18}F]FDG uptake in AIDS allows [^{18}F]FDG-PET to be used in treatment monitoring and the detection of AIDS-related complications. As yet there is insufficient evidence to establish the role of [^{18}F]FDG-PET in treatment monitoring or follow-up in TB, although preliminary data are encouraging.

Conclusion

Many nuclear medicine methods have been used over the last 40 years in FUO. Nowadays, ^{111}In- or ^{99m}Tc-labeled WBCs and ^{99m}Tc-labeled mAbs are indicated in patients with diagnostic clues towards infection, e.g. longstanding postoperative fever. In true FUO and in patients with no PDCs towards

Figure 16.7 (A) [^{18}F]FDG-PET and (B) [^{18}F]FDG-PET/CT fusion in a patient treated for septicemia with *S. pneumoniae*; this was responsible for meningitis, otitis media and mastoiditis. After treatment, fever persisted and inflammatory markers remained elevated; MRI showed residual fluid in the mastoid, of undetermined significance. The [^{18}F]FDG-PET/CT image clearly indicates a focus of increased metabolic activity in the mastoid bone, suggesting persistent infection.

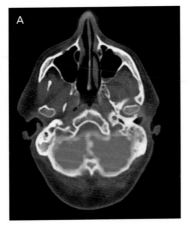
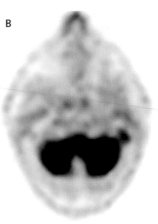

infection, [^{18}F]FDG-PET/CT is highly recommended as the method of choice [69]. This group encompasses not only patients in whom neoplasms, inflammatory disorders (e.g. vasculitis, sarcoidosis, systemic disease) and infections with limited neutrophil infiltrates (e.g. TB or opportunistic viral and fungal infections, notably in HIV-positive patients) will eventually be found, but also patients in whom [^{18}F]FDG-PET will be negative with a high negative predictive value. In these patients, who can account for up to 50% of the population studied, no final diagnosis will be found, but importantly, the prognosis is usually very good, even without treatment. The good diagnostic performances of [^{18}F]FDG-PET in such disorders suggest that it may also become a good tool for patient follow-up after therapy. This has been demonstrated in patients treated with steroids and other immunosuppressive therapies for vasculitis and in HIV-positive patients in whom a relationship between [^{18}F]FDG uptake and changes in retroviral load have been found. Other studies are needed to demonstrate the role of [^{18}F]FDG-PET in assessing response to therapy in FUO with other underlying disorders.

References

1. Petersdorf RG, Beeson PB. Fever of unexplained origin: report on 100 cases. *Medicine* 1961;40:1–30.
2. Larson EB, Featherstone HJ, Petersdorf RG. Fever of undetermined origin: diagnosis and follow up of 105 cases, 1970–1980. *Medicine* 1982;61:269–292.
3. Durack DT, Street AC. Fever of unknown origin-reexamined and redefined. *Curr Clin Top Infect Dis* 1991;11:35–51.
4. Arnow PM, Flaherty JP. Fever of unknown origin. *Lancet* 1997;350:575–580.
5. Bleeker-Rovers CP, Vos FJ, de Kleijn EM *et al.* A prospective multicenter study on fever of unknown origin: the yield of a structured diagnostic protocol. *Medicine* 2007;86:26–38.
6. Mourad O, Palda V, Detsky AS. A comprehensive evidence-based approach to fever of unknown origin. *Arch Intern Med* 2003;163:545–551.
7. Iikuni Y, Okada J, Kondo H, Kashiwazaki S. Current fever of unknown origin 1982–1992. *Intern Med* 1994;33:67–73.
8. de Kleijn EM, van Lier HJ, van der Meer JW. Fever of unknown origin (FUO). II. Diagnostic procedures in a prospective multicenter study of 167 patients. The Netherlands FUO Study Group. *Medicine* 1997;76: 401–414.
9. Knockaert DC, Vanderschueren S, Blockmans D. Fever of unknown origin in adults: 40 years on. *J Intern Med* 2003;253:263–275.
10. Ergönül O, Willke A, Azap A, Tekeli E. Revised definition of 'fever of unknown origin': limitations and opportunities. *J Infect* 2005;50:1–5.
11. Saltoglu N, Tasova Y, Midikli D, Aksu HS, Sanli A, Dündar IH. Fever of unknown origin in Turkey: evaluation of 87 cases during a nine-year-period of study. *J Infect* 2004;48:81–85.
12. Tabak F, Mert A, Celik AD *et al.* Fever of unknown origin in Turkey. *Infection* 2003;31:417–420.
13. Peters AM. Localising the cause of an undiagnosed fever. *Eur J Nucl Med* 1996;23:239–242.
14. Hilson AJ, Maisey MN. Gallium-67 scanning in pyrexia of unknown origin. *Br Med J* 1979;24:1330–1331.
15. Bleeker-Rovers CP, Vos FJ, Mudde AH *et al.* A prospective multi-centre study of the value of FDG-PET as part of a structured diagnostic protocol in patients with fever of unknown origin. *Eur J Nucl Med Mol Imaging* 2007;34:694–703.

16. ICRP. Radiation dose to patients from radiopharmaceuticals (addendum 2 to ICRP publication 53). *Ann ICRP* 1998;28:1–126.

17. Lavender JP, Lowe J, Barker JR, Burn JI, Chaudhri MA. Gallium 67 citrate scanning in neoplastic and inflammatory lesions. *Br J Radiol* 1971;44:361–366.

18. Knockaert DC, Mortelmans LA, De Roo MC, Bobbaers HJ. Clinical value of gallium-67 scintigraphy in evaluation of fever of unknown origin. *Clin Infect Dis* 1994;18:601–605.

19. Habib GS, Masri R, Ben-Haim S. The utility of gallium scintigraphy in the evaluation of fever of unknown origin. *Isr Med Assoc J* 2004;6:463–466.

20. Meller J, Altenvoerde G, Munzel U *et al*. Fever of unknown origin: prospective comparison of [^{18}F]FDG imaging with a double-head coincidence camera and gallium-67 citrate SPECT. *Eur J Nucl Med* 2000;27:1617–1625.

21. Blockmans D, Knockaert D, Maes A *et al*. Clinical value of [(18)F]fluoro-deoxyglucose positron emission tomography for patients with fever of unknown origin. *Clin Infect Dis* 2001;32:191–196.

22. Peters AM. The use of nuclear medicine in infections. *Br J Radiol* 1994;71:252–261.

23. de Kleijn EM, Oyen WJ, Claessens RA, Corstens FHM. Utility of scintigraphic methods in patients with fever of unknown origin. *Arch Intern Med* 1995;155:1989–1994.

24. Oyen WJG, Claessens RAMJ, van der Meer JWM, Corstens FHM. Detection of subacute infectious foci with In-111-labeled autologous leucocytes and In-111-labeled human nonspecific immunoglobulin G: A prospective comparative study. *J Nucl Med* 1991;32:1854–1860.

25. Oyen WJG, Claessens RAMJ, van Horn JR, van der Meer JWM, Corstens FHM. Scintigraphic detection of bone and joint infections with indium-111-labeled nonspecific polyclonal human immunoglobulin G. *J Nucl Med* 1990;31:403–412.

26. Datz FL, Anderson CE, Ahluwalia R *et al*. The efficacy of indium-111- polyclonal IgG for the detection of infection and inflammation. *J Nucl Med* 1994;35:74–83.

27. Meller J, Sahlmann CO, Gurocak O, Liersch T, Meller B. FDG-PET in patients with fever of unknown origin: the importance of diagnosing large vessel vasculitis. *Q J Nucl Med Mol Imaging* 2009;53:51–63.

28. Buscombe JR, Miller RF, Lui D, Ell PJ. Combined ^{67}Ga and ^{99Tcm}-human immunoglobulin imaging in human immunodeficiency virus-positive patients with fever of undetermined origin. *Nucl Med Commun* 1991;12:583–592.

29. Roca M, de Vries EF, Jamar F, Israel O, Signore A. Guidelines for the labelling of leucocytes with (111) In-oxine. Inflammation/Infection Taskgroup of the European Association of Nuclear Medicine. *Eur J Nucl Med Mol Imaging* 2010;37:835–841.

30. Schmidt KG, Rasmussen JW, Sørensen PG, Wedebye IM. Indium-111-granulocyte scintigraphy in the evaluation of patients with fever of undetermined origin. *Scand J Infect Dis* 1987;19:339–345.

31. Davies SG, Garvie NW. The role of indium-labelled leukocyte imaging in pyrexia of unknown origin. *Br J Radiol* 1990;63:850–854.

32. MacSweeney JE, Peters AM, Lavender JP. Indium labelled leucocyte scanning in pyrexia of unknown origin. *Clin Radiol* 1990;42:414–417.

33. Tudor GR, Finlay DB, Belton I. The value of indium-111-labelled leucocyte imaging and ultrasonography in the investigation of pyrexia of unknown origin. *Br J Radiol* 1997;70:918–922.

34. Seshadri N, Solanki CK, Balan K. Utility of ^{111}In-labelled leucocyte scintigraphy in patients with fever of unknown origin in an era of changing disease spectrum and investigational techniques. *Nucl Med Commun* 2008;29:277–282.

35. Kjaer A, Lebech AM, Eigtved A, Hojgaard L. Fever of unknown origin: prospective comparison of diagnostic value of ^{18}F-FDG PET and ^{111}In-granulocyte scintigraphy. *Eur J Nucl Med Mol Imaging* 2004;31:622–626.

36. de Vries EF, Roca M, Jamar F, Israel O, Signore A. Guidelines for the labelling of leucocytes with (99m) Tc-HMPAO. Inflammation/Infection Taskgroup of the European Association of Nuclear Medicine. *Eur J Nucl Med Mol Imaging* 2010;37:842–848.

37. Becker W, Dölkemeyer U, Gramatzki M, Schneider MU, Scheele J, Wolf F. Use of immunoscintigraphy in the diagnosis of fever of unknown origin. *Eur J Nucl Med* 1993;20:1078–1083.

38. Meller J, Ivancevic V, Conrad M, Gratz S, Munz DL, Becker W. Clinical value of immunoscintigraphy in patients with fever of unknown origin. *J Nucl Med* 1998;39:1248–1253.

39. ICRP. Radiation dose to patients from radiopharmaceuticals. Addendum 3 to ICRP Publication 53. ICRP Publication 106. *Ann ICRP* 2008;38:1–197.

40. Lorenzen J, Buchert R, Bohuslavizki KH. Value of FDG PET in patients with fever of unknown origin. *Nucl Med Commun* 2001;22:779–783.

41. Bleeker-Rovers CP, de Kleijn EM, Corstens FH, Van Der Meer JW, Oyen WJ. Clinical value of FDG PET in patients with fever of unknown origin and patients suspected of focal infection or inflammation. *Eur J Nucl Med Mol Imaging* 2004;31:29–37.

42. Buysschaert I, Vanderschueren S, Blockmans D, Mortelmans L, Knockaert D. Contribution of (18) fluoro-deoxyglucose positron emission tomography to the work-up of patients with fever of unknown origin. *Eur J Intern Med* 2004 15:151–156.

43. Keidar Z, Gurman-Balbir A, Gaitini D, Israel O. Fever of unknown origin: the role of ^{18}F-FDG PET/CT. *J Nucl Med* 2008;49:1980–1985.

44. Federici L, Blondet C, Imperiale A *et al*. Value of (18) F-FDG-PET/CT in patients with fever of unknown origin and unexplained prolonged inflammatory syndrome: a single centre analysis experience. *Int J Clin Pract* 2010;64:55–60.

45. Balink H, Collins J, Bruyn GA, Gemmel F. F-18 FDG PET/CT in the diagnosis of fever of unknown origin. *Clin Nucl Med* 2009;34:862–868.

46. Ferda J, Ferdová E, Záhlava J, Matejovic M, Kreuzberg B. Fever of unknown origin: A value of (18)F-FDG-PET/CT with integrated full diagnostic isotropic CT imaging. *Eur J Radiol* 2009;73:518–525.

47. Kei PL, Kok TY, Padhy AK, Ng DC, Goh AS. [^{18}F] FDG PET/CT in patients with fever of unknown origin: a local experience. *Nucl Med Commun* 2010;31: 788–792.

48. Pelosi E, Skanjeti A, Penna D, Arena V. Role of integrated PET/CT with [(18)F]-FDG in the management of patients with fever of unknown origin: a single-centre experience. *Radiol Med* 2011;116: 809–820.

49. Kubota K, Nakamoto Y, Tamaki N *et al*. FDG-PET for the diagnosis of fever of unknown origin: a Japanese multi-center study. *Ann Nucl Med* 2011;25: 355–364.

50. Dong MJ, Zhao K, Liu ZF, Wang GL, Yang SY, Zhou GJ. A meta-analysis of the value of fluorodeoxyglucose-PET/PET-CT in the evaluation of fever of unknown origin. *Eur J Radiol* 2011;80:834–844.

51. Jasper N, Däbritz J, Frosch M, Loeffler M, Weckesser M, Foell D. Diagnostic value of [(18)F]-FDG PET/CT in children with fever of unknown origin or unexplained signs of inflammation. *Eur J Nucl Med Mol Imaging* 2010;37:136–145.

52. Simons KS, Pickkers P, Bleeker-Rovers CP, Oyen WJ, van der Hoeven JG. F-18-fluorodeoxyglucose positron emission tomography combined with CT in critically ill patients with suspected infection. *Intensive Care Med* 2010;36:504–511.

53. Rabkin Z, Israel O, Keidar Z. Do hyperglycemia and diabetes affect the incidence of false-negative ^{18}F-FDG PET/CT studies in patients evaluated for infection or inflammation and cancer? A comparative analysis. *J Nucl Med* 2010;51:1015–1020.

54. Meller J, Sahlmann CO, Scheel AK. ^{18}F-FDG PET and PET/CT in fever of unknown origin. *J Nucl Med* 2007; 48:35–45.

55. Nishiyama Y, Yamamoto Y, Fukunaga K *et al*. Comparative evaluation of ^{18}F-FDG PET and ^{67}Ga scintigraphy in patients with sarcoidosis. *J Nucl Med* 2006;47:1571–1576.

56. Bonardel G, Carmoi T, Gontier E *et al*. Use of positron emission tomography in sarcoidosis. *Rev Med Interne* 2011;32:101–108.

57. Teirstein AS, Machac J, Almeida O, Lu P, Padilla ML, Iannuzzi MC. Results of 188 whole-body fluorodeoxyglucose positron emission tomography scans in 137 patients with sarcoidosis. *Chest* 2007;132: 1949–1953.

58. Keijsers RG, Verzijlbergen FJ, Oyen WJ *et al*. ^{18}F-FDG PET, genotype-corrected ACE and sIL-2R in newly diagnosed sarcoidosis. *Eur J Nucl Med Mol Imaging* 2009;36:1131–1137.

59. Bossert M, Prati C, Balblanc JC, Lohse A, Wendling D. Aortic involvement in giant cell arteritis: Current data. *Joint Bone Spine* 2011;78:246–251.

60. Sathekge M, Goethals I, Maes A, van de Wiele C. Positron emission tomography in patients suffering from HIV-1 infection. *Eur J Nucl Med Mol Imaging* 2009;36:1176–1184.

61. Sathekge M, Maes A, Kgomo M, Van de Wiele C. Fluorodeoxyglucose uptake by lymph nodes of HIV patients is inversely related to CD4 cell count. *Nucl Med Commun* 2010;31:137–140.

62. Bleeker-Rovers CP, Vos FJ, Corstens FH, Oyen WJ. Imaging of infectious diseases using [^{18}F] fluorodeoxyglucose PET. *Q J Nucl Med Mol Imaging* 2008;52: 17–29.

63. Lucignani G, Orunesu E, Cesari M *et al*. FDG-PET imaging in HIV-infected subjects: relation with therapy and immunovirological variables. *Eur J Nucl Med Mol Imaging* 2009;36:640–647.

64. Castaigne C, Tondeur M, de Wit S, Hildebrand M, Clumeck N, Dusart M. Clinical value of FDG-PET/CT for the diagnosis of human immunodeficiency virus-associated fever of unknown origin: a retrospective study. *Nucl Med Commun* 2009;30:41–47.

65. Sathekge M, Maes A, Kgomo M, Pottel H, Stolz A, Van De Wiele C. FDG uptake in lymph-nodes of HIV+ and tuberculosis patients: implications for cancer staging. *Q J Nucl Med Mol Imaging* 2010;54:698–703.

66. Sathekge M, Maes A, Kgomo M, Stoltz A, Pottel H, Van de Wiele C. Impact of FDG PET on the management of TBC treatment. A pilot study. *Nuklearmedizin* 2010;49:35–40.

67. Bouyadlou S, Conti PS. Unknown primary tumors. In: Conti PS, Cham DK. (eds) *PET-CT: A Case Based Approach*. New York: Springer Verlag, 2005.

68. Braun JJ, Kessler R, Constantinesco A, Imperiale A. ^{18}F-FDG PET/CT in sarcoidosis management: review and report of 20 cases. *Eur J Nucl Med Mol Imaging* 2008;35:1537–1543.

69. Glaudemans AW, Signore A. FDG-PET/CT in infections: the imaging method of choice? *Eur J Nucl Med Mol Imaging* 2010;37:1986–1991.

Clinical cases

Case 1

A 55-year-old male with an extensive medical history: right nephrectomy with renal transplantation for polycystic kidney disease, TB, inferior wall myocardial infarction, carcinoid tumor of the main bile duct treated surgically, known stable metastasis in liver segment IV.

He was admitted to the emergency room for long-standing hyperthermia and on admission his temperature was 40°C. His respiratory distress required assisted ventilation. Sepsis with *Escherichia coli*, *Klebsiella pneumoniae* and *Streptococcus bovis* was diagnosed and treated with broad-spectrum antibiotics.

After clinical stabilization, MRI, ^{111}In-labeled WBC scanning and [18F]FDG-PET imaging were performed in search of the responsible reservoir. PET showed, in addition to the known carcinoid metastasis in the liver (Figure 16.8), a definite hot spot with a photopenic center in the large photopenic zone of the polycystic left kidney, consistent with a cyst infection. ^{111}In-labeled WBC imaging confirmed a clear neutrophilic accumulation in this area (Figure 16.9A–D), while MRI showed an increased T1 signal consistent with a cyst infection (Figure 16.9E). The lesion that showed positive in liver segment IV on MRI appeared negative on ^{111}In-labeled WBC scanning. After antibiotic therapy, a left nephrectomy was performed to prevent further infection.

Teaching points

• The main difficulty with this patient was the identification of the origin of sepsis. With several past surgeries, infection of the renal graft, an angiocholitis due to the bile duct surgery, or a cyst infection of the remaining left kidney were all possible. Imaging procedures were able to identify the source of infection and to further adapt treatment.

• [18F]FDG-PET proved non-specific by showing equal uptake in both the liver segment IV lesion and the renal abscess, whereas ^{111}In-labeled WBCs were specific in identifying the abscess in the left polycystic kidney.

Case 2

A 66-year-old male with no relevant medical history was diagnosed with rectal cancer after a routine check-up.

Longstanding moderate fever was noted (37.5–38.5°C) A chest CT scan performed for staging purposes showed mediastinal and hilar lymph nodes. Carcinoembryonic antigen (CEA) was not increased, with a value of 9 ng/dL, and the CRP level and hemogram were normal.

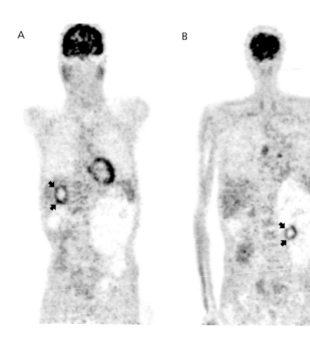

A

B

Figure 16.8 [18F]FDG-PET coronal views. (A) [18F]FDG uptake is seen in the known liver metastasis of the carcinoid tumor (arrows). (B) Peripheral uptake in a left kidney cyst (arrows) is seen. Note the photopenic area surrounding the infected cyst, corresponding to a large left polycystic kidney.

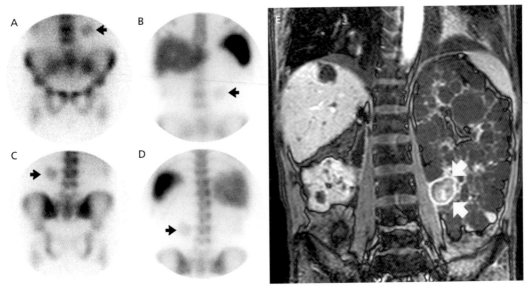

Figure 16.9 ^{111}In-labeled WBC scintigraphy (A–D) and coronal MRI T1 view (E) for the same patient as in Figure 16.8. The infected cyst shows accumulation of WBCs (A–D, black arrows), while the increased T1 MRI signal is consistent with an infected cyst (E, white arrows).

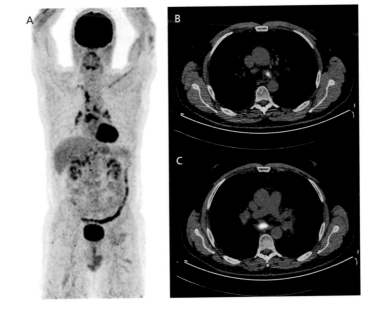

Figure 16.10 (A) Maximal intensity projection of [18F]FDG-PET showing uptake in mediastinal and hilar lymph nodes. Fusion [18F]FDG-PET/CT clearly located the lymph nodes, e.g. in the aortopulmonary window, mediastinal station 4L (B) and subcarinal lymph node, mediastinal station 7 (C).

[18F]FDG-PET/CT was then performed and showed intense uptake in the mediastinal and hilar lymph nodes (Figure 16.10). Mediastinoscopy finally demonstrated granulomatous inflammatory mediastinal lymph nodes consistent with sarcoidosis. No tumor cells were detected in these lymph nodes.

Teaching point

Inflammatory diseases can be misleading in the work-up of suspected neoplasia, as inflammatory lymph nodes show both CT and [18F]FDG-PET patterns of malignancy (i.e. increased size and [18F] FDG uptake).

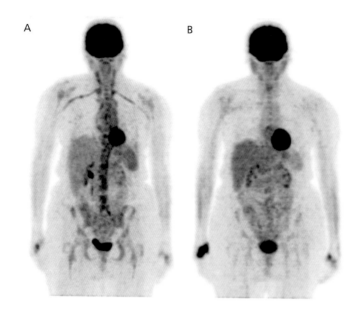

Figure 16.11 Maximal intensity projections of [^{18}F]FDG-PET (A) at the time of diagnosis and (B) after steroid treatment. Note the [^{18}F]FDG uptake by the large vessels and shoulders, which is highly suggestive of giant cell arteritis with scapular involvement (polymyalgia rheumatica).

Case 3

A 59-year-old female with a medical history of Lyme's disease and depression showed abdominal rash, asthenia and a moderate fever (37.7 °C). The patient did not report ocular or mandibular symptoms, but the asthenia was particularly intense with major impairment of scapular mobility.

She was referred to an infectious diseases' specialist, who ruled out any evidence of active infection by serial bacteriological specimens. Serology did not show any relevant clue (*Borrelia burgdorferi*, *Brucella melitensis*, *Chlamydia trachomatis*, *Mycoplasma pneumoniae*, *Coxiella burnetti*, syphilis, hepatitis A, B and C, and HIV were all negative); CRP (<0.1 mg/dL), WBC count (5790/µL) and markers of systemic diseases (ANF, Waaler-Roose, ANCA) were all normal.

Therefore, [^{18}F]FDG-PET/CT was performed to rule out polymyalgia rheumatica. [^{18}F]FDG-PET showed intense uptake in the aorta and large vessels and in the shoulders, which is consistent with GCA (Horton's disease) associated with rhizomelic involvement (Figure 16.11A). Following steroid therapy, [^{18}F]FDG-PET was repeated at 6 months from diagnosis and showed complete normalization of uptake (Figure 16.11B).

Teaching points

• Large vessel vasculitis can show various clinical presentations and sometimes only asthenia. [^{18}F]FDG-PET can be helpful in the diagnostic process.

• Normalization is rapid with treatment, indicating that patients should not be started on steroids before [^{18}F]FDG-PET is performed.

CHAPTER 17

Nuclear Medicine Imaging of Inflammatory Diseases

Marco Chianelli[1], Gaurav Malviya[2,3], Andor W.J.M. Glaudemans[2] and Alberto Signore[3]

[1]Regina Apostolorum Hospital, Albano, Rome, Italy
[2]University of Groningen, Groningen, The Netherlands
[3]"Sapienza" University, Rome, Italy

Introduction

Inflammatory diseases are a heterogeneous class of diseases characterized by chronic inflammation of the target organ. They are often relapsing and require life-long treatment. The so-called "aseptic chronic inflammatory diseases" include: autoimmune diseases, graft rejection, sarcoidosis, vasculitis, atherosclerosis and some degenerative diseases. In these patients it is very important to try and achieve specific immunosuppression to extinguish the immune process with the aim of halting the disease, preventing or delaying complications and avoiding disease relapse. It is important that, while attempting to improve the quality of life of these patients by means of anti-inflammatory drugs, side effects are reduced to a minimum by using specific immune therapies that block as selectively as possible the pathological mechanisms responsible for the disease.

New specific targeted therapies are being developed. Several clinical trials are being performed to assess the efficacy and safety of this new approach. All of them, however, rely largely on the clinical assessment of patients to evaluate the effect of treatment. An objective and reliable method to visualize directly the immune process underlying the individual disease would be valuable; specific diagnostic tests, furthermore, may allow the selection of patients to be treated.

Nowadays, nuclear medicine techniques are not often used for the diagnosis of chronic inflammatory diseases, but they do greatly contribute to the management and determination of the prognosis of the disease. Most importantly, nuclear medicine techniques are the most sensitive diagnostic modalities for the evaluation of disease activity. This is of paramount importance since, in most cases, therapeutic options are available and a prompt start to treatment may prevent disease or delay complications.

One of the most important steps in the study of autoimmune diseases has been the development of molecular nuclear medicine that, with the production of specific radiopharmaceuticals, has contributed to the identification of the immune process responsible for the individual disease. This is particularly important because new molecular

Diagnostic Imaging of Infections and Inflammatory Diseases: A Multidisciplinary Approach, First Edition. Edited by Alberto Signore and Ana María Quintero.
© 2014 John Wiley & Sons, Inc. Published 2014 by John Wiley & Sons, Inc.

therapeutic agents are being developed that specifically target and block inflammatory reactions. The referring physician not only obtains information on disease activity, but also on the nature of the process, and can, therefore, decide which treatment to start, when to start it and when to stop it or modify it.

Basic knowledge of the clinical problem

Th1- and Th2-type chronic inflammation

Persistence of an antigen maintains the production of selected cytokines by immune cells; these induce the differentiation of the effectors cells responsible for the specific immune response. Following the activation of T lymphocytes, their proliferation and maturation is regulated by the secretion of T-cell soluble mediators, called cytokines, and by the expression of specific cell-surface receptors.

It has become clear that the type of antigen determines the type of immune response. Amongst CD4+ T-helper lymphocytes, three different subsets exist, called Th1, Th2 and Th17. Each subset maintains the immune response but through the production of different cytokines. In particular, Th1 lymphocytes produce predominantly interleukin (IL)-2, tumor necrosis factor alpha (TNFα) and interferon-gamma (IFN-γ), and are particularly effective in stimulating a cellular immune response, whereas Th2 lymphocytes produce IL-4, IL-5, IL-6 and IL-10, and are particularly effective in stimulating B lymphocytes and eosinophils. It has been reported that IL-4 can inhibit Th1 lymphocytes and IFN-γ can inhibit Th2 lymphocytes. Th1 and Th2 lymphocytes also have different functions and respond differently to chemokines through different membrane receptors: Th1 cells express the chemokine receptor CCR5 (but not CCR3) and Th2 cells express the chemokine receptor CCR3 (but not CCR5) [1].

It has become clear that different inflammatory diseases are driven predominantly by a Th1/Th17 or a Th2 response. It is now possible, in an attempt to achieve a more selective immune suppression, to use treatments that induce a shift from Th1 to Th2 or vice versa, thereby changing the inflammation from a pathogenic type to a non-pathogenic one in the individual disease. Th1-mediated diseases would benefit from therapies that induce a shift towards Th2 and *vice versa*.

Since Th1 and Th2 cells express distinct sets of chemokine receptors, it is envisaged that, by using radiolabeled ligands that specifically bind to the different Th subsets, it may be possible to identify *in vivo* the occurrence of the two types of inflammation. With new therapeutic options, therefore, the challenge is not to verify whether the inflammation is active or not, but to identify the type of inflammation. In this field, molecular nuclear medicine can offer unique information.

Autoimmune diseases: types and classification

Almost all body tissues have been described as possible targets for an autoimmune reaction, the pathogenesis of which is still incompletely understood. Among the factors involved in the genesis of autoimmunity are lost thymic tolerance, failure of peripheral anergy against self-antigens and – in some cases – a cross-reaction with bacterial, viral and retroviral antigens. There is an undoubted genetic predisposition for autoimmune diseases, since they are associated with major histocompatibility complex (MHC) and non-MHC-related genes.

Several classifications of autoimmune diseases have been proposed, based on the clinical and pathogenetic findings; in particular, they can be classified as either systemic or organ-specific diseases, depending on whether the response is primarily against widespread or tissue-specific antigens. An important clinical characteristic of autoimmune diseases, that reflects the common genetic predisposition, is the associated high frequency of polyglandular autoimmune syndromes. This is particularly interesting because nuclear medicine techniques can visualize in a single test the possible involvement of multiple organs.

Histopathology of autoimmune diseases: rationale for using specific radioactive probes in molecular nuclear medicine

In autoimmune diseases, a distinctive chronic reaction is observed from the outset with little increased vascularity and permeability, and little or no neutrophil infiltration [2]. Autoimmune diseases give rise to a whole spectrum of different histological characteristics, ranging from a typical lymphocytic infiltration, as in thyroiditis, to a mixed infiltrating cell population consisting of T and B lymphocytes, plasma cells and neutrophils, as in rheumatoid arthritis, to a typically humoral-mediated reaction, as in systemic lupus erythematosus [3].

Cellular immunity is based on specific antigen recognition and is mediated by cytotoxic (CD8+) T lymphocytes, macrophages and natural killer (NK) cells, and coordinated by T helper (CD4++) lymphocytes. Following the specific interaction of lymphocytes with the antigen and appropriate co-stimulatory signals, a complex series of phosphorylation reactions causes the transcription of genes that result in lymphocyte proliferation and differentiation. The cell starts synthesizing RNA and moves from the G0 into the G1 phase of the mitotic cycle; proteins are synthesized, the cell enlarges and synthesis of IL-2 and the IL-2 receptor (IL-2R) begins. Transferrin receptors are synthesized after 14 hours, MHC class II molecules after 3–5 days and the very late activation antigen (VLA-4) after 7–14 days [3].

The endothelium undergoes major changes that facilitate and enhance the recruitment of inflammatory cells and molecules. Permeability is increased to facilitate diffusion of macromolecules; adhesion molecules, such as intercellular adhesion molecule (ICAM)-1, vascular cell adhesion molecule (VCAM) and E-selectins, are specifically expressed and bind to circulating granulocytes and lymphocytes, promoting active migration into inflamed tissues [4]. Somatostatin receptors have also been described on the endothelium of inflamed vessels [5]. The targeting of inflamed vessels is a further option for the diagnosis of immune processes.

Apoptosis is a term referring to the cytologically observable changes associated with a process of cellular self-destruction observed in all eukaryotes. It is also called programmed cell death because it requires controlled gene expression, which is activated in response to a variety of external or internal stimuli. This type of cell death involves cell activation through the engagement of cell surface receptors and subsequent signaling processes initiated by these receptors. During apoptosis, cells shrink, develop bubble-like blebs on their surface, have the chromatin in their nucleus degraded and break into small, membrane-wrapped fragments. One of the earliest events is the exposure on the surface membrane of phosphatidylserine, which is normally hidden within the plasma membrane. This is bound by receptors on phagocytic cells like macrophages and dendritic cells that engulf cell fragments.

Since intracellular contents are not released from apoptotic cells and their fragments, this process is not accompanied by inflammation and as a result it can be regarded as an injury-limiting mode of cell disposal. Apoptotic processes are physiologically observed during embryonal development, morphogenesis, metamorphosis, in endocrine tissue atrophy, during the normal turnover of tissues and during tumor regression. Apoptosis also provides a defense mechanism against viruses by reducing virus spread through the rapid death of virus-infected cells and also eliminates cells with DNA damage. Apoptotic cell death can be triggered by a variety of stimuli, including increased levels of oxidants within the cell, gamma irradiation, glucocorticoids or cytotoxic drugs [6,7].

During inflammatory processes, cytotoxic T lymphocytes secrete TNFα and TNFβ, which, after binding to the TNF receptor, mediate apoptosis. Alternatively, when cytotoxic T cells bind to their target, they produce more Fas ligand (FasL) at their surface. This binds with the Fas (also called CD95) on the surface of the target cell, leading to its death by apoptosis. Fas and the TNF receptor are integral membrane proteins with their receptor domains exposed at the surface of the cell.

Apoptosis normally occurs in autoimmune diseases and organ transplantation and even in atherosclerotic plaques. Detection of apoptosis, therefore, in autoimmune diseases reveals important information on the ultimate effect of the inflammatory process on the target organ and can be very important in the assessment of the efficacy of treatment.

Graft rejection

Acute allograft rejection is one of the major complications that may occur in transplanted patients. Histopathological lesions, observed in acute rejection, show perivascular and interstitial mononuclear cell infiltrates in the allograft [8]. Later, there is a T-cell dependent lymphocytic infiltration, which is driven by IL-2, among others. The first episode of acute rejection generally occurs between 2 days and 1 week after surgery. After the first year, the major cause of death is the bronchiolitis obliterans syndrome (BOS). This is characterized histologically by fibrous obliteration of the small- to medium-sized bronchioles and is thought to represent a manifestation of chronic allograft rejection [8].

Sarcoidosis

Granuloma formation in sarcoidosis is caused by an excessive immunological response to an infectious agent, organic particle or inorganic agent. The development of the epitheloid cell granuloma is based on three phases [9]. First, the granuloma formation is initiated by the incorporation of the unknown antigen by antigen-presenting cells (APCs). Then the antigen is attached to a MHC class II molecule and presented to the naïve CD4+ T lymphocytes. In the third phase, under the influence of IL-12 and IL-18, the CD4+ T lymphocytes will be activated and differentiate into Th1 cells, macrophages are recruited in the center of the granuloma and surrounded by a rim of lymphocytes and fibroblasts [10]. The continuous presentation of the antigen by alveolar macrophages to Th1 cells results in the formation of these granulomas. The alveolar macrophage releases IL-1, IL-6, IL-12, macrophage inflammatory protein-1 (MIP-1), monocyte chemotactic protein-1 (MCP-1) and, above all, TNFα. This specific cytokine has a crucial role in granuloma development.

The Th1 response is mainly induced by IL-12. Activated Th1 cells predominantly secrete IL-2 and IFN-γ, which also have a pivotal role in the granulomatous process. Additionally, the released chemokines boost the formation of the granuloma by the recruitment and proliferation of monocytes/macrophages and T cells.

The granulomatous inflammation may disappear without residual scarring, remain stable, or lead to fibrosis with permanent damage to the affected tissue. Different immune responses are thought to determine the varying disease course. Elimination of the eliciting factor and subsequent downregulation of the immune response might result in the spontaneous resolution of the granuloma. In case of an inadequate Th1 response, Th2 cells are activated to more effectively eliminate the antigen [11]. However, the switch from a Th1 to Th2 response occurs in patients developing chronic sarcoidosis, potentially followed by fibrosis [12].

Vasculitidis

The histopathology of vasculitidis consists of an inflammatory infiltrate in all three tunicas of the arterial wall, with giant cells forming granulomas in the media, particularly at the intima–media border. Several lines of evidence indicate that vasculitis is a T-cell mediated disease. The infiltrate in the arterial wall consists primarily of T lymphocytes and macrophages, with few to no B lymphocytes. The T lymphocytes are predominantly of the CD4+ phenotype, with the highest number of cells found in the adventitia, followed by the intima, whereas few lymphocytes are detected in the media. T lymphocytes infiltrating vasculitic lesions show signs of activation, such as MHC class II and CD25 (IL-2 receptor) expression. The Th1 type is thought to play the most important role. IFN-γ is a major factor in the activation of macrophages in vasculitic lesions and these are the major source of a variety of cytokines, including IL-1β, IL-6, TNFα, transforming growth factor (TGF) β and IL-32 [13].

Atherosclerosis

The exact mechanisms by which atherogenic factors act are only partially understood. However, there are indications that they primarily alter the protective function of the endothelium, thus favoring lipid and monocyte/macrophage deposition into the vascular wall. In the first step, i.e. the formation of stable plaque, an innate immune response plays a pivotal role in determining the evolution of the lesion. In particular, monocytes/macrophages overload oxidized low density lipoprotein (oxLDL) via scavenger receptors and perpetuate the local inflammatory response secreting cytokines, degrading enzymes (matrix metalloproteinases), as well as growth factors that stimulate smooth muscle cell migration and proliferation.

The microenvironment of the plaque could elicit an adaptive immune response that determines the selective recruitment of inflammatory cells. At this stage, lymphocytes, instead of macrophages, orchestrate the immune response. The switch to the selective recruitment of Th1 lymphocytes represents a key step in the development of plaque vulnerability/disruption. IFN-γ strongly inhibits the proliferation of smooth muscle cells and the production of interstitial collagens by vascular smooth muscle cells, thereby affecting the stability of the fibrous cap [14].

The clinical questions

The clinical diagnosis of chronic inflammatory diseases is commonly made when symptoms of target tissue hypofunction appear. Thyroid Graves' disease is an exception, since the presence of antithyrotropin receptor (anti-TSHr) antibodies stimulates the thyroid function and therefore, an early diagnosis of hyperthyroidism can be made and therapy started before the thyroid is destroyed by infiltrating lymphocytes.

Immunologically, autoimmune diseases are quite heterogeneous. In some cases there is a predominance of humoral immunity (i.e. production of autoantibodies) and in others of cellular immunity (i.e. a decrease in circulating T-suppressor cells, an increase in activated T cells and mononuclear cell infiltration of the target tissue). However, the same disease in different subjects may have different involvement of the two compartments.

In most organ-specific autoimmune diseases, therefore, the detection of lymphocytes infiltrating the target tissue represents an important additional marker, together with the measurement of circulating autoantibody titer, for early diagnosis, early treatment and therapy follow-up. For histological examination, tissue specimens can be obtained from the thyroid, gut, joints, skin and kidney, but for other tissues (e.g. the parathyroid, adrenals, pancreas, gonads, pituitary gland, brain, etc.), biopsies can be difficult to obtain.

The same considerations can be made for graft rejection, sarcoidosis, vasculitis and atherosclerosis. Patients receiving organ transplantation are constantly followed up by evaluating organ/tissue function and with regular biopsies. Nevertheless, an acute or chronic rejection is often unpredictable. Sarcoidosis, vasculitis and atherosclerosis are often only detected very late when complications or severe symptoms appear.

In all these diseases, clinicians want to know the severity and extent of lymphocytic infiltration, as this will guide therapy decision-making and evaluates the efficacy of immune therapy. Therefore, the imaging of infiltrating lymphocytes in tissues is an important goal for nuclear medicine.

A particular indication for nuclear medicine in this field could be the investigation of healthy siblings of affected patients or subjects genetically at risk in order to predict and eventually prevent clinical onset of the disease.

Methodological considerations

As mentioned above, most organ-specific autoimmune diseases are characterized by a chronic infil-

tration of the target tissue by mononuclear cells, with little or no hemodynamic change and few symptoms of inflammation. Tissue mononuclear cell infiltration precedes and persists until target cells are destroyed and symptoms of hypofunction appear. Thus, functional imaging of the tissue is generally not useful for early diagnosis. It may just support the clinical diagnosis (i.e. decreased iodine uptake in Hashimoto's thyroiditis) or be used in some cases for therapy follow-up (i.e. liver colloid scintigraphy in chronic hepatitis). In contrast, it has a relevant diagnostic and therapeutic importance because of the possibility of detecting and quantifying the tissue mononuclear cell infiltration (i.e. what causes the autoimmune disease). Low molecular weight radiolabeled receptor ligands should be used – they can pass through the intact capillary endothelium and bind specifically to infiltrating cells. Radiolabeled granulocytes cannot be used for the detection of tissues infiltrated by mononuclear cells. However, in some autoimmune diseases, such as Crohn's disease and rheumatoid arthritis, typical signs of acute inflammation coexist with chronic lymphocytic infiltration. In these cases, radiolabeled granulocytes or mixed leukocytes can be used. Other techniques can also be employed, such as the use of macromolecules like nanocolloids and non-specific human immunoglobulin (HIG) that accumulate at sites of acute inflammation as a result of non-specific extravasation. A brief description of the most relevant radiopharmaceuticals for the study of inflammatory and autoimmune diseases will follow.

This chapter reviews molecular imaging by nuclear medicine techniques and non-specific techniques are not considered.

Normal findings and artifacts

Radiolabeled autologous lymphocytes

Several studies have reported the use of ^{111}In-labeled lymphocytes in normal subjects and in patients with malignancies. Good results were obtained in patients with hematological tumors and organ-specific autoimmune diseases [15–17]. However, their use was discontinued when *in vitro* studies reported that lymphocytes were highly sensitive to radiation damage [18,19].

Radiolabeled non-specific human immunoglobulins

The use of radiolabeled non-specific HIGs has been introduced for detecting sites of inflammation/infection [20]. They produce no allergic reactions or any other side effects and are commercially available in a ready-to-use kit form. Although their mechanism(s) of action has not been completely clarified, their accumulation seems to be mainly non-specific as a result of leakage into the inflamed site.

They are available labeled with ^{99m}Tc or ^{111}In. The mechanism of accumulation is the same for both radiopharmaceuticals and their biodistribution is similar. Both accumulate in the liver and have slow kinetics. Diagnostic images are usually acquired at late time points (6–24 hours). However, compared with ^{99m}Tc-HIG, the use of ^{111}In-HIG results in a higher concentration in inflamed tissue, due to accumulation of the free ^{111}In that results from the local metabolism of ^{111}In-HIG.

The major indication for the use of radiolabeled HIGs is the study of inflamed/infected joints and/or bone, for which good results have been obtained [21].

Radiolabeled antibodies against granulocyte or lymphocyte antigens

Radiolabeled monoclonal antibodies (mAbs) have a long plasma half-life and give a high background radioactivity that decreases slowly with time. A long interval (6–24 hours) is usually required between the administration of the labeled mAb and the acquisition of images in order to achieve a good target-to-background ratio. Some of them are of heterologous origin and may induce the production of human antimurine antibodies (HAMAs) with the possible development of allergic reactions, anti-idiotypic antibodies and altered pharmacokinetics.

Radiolabeled antibodies recognizing lymphocyte antigens, such as CD3 or CD4, have been used for the study of autoimmune diseases [22,23]. BW 250/183 is a mAb recognizing the non-specific cross-reacting antigen 95 (NCA95) that is expressed on human granulocytes, pro-myelocytes and myelocytes. It is commercially available and provided as a ready-to-use kit for ^{99m}Tc labeling. Localization of inflammatory processes is thought to be mediated by migration of circulating radiolabeled granulocytes and non-specific extravasation of the free antibody into the inflamed focus. Following binding to bone marrow (55%), liver (10%), spleen (6%) and peripheral organs, the antibody is rapidly cleared from the circulation and low values of circulating radioactive mAbs are obtained [24].

Another commercially available stage-specific embryonic antigen 1 (SSEA-1) murine mAb, called ^{99m}Tc-fanolesomab (LeuTech) and an IgM, binds with high affinity to the CD15 antigen expressed on neutrophils. Scintigraphy with ^{99m}Tc-SSEA-1 has been proposed for diagnostic purposes in equivocal cases of appendicitis. A study was performed in 25 diabetic patients for diagnosis of pedal ulcers. Reported sensitivity, specificity and accuracy of the radiolabeled mAb were 90%, 67% and 76%, respectively [25]. In another study, the diagnostic accuracy was similar to that for labeled white blood cell (WBC) scintigraphy [26]. A transient neutropenia has been noted after the use of ^{99m}Tc-SSEA-1; nevertheless, in most cases, this does not represent a clinical problem and does not impair image quality. Unfortunately, as a consequence of serious and potentially fatal cardiopulmonary reactions associated with its use, ^{99m}Tc-SSEA-1 has been suspended from the market.

Several patient studies have also been performed with ^{99m}Tc-labeled sulesomab (Leukoscan, Immunomedics GmbH, Germany), an antigranulocyte (anti-G), murine IgG1 Fab' fragment of anti-NCA-90 antibody. Immunoscintigraphy with ^{99m}Tc-sulesomab enables rapid localization of osteomyelitis, with a negligible HAMA response rate and accuracy comparable to WBC scintigraphy. Encouraging results have been obtained in the detection of suspected endocarditis [27] and appendicitis [28]. In a large study, 122 diabetic patients with foot ulcers were evaluated with radiolabeled sulesomab scintigraphy [29]. In this study, the labeled mAb fragment showed a high sensitivity of 91%, but specificity of only 56% for the reasons mentioned at the beginning of this chapter (i.e. long plasma half-life and high specific uptake in inflammatory lesions). Another study using SPECT with the radiolabeled anti-G mAb was performed in patients with infected endocarditis. The authors reported 71% sensitivity and 94% specificity for detection, while, together with transesophageal echocardiography, it accurately identified all patients with infected endocarditis, but missed the diagnosis in patients receiving long-term antibiotic therapy [27].

Radiolabeled monoclonal antibodies against TNFα

Two mAbs directed against TNFα have been developed, infliximab and adalimumab. Infliximab (Remicade®; Jansen Biotech Inc, USA) is a chimeric IgG1 mAb with a murine variable (Fv) domain of mouse antihuman TNFα antibody and constant (Fc) sequences of human IgG1, produced by recombinant cell culture technique. Adalimumab (Humira®; Abbott Laboratories, USA) is the first "fully human" antibody against TNFα, engineered using phase display technology. It is a recombinant human monoclonal IgG1 antibody, composed of two kappa light chains (24 kDa each) and two IgG1 heavy chains (49 kDa each), expressed in Chinese hamster ovary cells and less immunogenic than infliximab [30].

Both infliximab and adalimumab recognize and bind both soluble and membrane-bound TNFα with high avidity and high affinity ($K_a = 1 \times 10^{10}$/M), forming stable non-dissociating immune complexes [31,32], and mediate a powerful anti-inflammatory effect. They are currently used for the treatment of moderate-to-severe active rheumatoid arthritis, ankylosing spondylitis, psoriatic arthritis and (infliximab only) Crohn's disease and ulcerative colitis.

Radiolabeled monoclonal antibodies against CD20

Rituximab (Rituxan®, Genentech, USA) was the first chimeric mAb approved in 1997 for the treatment of malignancies and in 2006 FDA approved for the treatment of patients with active rheumatoid arthritis who do not respond to one or more TNF antagonist therapies. Rituximab is a genetically engineered chimeric murine/human mAb against the CD20 antigen found on the surface of normal and malignant B lymphocytes but not expressed on hemopoietic stem cells [33,34]. Rituximab consists of IgG1 kappa containing variable region sequences of murine light chains (213 amino acids) and heavy chains (451 amino acids) and human constant region sequences [33].

In vivo, rituximab induces depletion of both normal and malignant B cells and down-regulates the production of autoantibodies, rheumatoid factor (RF), T-cell activation and pro-inflammatory cytokine production [34,35].

Radiolabeled monoclonal antibodies against CD3

A humanized non-FcR-binding derivative of the anti-human CD3 mAb, OKT3, can induce generalized immunosuppression in patients with psoriatic arthritis [36,37]. In this mAb, two alanine mutations (amino acids 234 and 235) have been introduced to prevent FcR binding. The complementarity defining region (CDR) of OKT3 is engrafted onto a human IgG1 backbone to give a low immunogenic profile. This antibody can modulate the CD3–T-cell receptor complex, induce clonal anergy and/or induce of regulatory T lymphocytes.

Visilizumab (Nuvion®, Protein Design Labs, USA), a new generation of genetically engineered anti-CD3 mAb, has been developed by grafting murine CDRs derived from a M291 hybridoma into a human non-CDR region of IgG2 and introducing non-FcR-binding mutations at amino acid residues 234 and 237 (Val → Ala) into the IgG2 Fc portion [38]. This non-FcR-binding humanized mAb is directed towards the CD3 antigen on T lymphocytes and binds with high specificity and high avidity ($K_a = 0.5 \times 10^9$/M) [39]. Non-FcR-binding mAbs do not activate resting T lymphocytes [40] and have limited potential for inducing cytokine release and acute toxicity *in vivo* [41]. Visilizumab has been proposed for the treatment of several autoimmune diseases.

Radiolabeled monoclonal antibodies against CD4

CD4 is a 55-kDa monomeric membrane glycoprotein expressed on T-lineage cells, including the majority of thymocytes and a subset of peripheral T lymphocytes and monocytes. The extracellular domains of CD4 bind to the conserved regions of MHC II molecules on APCs. CD4+ T lymphocytes constitute the helper subset which regulates T and B lymphocyte function during T-cell-dependent responses. CD4+ T cells and their cytokine products play an important role in rheumatoid arthritis [42]. A number of anti-CD4 monoclonal antibodies are available for the management of rheumatoid arthritis and other autoimmune diseases, including murine and primatized CD4 mAbs [43].

Radiolabeled monoclonal antibodies against CD25

CD25 is also called the IL-2 receptor alpha chain (the Tac subunit). High CD25 expression is associated with advanced cutaneous T-cell lymphoma and with clinical response to denileukin–diftitox therapy, a recombinant fusion protein of diphtheria toxin and IL-2, which binds to CD25. It is expressed by activated B lymphocytes, macrophages, some thymocytes, some myeloid precursors and some oligodendrocytes.

Daclizumab (Zenapax®; Hoffman-La Roche, Switzerland) is a humanized IgG1 mAb that specifically binds to the Tac subunit (CD25) of the high-affinity IL-2 receptor complex, inhibiting the binding of IL-2 and the cascade of pro-inflammatory events involved in organ transplant rejection and several autoimmune diseases. Similarly, basiliximab (Simulect®; Novartis Pharma, USA) is a chimeric IgG1 mAb, produced by recombinant DNA technology, against the IL-2 receptor (CD25) expressed on T lymphocytes. Basiliximab has a molecular weight of 144 kDa and it binds with high affinity ($K_a = 1 \times 10^{10}$/M) to the alpha chain of the high-affinity IL-2 receptor complex. Interestingly, CD25 antigen is expressed on activated but not on resting T lymphocytes. Anti-CD25 mAbs and their fragments have been radiolabeled with ^{67}Ga, ^{211}At, ^{212}Bi, ^{125}I, ^{99m}Tc, ^{111}In, ^{88}Y and ^{18}F for different diagnostic and therapeutic purposes. Several studies in animals as well as in humans have demonstrated the complete blockade of IL-2 receptors with anti-CD25 mAbs [44–48].

Radiolabeled monoclonal antibodies against CD56 (anti-NCAM)

CD56, also called neural cell adhesion molecule (NCAM), is a homophilic binding glycoprotein expressed on the surface of neurons, glia, skeletal muscle and natural killer cells. It is thought to induce neurite outgrowth via the fibroblast growth factor receptor and acts upon the p59Fyn signaling pathway. NCAM has been implicated as having a role in cell–cell adhesion, neurite outgrowth, synaptic plasticity and learning and memory. Several anti-NCAM antibodies, including 123C3, NY3D11, ERIC-1, NK1NBL1 and C218 have been developed and radiolabeled to image small cell lung cancer and relapsed malignant gliomas [49–53].

Radiolabeled monoclonal antibodies against HLA-DR

Human leukocyte antigen (HLA) class II antigens are highly expressed throughout B-cell development and differentiation, and are known to play important roles in controlling cell cycling and proliferation. In humans, MHC class II genes, which encode for HLA-DR, DQ and DP antigens, are expressed mainly on B lymphocytes and plasma cells, but also on activated T lymphocytes (but not those in the resting state), macrophages, monocytes, dendritic cells, activated NK cells and progenitor hemopoietic cells. Triggering HLA class II antigens on B lymphocytes mediates homotypic cell aggregation, inhibits cell proliferation and immunoglobulin secretion and induces cell-surface expression of co-stimulatory molecules. HLA-DR molecules are composed of α (35 kDa) and β (28 kDa) subunits. Each subunit contains two extracellular domains, a membrane-spanning domain and a cytoplasmic tail. In the mouse, there are two subclasses, H2-A (HLA-DQ homolog) and H2-E (HLA-DR homolog) and both are functional [54,55]. The HLA-DR protein is an intermediate activation antigen that is expressed on the surface of CD4+ and CD8+ T cells in the course of lymphocyte activation.

Recently, a fully humanized IgG4 mAb, 1D09C3, was discovered by screening the Morphosys Human Combinatorial Antibody Library (Hu-CAL), a diverse library of single-chain antibody variable fragments, and constructed by combining highly variable CDRs [56].

Radiolabeled monoclonal antibodies against CD19

CD19 is a phosphoglycoprotein that forms the antigen receptor complex on B lymphocytes in conjunction with CD21 and CD81, also called surface immunoglobulin-associated molecules (sIgs). It primarily acts as a co-receptor, transduces signals initiated through the antigen receptor of B lymphocytes [57] and decreases the threshold for antigen receptor-dependent stimulation. It has also been shown to have another important role in the early antigen-independent stages of B-cell development [58]; it facilitates the pro-B/pre-B transition. CD19 is considered a pan B-cell antigen and is present on the earliest recognizable B-lineage cells through to the B-cell blasts, but is lost on their maturation to plasma cells. It is indeed the first B-cell antigen after HLA-DR to be expressed and is also expressed on follicular dendritic cells.

Anti-CD19 mAbs also have potentially wider applications for other B-cell hematological malignancies that are refractory to currently available treatment, but further studies are required [59,60].

Radiolabeled monoclonal antibodies against CD22

The CD22 antigen is a B-lymphocyte-restricted 135-kDa type I transmembrane sialoglycoprotein of the immunoglobulin superfamily. It is initially present in the cytoplasm of developing B cells but is later expressed on the surface during B-cell maturation and once IgD expression occurs [61]. Most circulating IgM+, IgD+ cells express CD22, also strongly expressed in follicular (primary and secondary B-cell zones), mantle and marginal zone B cells, but is only weakly expressed in germinal (activated or differentiating) B cells. In B-cell malignancies, CD22 have been observed in 60–80% or more of samples evaluated [62]. When bound by ligand or antibody, CD22 is rapidly internalized within hours. The function of CD22 is not entirely clear, but it appears to be involved in the regulation of B-cell function and survival, CD19 and B-cell antigen receptor (BCR) signal transduction and B-cell receptor-induced cell death. It is implicated through these roles in the modulation of humoral immunity and in the growth of malignant B cells, suggesting that it may have utility as a target for therapeutic antilymphoma antibodies [63,64].

Murine and humanized forms of anti-CD22 antibodies have been used in combination with different radionuclides. The most studied and promising is epratuzumab, a humanized IgG1 mAb directed against the CD22 antigen. The murine LL2 antibody was re-engineered into the humanized antibody (hLL2) [65]. Several studies have been conducted with both murine and humanized radiolabeled (^{131}I, ^{90}Y and ^{186}Re) forms of LL2. In a review of mAbs for hematological malignancies, Castillo et al. described and compared the efficacy, advantages and disadvantages of the different isotopes used to radiolabel LL2 [66].

Bectumomab is a mouse anti-CD22 mAb that has been radiolabeled with ^{99m}Tc (IMMU-LL2, Lymphoscan®). The efficacy of this radiolabeled mAb was retrospectively examined in the staging of recurrent or newly diagnosed non-Hodgkin's lymphoma (NHL) and to assess targeting before radioimmunotherapy. The study concluded that bectumomab shows promise as a pre-radioimmunotherapy probe

for targeting B-cell NHL. However, as a purely diagnostic agent, its performance was variable [67].

Radiolabeled monoclonal antibodies against CD2

CD2 is a 50-kDa transmembrane protein belonging to the immunoglobulin superfamily which participates in the immune response. Together with its ligands, it is involved in the formation of cell–cell contacts between APCs or cytotoxic lymphocytes and their target cells. It also participates in many T-cell interactions and activation, as observed in the thymus between thymocytes and epithelial cells [68].

Two mAbs and their F(ab')$_2$ fragments that target CD2 and CD5 were labeled with ^{131}I and intravenously injected into nude mice bearing a solid subcutaneous human T-cell leukemia line xenograft [69]. Both mAbs, anti-CD2 and anti-CD5, yielded a satisfactory mean tumor to whole-body ratio and, moreover, this ratio was further increased (approximately three times) for both the mAbs when their F(ab')$_2$ fragments were used.

Siplizumab is a novel human IgG1 mAb directed at CD2. In recent clinical trials, this agent has exhibited an acceptable safety profile, potent immunomodulatory effects and selective suppression of the function of T and NK cells in adult patients with plaque psoriasis, renal allograft recipients and acute graft-versus-host disease (GVHD), when administered in multiple intravenous or subcutaneous doses [70,71]. Therefore, if radiolabeled, this mAb may provide a useful tool for molecular imaging and therapy decision-making.

Radiolabeled monoclonal antibodies against CD5

CD5 is a 67-kDa member of the scavenger receptor cysteine-rich (SRCR) receptor glycoprotein family, expressed very early in cell ontogeny in the thymus where it plays a role in thymocyte maturation. It is also present on most peripheral T lymphocytes and is implicated in their activation and proliferation, acting as a co-stimulator [72,73].

A mAb recognizing Ly1, the murine homolog of CD5, was labeled with ^{90}Y and used in the mouse model in the treatment of active GVHD [74]. Another anti-CD5 antibody, T101, was radiolabeled with ^{111}In and ^{90}Y for imaging and therapy, respectively [75].

Radiolabeled monoclonal antibodies against CD45

CD45 is a protein tyrosine phosphatase (PTP) located in hematopoietic cells other than erythrocytes and platelets. CD45 is also called the common leukocyte antigen. It is the most broadly expressed hematopoietic marker with approximately 200 000 non-internalizing copies on the surface of each cell. Different isoforms of CD45 are found on cells of different lineages and during development of cells of a particular lineage. Higher molecular mass forms of the molecule (220–240 kDa) are found on B cells and a subpopulation of CD8+ T cells. Lower molecular mass forms are expressed on T cells and thymocytes. Specific mAbs that react with any particular subsets or single isoforms of the protein have helped to define functional subsets of Th cells in the rat and human.

The suitability of using a high affinity (K_d = 1.1 nM) anti-CD45 mAb, AHN-12, for delivering the high energy emitting isotope ^{90}Y to lymphohematopoietic target cells *in vivo* was investigated. The authors concluded that radiolabeled anti-CD45 antibody can be used to deliver radiation selectively to lymphohematopoietic tissue [76] and thus, this agent may be used to improve treatment of hematopoietic malignancies. Recently, another study evaluated the biodistribution of ^{111}In-labeled anti-CD45 antibody in humans using the rat IgG2a mAb YAML568 that recognizes a common CD45 epitope present on all human leukocytes [77].

Radiolabeled cytokines

The use of radiolabeled cytokines is a new field in molecular nuclear medicine. Their use allows immune processes to be studied *in vivo* and, by contributing to the molecular characterization of diseased tissues, they provide relevant information for the clinical management of patients.

As the pathophysiology of the individual underlying diseases differs, so does the cytokine network involved. Therefore, a cytokine suitable for the study of all pathological conditions does not exist. The optimal cytokine eligible for disease and stage-specific diagnosis will change according to the pathophysiological mechanisms operating in different diseases and to the different clinical stages of a given disease.

In immune-mediated pathologies, radiolabeled cytokines contribute to the differential diagnosis by confirming the immune nature of the disease, and to the study of the localization, severity and extent of the immune process. The major indication is the study of disease activity for the selection of patients eligible for treatment and for therapy follow-up.

The use of radiolabeled cytokines for diagnostic purposes is safe. Although several cytokines have undesirable biological effects at very low doses, radiolabeled cytokines are used in very small amounts (a few micrograms) and generally do not induce side effects. They are human in origin and produced by recombinant DNA technology, and are not immunogenic even if used on repeated occasions for follow-up studies [78].

The use of cytokines is easy and effective. Due to their low molecular weight, they are rapidly cleared from plasma via the kidneys and easily concentrate in affected tissues infiltrated by inflammatory cells. Areas of pathological uptake are easily differentiated from the background radioactivity of the body within a few hours after the injection [79].

IL-1 is a proinflammatory cytokine with a high affinity for a specific receptor expressed on monocytes and lymphocytes. It was one of the first cytokines developed for the imaging of acute inflammation. Labeled with ^{123}I or ^{125}I, IL-1 was tested in different animal models of infection or sterile inflammation [80]. There was a highly specific uptake at the infection site, but due to side effects (hypotension, headache) even at low doses, the radioiodinated IL-1 has never been trialed in humans. Consequently, a radiolabeled IL-1 receptor antagonist (IL1 RA) was developed, with the same binding affinity for IL-1 receptors, but without any biological activity. However, in mice the uptake of IL1 RA by abscess was much lower than that of IL-1 because of interaction with serum proteins [81]. This was also seen in a rabbit infection model, although radiolabeled IL1 RA in the infectious focus could be observed [82].

IL-2 is a single-chain glycoprotein, synthesized and secreted *in vivo* by T lymphocytes after specific antigen stimulation [83]. Its specific receptor is expressed on activated T lymphocytes. IL-2 maintains the immune response by inducing the long-term proliferation of activated T lymphocytes, and by stimulating the proliferation and differentiation of NK cells, B lymphocytes and macrophages [84]. Infiltrating lymphocytes are activated only after interaction with the antigen. As a consequence, cell activation is an asynchronous process and follows a gradient of antigen concentration. In inflammatory foci, activated lymphocytes express IL-2R and therefore become a target for radiolabeled IL-2, whereas under physiological conditions the expression of IL-2R in lymphoid tissues is negligible [85,86]. Peripheral blood cells do not express IL-2R in the course of inflammatory diseases; thus, there is very low binding of radiolabeled IL-2 to circulating lymphocytes, i.e. low levels of background radioactivity. The transient expression of IL-2R is an early lymphocyte activation marker. However, during the entire immune process, some lymphocytes activate and drive the inflammatory reaction until the antigen is completely eliminated.

Radiolabeled IL-2 allows the visualization of both lymphocytic infiltration and T-lymphocyte activation. Evaluation of the activity of immune-mediated processes is feasible through scintigraphy with this radiopharmaceutical. IL-2 has been labeled with ^{35}S and ^{125}I, and tested *in vitro* [87,88]. Biodistribution in rats has also been studied using ^{131}I-labeled IL-2 [89].

The reliability of ^{123}I-IL-2 for the *in vivo* detection of lymphocytic infiltration has been tested in animal models of human autoimmune diabetes, in bio-Breeding Worcester (BB/W) rats, in non-obese diabetic (NOD) mice [90,91] and in rats with renal allografts [92]. Studies in healthy volunteers and patients have shown no significant biological effects at the low doses (20–30 ng) used for imaging [93]. Inflammatory bowel diseases [94,95], autoimmune thyroid diseases, insulin-dependent diabetes [96,97], melanoma [98] and other pathologies have been investigated in over 1000 patients.

Currently, the best approach for imaging chronic inflammation is the use of labeled IL-2, although it binds to both Th1 and Th2 cells.

IL-8 is a chemotactic cytokine that binds with a high affinity to receptors expressed on neutrophils. It plays an important role in cell recruitment during acute inflammation. Various animal models have shown specific and rapid accumulation of ^{99m}Tc-IL-8 in infectious and inflammatory foci [99,100]. Injection was well tolerated and ^{99m}Tc-IL-8 scintigraphy appears to be a promising new tool for the detection of infections in patients as early as 4 hours after injection [101], but it has yet to be tested in inflammatory diseases.

Radiolabeled peptides

Radiolabeled peptides are a promising class of radiopharmaceuticals with diagnostic potential in several pathological conditions. Compared to larger molecules, like proteins and mAbs, peptides exhibit a rapid uptake by target tissues with good penetration into them and usually rapid plasma clearance due to the renal excretion. This biodistribution is particularly important for the study of most autoimmune diseases where hemodynamic changes are minimal and passive diffusion of macromolecules is very limited. Following intravenous injection, radiolabeled peptides accumulate in target tissues and organs by binding to specific receptors. They act as "probes" for the detection of target cells through external detection of body radioactivity with gamma-cameras, gamma-probes or PET scanners. Several radiolabeled peptides have been used so far in oncology, neurology, metabolism and inflammation [102].

Somatostatin receptors (SSRs) are expressed on both activated lymphocytes and inflamed vascular endothelium. Somatostatin receptor scintigraphy (SRS) has been used to demonstrate the presence of inflammation and also provides the rationale for the use of unlabeled somatostatin for the treatment of the disease in selected positive patients. Hyperexpression of SSRs has been found in intestinal samples from patients with active ulcerative colitis and Crohn's disease. SSRs were localized to intramural veins but were not detected in non-inflamed control intestine [5]. SSRs were reported *in vitro* in patients with active rheumatoid arthritis [103]. SRS is applicable in imaging of chronic inflammation, but is unsuitable for visualization of acute infectious diseases [104].

Radiolabeled somatostatin analogs have been extensively used for the detection of neuroendocrine tumors [105]. The most commonly used analog is ^{111}In-[D-Phe^1]-pentetreotide (Octreoscan), a small octapeptide that binds with high affinity to the somatostatin type 2 receptor expressed on the cell membrane of target tissues. It has no side effects. Several analogs have been synthesized and are currently used in routine clinical practice. A recent analog that has been used in autoimmune diseases is ^{99m}Tc-HYNIC-[D-Phe1,Tyr3]-octreotide (^{99m}Tc-HYNIC-TOC) [106].

Radiopharmaceuticals for apoptosis imaging

Radiolabeled annexin-V, an endogenous human protein, binds phosphatidylserine with high affinity. This allows the non-invasive assessment of the early stage of apoptosis, before DNA degradation and membrane vesicle formation, thereby providing information about disease progression or regression and about the efficacy of a therapy for inhibition or induction of cell death. This technique is unable to distinguish apoptosis from necrosis, because phosphatidylserine is externalized during both processes, but the information acquired is of fundamental importance in clinical practice.

A recent study has tested the reliability of ^{99m}Tc-HYNIC-annexin-V in the study of fulminant hepatic apoptosis induced by anti-Fas antibody injection in BALB/c mice. In control animals the radiopharmaceutical visualized only the kidney, whereas in mice affected by fulminant hepatitis the liver was clearly visualized at 1 hour, with increased uptake up to 2 hours and concomitant decreased renal activity [107].

The usefulness of ^{99m}Tc-HYNIC-annexin-V to image apoptotic processes *in vivo* has been evaluated in mice given dexamethasone to induce thymic apoptosis; in wild-type mice treated with anti-Fas antibody to produce massive apoptosis similar to fulminant hepatitis; and in Fas-defective mice (*lrp/ lrp*) in which no hepatic apoptosis is induced by the administration of anti-Fas antibody [108].

A recent study described the use of ^{99m}Tc-annexin-V in an experimental model of rheumatoid arthritis. Results showed that radiolabeled annexin-V accumulated with high target-to-background values in the affected joints. Annexin-V uptake significantly decreased after steroid treatment [109].

[^{18}F]FDG for imaging cell metabolism

It is well known that activated lymphocytes and monocytes as well as granulocytes show uptake of fluorodeoxyglucose (FDG) as these cells use glucose as an energy source only after activation during the metabolic burst and thus during inflammatory reactions. Transport of FDG across the cellular membrane is mediated by the glucose transporter (GLUT) proteins that are present on the cell membrane of lymphocytes and monocytes. Intracellularly, FDG is phosphorylated to FDG-6-phosphate by hexokinase and the phosphorylated molecule remains trapped inside the cell, unlike phosphorylated glucose that enters the glycolysis cycle. FDG is taken up by a variety of cells that are metabolically active during inflammation (endothelial cells, granulocytes, connective tissue cells, etc.) and also by neoplastic cells. [^{18}F]FDG should therefore be considered a non-specific radiopharmaceutical for imaging inflammation and it may lead to false-positive results. Several recent studies with [^{18}F]FDG positron emission tomography ([^{18}F]FDG-PET) have demonstrated promising results for imaging in different inflammatory diseases, including vasculitis, Crohn's disease, sarcoidosis and rheumatoid arthritis.

^{11}C-PK11195 for monocyte imaging

The need for a specific monocyte/macrophage-binding radiopharmaceutical has led to research into several receptors that target these cells. In particular, benzodiazepine receptors are expressed on microglia and monocytes. ^{11}C-PK11195 is a new PET radiopharmaceutical for imaging peripheral benzodiazepine receptors (PBR), but originally developed for measuring inflammation-induced microglia activation. PET with ^{11}C-PK11195 [(R)-N-methyl-N-(1-methylpropyl)-1-(2-chlorophenyl) isoquinoline-3-carboxamide] has been successfully applied in patients with viral encephalitis, e.g. herpes simplex virus (HSV) encephalitis, Rasmussen's encephalitis and acquired immunodeficiency syndrome (AIDS) [110–112]. In patients suffering from multiple sclerosis, enhanced ^{11}C-PK11195 uptake seems to correlate with new lesions, whereas old lesions show little radiopharmaceutical uptake [113]. Focal ^{11}C-PK11195 binding by structures that appeared normal by MRI and asymmetric increased radiopharmaceutical uptake in the thalamus and brain stem were also observed. T2-weighted MRI lesions showed an increase in ^{11}C-PK11195 uptake during relapse [114]. Similarly, ^{11}C-PK11195-PET has been proposed for imaging monocytes in rheumatoid arthritis [115,116].

Pathological findings and significance

The use of nuclear medicine techniques will be reviewed in those autoimmune diseases in which their role in diagnosis and follow-up is clearly established, including sarcoidosis, vasculitis and atherosclerosis.

Rheumatoid arthritis

Rheumatoid arthritis is a chronic autoimmune disease characterized by severe short- and long-term complications of the joints. Chronic mononuclear cell infiltration of the synovial membrane and subsequent erosion of cartilage and bone lead to joint ankylosis. The typical hemodynamic changes of acute inflammation and the persistence of the chronic infiltrate are both present. The specific and non-specific signs of inflammation are normally used for the clinical diagnosis and follow-up of the disease. Systemic treatment with anti-inflammatory drugs (steroidal and non-steroidal) is commonly employed for relief of symptoms and to delay disease progression. Treatment is usually life-long and is accompanied by several side effects. Local therapy is also used and has the advantages of higher local concentrations and fewer side effects.

It would be very useful for the prevention of disease progression to be able to diagnose affected joints before they become clinically evident; this would allow local therapies to be applied before complications develop. Rheumatoid arthritis has been extensively studied by nuclear medicine techniques and all the radiopharmaceuticals tested have been shown to accumulate in the inflamed joints [117].

In a comparative study, [99mTc]-HIG, [99mTc]-nanocolloid and [99mTc]-HMPAO-labeled WBCs showed similar diagnostic accuracy [118]. The use of a [99mTc]-labeled mAb (OKT3) has been described in patients with rheumatoid arthritis; the accumulation of the radiolabeled mAb correlated with the intensity of the inflammation and also detected active joints that were clinically asymptomatic [23]. The use of this antibody was, however, associated with side effects due to the release of cytokines following binding of the mAb to the CD3 molecule. [99mTc]-labeled anti-CD3 has recently been used for monitoring synovitis in patients with rheumatoid arthritis [119].

Anti-CD4 radiolabeled antibodies also have been used in patients with rheumatoid arthritis. In a comparative study of anti-CD4 and [99mTc]-labeled polyclonal HIGs, both preparations showed similar accumulation in inflamed joints. However, the anti-CD4 antibody showed a higher target-to-background ratio owing to the faster clearance of background radioactivity as a result of greater binding to the liver and the spleen [22].

Several studies have been performed in rheumatoid arthritis patients using anti-CD4 mAbs. A [99mTc]-labeled CD4-specific antibody scintigraphic study was performed by Becker et al. in six patients

with active, severe rheumatoid arthritis [120]. The CD4 mAb was labeled with [99mTc] by a direct method using 2-mercaptoethanol. Each patient received a sub-therapeutic dose of 200–300 μg of [99mTc]-labeled CD4 specific antibody (555 MBq) and then examined at 1.5, 4 and 24 hours post injection of the radiopharmaceutical. The localization of diseased joints correlated with clinical signs, early methylene diphosphonate (MDP) scan and late bone scan, but had higher specificity and sensitivity in early joint disease.

Kinne et al. performed a direct comparison between radiolabeled anti-CD4 mAb and non-specific HIG for imaging inflamed joints in rheumatoid arthritis patients. Eight patients with active or severe rheumatoid arthritis were intravenously injected with a sub-therapeutic dose of 200–300 μg (370–550 MBq) of [99mTc]-murine anti-human CD4 mAb or 1 mg (370 MBq) of polyclonal HIG. Whole-body and joint-specific scintigraphic images were acquired at 1, 4 and 24 hours post injection. The anti-CD4 mAb showed better detection of inflammatory infiltrates rich in CD4-positive cells [22].

A mAb against E-selectin labeled with [111In] has been studied in an animal model of rheumatoid arthritis and in rheumatoid arthritis patients [121,122]. Keelan et al. performed an in vivo study in an animal model with [111In]-labeled anti-E-selectin mAb (1.2B6) to assess the imaging potential of the antibody [123]. The accumulation of intravenously injected [111In]-labeled mAb was compared to that of the [111In]-control antibody in the pig arthritis model. This study demonstrated higher accumulation of [111In]-anti-E-seletin antibody in the synovitis. A comparative study was also performed by Jamar et al. between [99mTc]-HIG, an established radiopharmaceutical for arthritis imaging, and [111In]-labeled anti-E-selectin mAb in 11 patients with active rheumatoid arthritis [124]. Each patient underwent [99mTc]-HIG scintigraphy followed within 5 days by [111In]-labeled anti-E-selectin antibody scintigraphy. Scintigraphic imaging was performed at 4 hours and 20–24 hours post injection of 555 MBq of [99mTc]-HIG or 15 MBq of [111In]-anti-E-selectin mAb. Scintigraphic results were compared with clinical scores of joint involvement. Net [111In] counts over joints increased significantly between 4 hours and 24 hours (mean change of 54% ± 40%). Moreover, the images obtained with [111In]-labeled anti-E-selectin mAb demonstrated much less vascular activity than those obtained with [99mTc]-labeled non-specific immunoglobulin. The study revealed that radioimmunoscintigraphy using [111In]-labeled anti-E-selectin was more sensitive, effective and specific than [99mTc]-HIG scintigraphy to assess the rheumatoid arthritis activity and identify the active synovitis.

An anti-CD3 murine mAb, OKT-3 (Ortho Pharma; Muromonab, IgG2a) labeled with [99mTc] ([99mTc]-OKT-3) was intravenously injected into seven rheumatoid arthritis and two psoriatic arthritis patients, each patient receiving a total dose of 5 mCi [23]. Anterior and posterior whole-body scans and specific regional imaging were commenced 20 minutes after the injection. The study showed that all 34 joints with moderate-to-severe pain had moderate-to-marked uptake of radioactivity and the authors concluded that [99mTc]-OKT-3 imaging could be useful in monitoring therapeutic effectiveness in rheumatoid arthritis.

We have recently radiolabeled visilizumab (Nuvion®) with [99mTc] [125]. This [99mTc]-labeled anti-CD3 mAb may be a useful tool for *in vivo* imaging of inflammation and the early follow-up of the efficacy of therapy, as well as providing a rationale for therapy with visilizumab.

Recently, Beckers *et al.* performed a study using FDG-PET in 16 patients with active rheumatoid arthritis [126]. They found PET was positive in 69% of the knees, while magnetic resonance imaging (MRI) and ultrasound (US) were positive in 69% and 75%, respectively. A study demonstrated that visual identification of rheumatoid arthritis knee synovitis by FDG-PET correlated with the visual identification with MRI and US. The standardized uptake values (SUVs) also correlated with serum C-reactive protein (CRP) and matrix metalloproteinase-3 (MMP-3) levels.

Chianelli *et al.* showed that [99mTc]-HYNIC-TOC can be successfully used to monitor the disease activity in the joints of patients with rheumatoid arthritis (Figure 17.1) and to follow-up the efficacy of therapy [106].

[123I]-IL-1 RA has been studied in patients with rheumatoid arthritis to assess whether it is suitable for scintigraphic visualization of synovitis. [123I]-IL-1 RA was able to image inflamed joints but autoradiographic studies did not indicate that the joint accumulation of radiolabeled IL-1 RA was due to specific IL-1 receptor targeting [127]. The uptake behavior

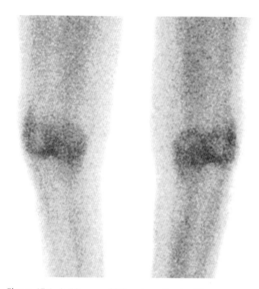

Figure 17.1 A 52-year-old female patient with rheumatoid arthritis. Images of the knees taken 1 hour after the injection of 370 MBq of [99mTc]-HYNIC-TOC. Somatostatin receptors expressed on the surface of activated lymphocytes are detected in the inflamed joints.

was similar to those of non-specific labeled agents, so it seems that radiolabeled IL-1 RA is not suitable for scintigraphic detection of inflammation.

Sjögren syndrome

Sjögren syndrome is characterized by dry mouth and dry eyes (sicca syndrome) as a result of the autoimmune destruction of the salivary and lacrimal glands. Specific autoantibodies (anti-SSA and anti-SSB) are detectable in the peripheral blood, but diagnosis is based on biopsy and/or salivary gland hypofunction as detected by scintigraphy and the Schirmer test (EULAR). New immunological treatments are being tested for Sjögren syndrome (infliximab, rituximab) and it would be useful to have a diagnostic test capable of detecting infiltrated glands that could be used for therapy selection and monitoring.

In a study in asymptomatic Sjögren syndrome patients, salivary gland scintigraphy with [99mTc]-IL-2 showed clear pathological uptake in patients with biopsy-proven infiltrated glands. No correlation was found with anti-SSA and anti-SSB antibodies. It was possible to demonstrate the presence of associated thyroid autoimmunity with the same [99mTc]-IL-2 [128].

Crohn's disease

Crohn's disease is characterized by a chronic mononuclear cell infiltration of the intestinal wall and hypertrophy of local lymphoid tissues [129]. Immune erosion of the intestinal wall may lead to severe complications of the affected bowel, such as stenosis and ulceration, which may require surgical resection. In over 70% of patients, relapse of the disease is noted within 1 year after the intervention. In the early relapse phase, symptoms are infrequent and non-specific and conventional barium X-ray examinations are negative. Since effective therapies are available, early diagnosis of relapse might allow prompt initiation of therapy to prevent the onset of complications and the need for further surgical resection [130].

Good results are obtained in Crohn's disease with radiolabeled autologous WBCs for preoperative evaluation of disease extent and for early diagnosis of relapse [131]. If ^{111}In-labeled WBCs are used, the severity of the inflammatory process can also be quantified by measuring the percentage of radioactivity excreted in the stools as a result of the migration of radiolabeled WBCs into the intestinal lumen. In normal subjects, this is less than 2% in the 4 days after the scan. Affected bowel is usually detected 3 hours after the injection.

The BW 250/183 mAb has shown good results in the study of chronic inflammatory bowel disease. Accumulation increased over the 24 hours following the injection, but there was no excretion of the radiolabel into the intestinal lumen and quantitative studies could not be performed. In a recent study, [123]1-IL-2 was successfully used in patients with Crohn's disease for the detection of bowel-infiltrating lymphocytes [91]. Nanocolloids cannot be reliably used for the study of gastrointestinal inflammation, probably owing to their slow and low uptake and also due to the physiological intestinal excretion of the tracer [132].

In a recent comparative study between ^{99m}Tc-IL-2 and ^{99m}Tc-HMPAO granulocytes in patients with inactive Crohn's disease, radiolabeled IL-2 and radiolabeled granulocytes in most cases accumulated in different areas, indicating that the two techniques detect different types of inflammation. Both techniques were characterized by high negative predictive values, but ^{99m}Tc-IL-2 was also characterized by a better correlation with time to relapse [133]. The use of ^{99m}Tc-anti-TNFα in Crohn's disease has also been proposed for therapy decision-making and biological therapy follow-up, but the uptake of this radiopharmaceutical in the gut wall has been shown to be minimal and not to correlate with the response to therapy [134].

Autoimmune thyroid diseases

Autoimmune thyroid diseases, including Graves' disease, primary myxedema and Hashimoto's thyroiditis, appear to have certain aspects of their pathogenesis and clinical course in common. Evidence of humoral immunity is provided in all of these disorders by the presence of antibodies against thyroid peroxidase (formerly known as microsomal antigen) and often against thyroglobulin. Titers tend to be highest in Hashimoto's disease and lowest in primary hypothyroidism at the time of diagnosis. More specific to Graves' disease are circulating autoantibodies that are capable of binding to the thyroid-stimulating hormone receptor (TSHr) on the surface of thyroid cells and stimulate cell growth and hormone production. However, these factors are also sometimes found in the serum of patients with Hashimoto's disease. Graves' disease, primary myxedema and Hashimoto's thyroiditis all share evidence of cell-mediated immunity against thyroid antigens and are characterized by a varying degree of infiltration by lymphocytes and plasma cells. The infiltrating cells collect in aggregates, forming lymphoid follicles with germinal centers [135,136].

Exophthalmos is a frequent manifestation of Graves' disease that may lead to severe complications. It is caused by muscle hypertrophy and lymphocytic infiltration of the retro-orbital space, which may eventually develop into fibrosis. Exophthalmos is usually treated with corticosteroids and/or cyclosporine, or by local X-ray therapy. It would be extremely useful to be able to determine the activity of the disease and to differentiate between active infiltration and fibrosis, because of the difference in their treatment.

Current diagnosis of thyroid autoimmunity is based on the detection of autoantibodies (anti-TSHr, anti-TPO and anti-TG), clinical signs and symptoms. However, the relationship between these autoantibodies and disease activity is still unclear and it is generally believed that the activity of the autoimmune process is determined by the intensity of intrathyroidal lymphocytic infiltration. *In vivo* measurement of thyroid cellular infiltration, particularly in patients with undetectable serum thyroid autoantibodies, would be the ideal approach for evaluating disease activity, determining the need for therapy and monitoring the efficacy of treatment.

Accumulation of ^{111}In-labeled lymphocytes has been shown in the thyroid glands of patients with Hashimoto's thyroiditis and primary myxedema, but not in patients with Graves' disease [12].

The use of ^{111}In-octreotide has also been investigated in patients with Graves' disease and a positive correlation between disease activity and accumulation of the agent in the thyroid and retro-orbital space of patients with exophthalmos has been reported [137,138]. However, these findings have not been confirmed by other investigators [139,140]. Further studies are required to help elucidate the potential value of this radiopharmaceutical in Graves' disease. A hypothesis has been formulated on the mechanisms of accumulation of octreotide: uptake occurs in the early stage of Graves' ophthalmopathy when active infiltration is present, but in the later stage there is fibroblastic activity with subsequent fibrosis in the retro-orbital region without expression of somatostatin receptors [141,142].

Activated lymphocytes express somatostatin receptors during the active phase of thyroid eye disease, permitting ^{111}In-pentetreotide scintigraphy. ^{111}In-pentetreotide orbital scintigraphy has been studied in patients with severe ophthalmopathy caused by Graves' disease, Hashimoto's thyroiditis, or Means' syndrome. The authors concluded that ^{111}In-pentetreotide scintigraphy allows patients to be selected for octreotide therapy, which seems to be adequate in active, moderately severe thyroid eye disease, especially when it involves soft tissues [143,144].

In a recent study in patients with Hashimoto's thyroiditis, it was possible to visualize the presence of activated lymphocytes with gamma-camera imaging using ^{99m}Tc-IL-2. No correlation was detected between the degree of thyroid accumulation of ^{99m}Tc-IL-2 and the autoantibody titer [93]. This interesting finding suggests that the humoral immunity and cell-mediated immunity are not directly related and that both should be evaluated in the assessment of disease activity.

Type 1 diabetes mellitus

Type 1 (insulin-dependent) diabetes mellitus (IDDM) is characterized by the autoimmune destruction of insulin-secreting ß-cells, mediated by mononuclear cells. Chronic lymphocytic infiltration of ß-cells is observed in two animal models of IDDM (the BB rat and NOD mouse) long before the onset of hyperglycemia and this persists until the clinical onset of disease [145]. In humans, lymphocytic infiltration of the endocrine pancreas is observed in patients soon after the diagnosis of diabetes [146] and a preclinical period of infiltration is thought to be present long before the clinical onset of the disease [147]. Indirect signs of the ongoing autoimmune process include the appearance in the peripheral blood of islet cell antibodies (ICAs), insulin autoantibodies (IAAs) and other circulating markers [148,149]. Their relation to the underlying autoimmune process, however, is unknown and it is noteworthy that a significant number of subjects with autoantibodies do not develop clinical diabetes [150]. The detection of lymphocytic infiltration before the clinical onset of disease could be used to select patients for preventive therapeutic trials and in the monitoring of the efficacy of therapy regimens.

There have been attempts to detect pancreatic lymphocytic infiltration using autologous radiolabeled lymphocytes. Kaldany et al. [16] attempted to image the infiltrated pancreas in a few newly diagnosed patients, but results were neither convincing nor conclusive. Gallina et al. [151] showed that ^{111}In-labeled lymphocytes did not visualize the infiltrated pancreas in BB rats. This might be explained by the pathophysiology of the immune process that leads to ß-cell destruction. It is a slowly progressive phenomenon that is thought to be operative for years before the clinical diagnosis; moreover, infiltrating cells are thought to be generated by *in situ* clonal expansion and not through migration from the peripheral blood. A more recent study on pancreas sections obtained from newly diagnosed diabetic patients showed typical findings of cell-mediated immunity: among the infiltrating cells, over 80% were lymphocytes, the majority of which were CD8+ positive; moreover, there was no accumulation of IgG or C3 in the infiltrated islets of Langerhans and, of a panel of adhesion molecules studied, only ICAM-1 was moderately hyperexpressed on very few endothelial cells [152]. The lack of hemodynamic changes and of endothelial activation supports the *in-situ* clonal expansion hypothesis and provides an explanation for the failure of autologous lymphocytes to migrate to and therefore visualize the infiltrated pancreas in this pathological condition.

^{123}I-IL-2 has been tested in animal models of human autoimmune diabetes (BB/W rats and NOD mice) [90]. These studies in pre-diabetic animals showed uptake and retention of ^{123}I-IL-2 in the pancreatic region between 5 and 15 minutes after injection. These data were confirmed by various experiments such as single-organ counting after sacrifice of the animals; also, autoradiography revealed that radioactivity was associated with infiltrating cells bearing IL-2R. Histological examination of pancreata revealed a positive correlation between radioactivity and the degree of lymphocytic infiltration. A preliminary study with radiolabeled IL-2 in high-risk subjects showed that this technique may be useful for early diagnosis of pancreatic infiltration and, possibly, for monitoring the efficacy of preventive treatments [97].

[18F]FDG-PET does not seem to be suitable for the detection of every inflammation, including insulitis in the pancreas of diabetic patients. Although *ex vivo* studies in NOD mice demonstrated enhanced [18F]FDG uptake in islets of Langerhans affected by insulitis, the relatively small difference between diseased and healthy islets, the small size of the islets and the limited resolution of the PET camera will most likely preclude successful application of this modality in diabetes [153]. No other validated PET radiopharmaceuticals for imaging of peripheral inflammation are available and thus more sensitive radiopharmaceuticals for PET imaging of insulitis are urgently awaited.

Sarcoidosis

Sarcoidosis is a multisystem granulomatous disease that affects predominantly the lungs and associated lymph nodes, but can involve virtually any organ. Systemic symptoms such as fatigue, night sweats and weight loss are common. Abnormalities on chest X-rays are found in more than 90% of patients with pulmonary sarcoidosis, including bilateral hilar and mediastinal lymphadenopathy with or without lung parenchymal infiltrates or interstitial

disease. Despite decades of research, the etiology of sarcoidosis is still unknown. The current hypothesis is that environmental factors trigger an immunological response that results in granuloma formation. APCs, in addition to producing high levels of TNFα, secrete IL-12, IL-15, IL-18, MCP-1, MIP-1 and granulocyte macrophage colony-stimulating factor (GM-CSF). All these factors activate CD4+ T cells to differentiate into Th1 cells and secrete IL-2, TNFα and IFN-γ. This leads to the interaction of CD4+ T cells with APCs to initiate the formation of granulomas. Sarcoidal granulomas may persist, resolve, or lead to fibrosis. Alveolar macrophages that are activated in the context of a Th2 cell response appear to stimulate fibroblast proliferation and collagen production, leading to progressive fibrosis [154]. These findings have stimulated researchers to use radiolabeled anti-TNFα antibodies to image TNFα production in the lungs and to follow-up the efficacy of specific treatments with biological anti-TNFα (Figure 17.2).

The diagnosis of sarcoidosis is established on the basis of compatible clinical and radiological findings, supported by histological evidence in one or more organs of non-caseating epithelioid cell granulomas in the absence of organisms or particles.

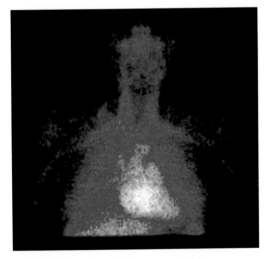

Figure 17.2 A patient with known sarcoidosis. Scintigraphy (anterior chest view) obtained 24 hours after IV injection of 400 MBq of [99mTc]-adalimumab shows the presence of TNFα in the inflamed lungs, thereby providing a rationale for therapy with unlabeled anti-TNFα monoclonal antibodies.

Nuclear medicine can be of value in the accurate assessment of disease activity, in evaluating extrapulmonary sites of sarcoidosis and in evaluating the efficacy of therapy.

The most widely used SPECT radiopharmaceuticals are ^{67}Ga-citrate and ^{99m}Tc or ^{111}In-octreotide for somatostatin receptor (SSR) imaging. Over the last decade, FDG-PET has been studied in a relatively large number of patients with sarcoidosis. FDG-PET provides valuable information on pulmonary and extrapulmonary sarcoidosis (Figures 17.3 and 17.4). There is a high uptake of [^{18}F]FDG by sarcoid granulomas, which typically appear as active lymph nodes in the mediastinum and hilar regions. [^{18}F]FDG-PET appears to be superior to ^{67}Ga-citrate scans for detecting pulmonary and extrapulmonary lesions in patients with sarcoidosis [155]. [^{18}F]FDG uptake was also described in cases of sarcoid lesions involving the brain, bones, bone marrow, muscles and skin [156].

A disadvantage of this technique is that [^{18}F]FDG uptake patterns in sarcoidosis can mimic lymph node involvement by malignancy. As a consequence, [^{18}F]FDG-PET may not be that useful as a definitive tool for the initial diagnosis of this disease, but has very good potential for monitoring the efficacy of therapy and for detecting disease relapse.

Another localization of sarcoidosis can be the heart. Cardiac involvement is difficult to determine, though this is crucial because it is the major cause of sarcoidosis-related death. [^{18}F]FDG-PET can be of value in the evaluation of cardiac sarcoidosis activity. The normal fasting period (6 hours) for [^{18}F]FDG-PET has to be prolonged to avoid physiological uptake in the heart and to shift myocardial cells from glucose metabolism to anaerobic metabolism [157].

There have also been reports in the literature describing other PET radiopharmaceuticals for assessing disease activity in sarcoidosis. Uptake of ^{11}C-methionine was an accidental finding in granulomatous lesions [158]. ^{11}C-methionine was evaluated along with [^{18}F]FDG in patients with sarcoidosis in a prospective study. From the ratio of [^{18}F]FDG-to-methionine uptake in pretreatment evaluation it is possible to predict the post-therapy outcome. This ratio could reflect the differential granulomatous states in this disease [159]. [^{18}F]Deoxyfluorothymidine ([^{18}F]FLT) was studied and compared with [^{18}F]FDG. [^{18}F]FLT uptake was specific for malignant

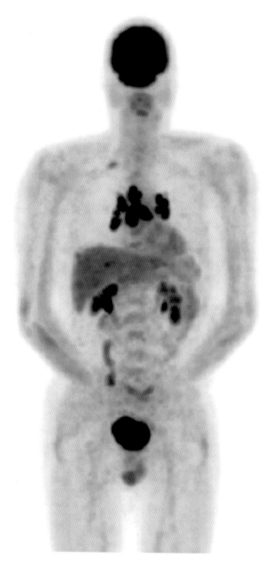

Figure 17.3 A patient with cough, tiredness and fever. Enlarged hili were seen on chest X-ray (not shown) and multiple enlarged mediastinal and hilar lymph nodes on CT scan (also not shown). [^{18}F]FDG-PET shows intense uptake in the mediastinal and hilar lymph nodes without intrapulmonary lesions. This pattern is typical for sarcoidosis, which was confirmed with histology.

lesions and revealed fewer false-positive finding in patients with sarcoidosis [160]. However, this means that [^{18}F]FLT is unsuitable as a diagnostic tool for sarcoidosis.

In summary, [^{18}F]FDG-PET is a valuable tool in sarcoidosis for the evaluation of extrapulmonary lesions, the diagnosis of cardiac involvement and

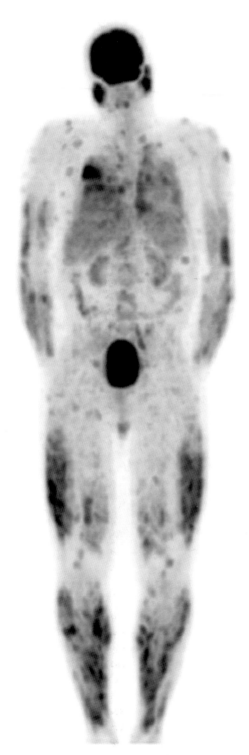

Figure 17.4 A patient with known pulmonary sarcoidosis. She also had muscle complaints. [^{18}F] FDG-PET shows extensive sarcoid disease with intrapulmonary lesions and multiple skin lesions.

the evaluation of efficacy of therapy. However, as a diagnostic tool it is rather non-specific due to the fact that it is not possible to distinguish between sarcoidosis and malignancies. When the hypothesis about the pathophysiology of sarcoidosis is proven, many new targets for the imaging of sarcoidosis may become available.

Vasculitis

The systemic vasculitides are a complex and often serious group of disorders which, while uncommon, require careful management in order to ensure optimal outcome. In most cases there is no known cause. Multisystem disease is likely to be fatal without judicious use of immunosuppression. A prompt diagnosis is necessary to preserve organ function. Comprehensive and repeated disease assessment is a necessary basis for planning therapy and modifying treatment protocols according to response. Therapies typically include glucocorticoids, especially for small and medium diseased vessels [161].

The diagnosis of large vessel vasculitis remains a challenge, especially in patients presenting with non-specific symptoms and laboratory tests. Standard diagnostic procedures include biopsy, angiography, US and magnetic resonance angiography. These procedures are either invasive, operator dependent or detect only morphological changes which occur mainly in the later stages of the disease. In contrast, PET is an operator-independent, non-invasive metabolic imaging modality based on the regional distribution of the glucose analog FDG. Today, [^{18}F]FDG-PET plays a major role in the management of oncology patients. However, activated inflammatory cells also overexpress GLUTs and accumulate increased amounts of glucose and structurally-related substances such as [^{18}F]FDG (Figure 17.5).

Remarkable images of patients with active vasculitis have been generated through [^{18}F]FDG-PET scans and initial studies indicate that [^{18}F]-FDG-PET may be useful for imaging giant cell arteritis and Takayasu's arteritis. Large vessel involvement is found on [^{18}F]FDG-PET scanning in about 83% of patients with giant cell arteritis. Vascular [^{18}F]FDG uptake is found especially in the subclavian arteries (74%), but also in the aorta ($\geq$50%) and femoral arteries (37%). The common [^{18}F]FDG uptake pattern found in giant cell arteritis is linear and

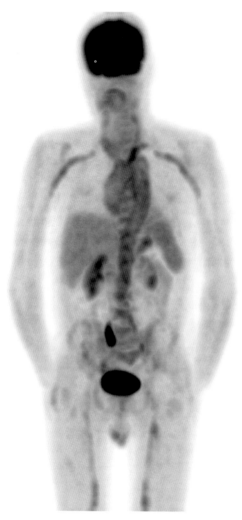

Figure 17.5 [^{18}F]FDG-PET in a 60-year-old male patient with a 6-month history of fever of unknown origin. No explanation for the fever was found on chest X-ray, CT scan or US (not shown). The patient's erythrocyte sedimentation rate (ESR) was 113 mm/h and CRP level was 12.1 mg/dL. This [^{18}F]FDG-PET image shows high uptake in the carotid arteries, subclavian arteries, aorta and iliac and femoral arteries. Pathology confirmed giant cell arteritis. The patient was treated with prednisone and his fever resolved.

continuous, and thoracic vessels are most frequently affected, followed by the abdominal vessels. The common [^{18}F]FDG uptake pattern in the early phases of Takayasu's arteritis is also linear and continuous, while in late phases it becomes patchy rather than continuous. Recent [^{18}F]FDG-PET studies have shown sensitivities between 56% and

100% for detecting giant cell arteritis and between 83% and 100% for detecting Takayasu's arteritis. [^{18}F]FDG-PET and MRI in comparative studies showed similar sensitivities, but [^{18}F]FDG-PET has been shown to identify significantly more affected vascular regions. Furthermore, [^{18}F]FDG-PET has shown value in predicting the development of complications (Figure 17.6), e.g. thoracic aortic dilatation in patients with giant cell arteritis, and the ability to demonstrate response after successful initiation of immunosuppressive treatment [162].

Atherosclerosis

Many radiopharmaceuticals have been developed with the molecules and cells involved in atherogenesis in mind. These radiopharmaceuticals can be divided into three major groups, based on their target cells: for imaging atherosclerotic components, for imaging thrombosis and for imaging inflammation. In particular, several cytokines, chemokines and their receptors, which are responsible for early events in atherosclerosis, can be directly or indirectly labeled with radionuclides to allow the imaging of vulnerable atherosclerotic lesions [14].

Monocytes and macrophages, the predominant cell types in acute and chronic inflammation, are attracted to and activated by MCP-1. ^{125}I-MCP-1 has been tested in normal mice and in atheroma-rich rabbits and the uptake shown to correlate with the number of macrophages per unit area [163]. Radiolabeled MCP-1 may be a useful radiopharmaceutical for imaging monocyte/macrophage-rich atherosclerotic lesions at the stage of subacute inflammation.

IL-2R-positive cells play a crucial role in atherosclerosis [164] and both ^{99m}Tc- and ^{123}I-IL-2 have been proposed for atherosclerosis imaging [165]. Higher serum IL-2 levels are associated with increased carotid artery intima–media thickness (IMT), a predictor of stroke and vascular disease [166]. ^{99m}Tc-IL-2 is therefore also used for imaging carotid atherosclerosis in humans (Figure 17.7). Fourteen patients (16 plaques) who were eligible for endarterectomy underwent ^{99m}Tc-IL-2 scintigraphy before surgery. Another nine patients (13 plaques) received atorvastatin or a standard hypocholesterolemic diet and scintigraphy was performed before and after 3 months of treatment. The accumulation of ^{99m}Tc-IL-2 in vulnerable carotid plaques corre-

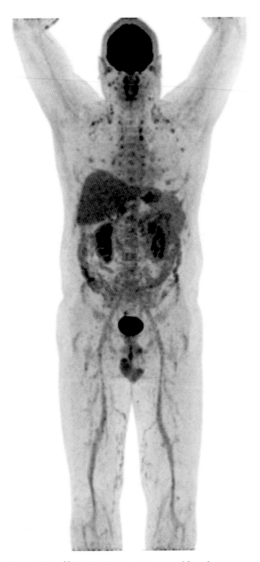

Figure 17.6 [^{18}F]FDG-PET in a 35-year-old male patient with known polychondritis. Despite treatment for the polychondritis, the patient was still experiencing fever and pain. Blood parameters were normal. This [^{18}F] FDG-PET image shows uptake in chondral structures (nose, ears, costochondral joints), but also high uptake in the iliac and femoral arteries, including all branches. Polychondritis can be associated with vasculitis; in this case of the peripheral vasculature including all small branches.

lated with the number of IL-2R-positive cells within the plaques (measured *ex vivo* by histology). Also, the amount of ^{99m}Tc-IL-2 within the plaques was influenced by lipid-lowering treatment with a statin [165]. Thus, ^{99m}Tc-IL-2 is a very promising radiop-

harmaceutical that could provide useful information for the identification of infiltrated vulnerable plaques at risk of rupture. There are no significant biological side effects at the low dose used for imaging purposes. However, ^{99m}Tc-IL-2 is not yet commercially available and a major drawback is the complexity of the labeling procedure in in-house preparation.

All the above-mentioned radiopharmaceuticals are for SPECT. The PET radiopharmaceutical [^{18}F] FDG has the possible advantage that it can provide absolute quantification and better resolution than the SPECT radiopharmaceutical. As [^{18}F]FDG is a glucose analog that is trapped in cells in proportion to the cells' metabolic activity, it is retained within plaque macrophages more avidly than within other plaque elements [167]. Good reproducibility was reported in a group of patients who underwent carotid artery and aortic imaging, with high inter- and intra-observer agreement and low variability of [^{18}F]FDG uptake over 2 weeks [168]. Results in the iliac and femoral arteries were also highly reproducible, although [^{18}F]FDG uptake in the carotid arteries was significantly higher than in both iliac and femoral vessels [169]. In 30% of patients with documented carotid atherosclerosis, inflammation was detected by [^{18}F]FDG-PET imaging. This raises the possibility that this non-invasive metabolic imaging modality could be useful in the risk stratification of patients and the selection of appropriate therapy. Large prospective studies are necessary to determine if the detection of inflamed plaque by FDG-PET is useful for predicting future cardiovascular disease [170].

Role for therapy follow-up and patient management

Rheumatoid arthritis

Conti *et al.* used the anti-TNFα mAb infliximab (Rimicade®) labeled with ^{99m}Tc to assess the degree of TNFα-mediated inflammation in the affected joints of patients with arthritis [171]. Patients underwent scintigraphic examination with ^{99m}Tc-infliximab before and 4 months after intra-articular infliximab therapy. Planar images of the inflamed joint were acquired at 6 hours and 24 hours post injection of infliximab (15 mCi). Intense accumulation of ^{99m}Tc-infliximab was seen in the affected knee, probably reflecting the high levels of intralesional TNFα.

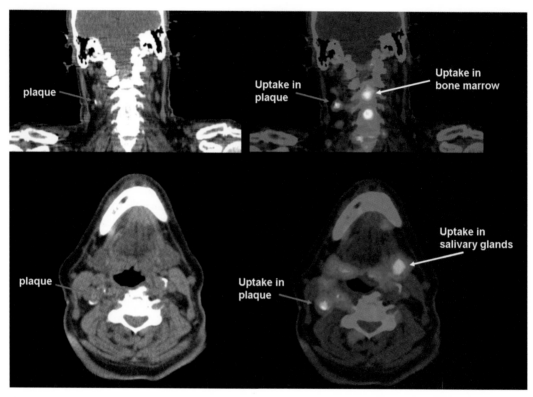

Figure 17.7 A 70-year-old male patient who presented with loss of power of the left hand and arm. Duplex US of the carotid arteries revealed a 70–90% stenosis in the right carotid artery and a 50–70% stenosis in the left carotid artery (not shown). Scintigraphy 1 hour after IV injection of 195 MBq of ^{99m}Tc-IL-2 showed uptake of IL-2 by the plaque in the right carotid artery; there was no uptake by the left carotid artery (upper row: coronal views of the CT and fused SPECT/CT; lower row: transaxial views of the CT and fused SPECT/CT). Uptake of IL-2 by the plaque on the right side is associated with inflammation around the plaque and, as a consequence, the plaque is vulnerable.

The anti-TNFα mAb adalimumab (Humira®) has been labeled with ^{99m}Tc using the indirect radiolabeling method described by Abrams *et al.* [172]. Barrera *et al.* performed a scintigraphic imaging study in ten patients with active rheumatoid arthritis to assess the sensitivity and biodistribution of systemically administered ^{99m}Tc-anti-TNF mAb [173]. All the patients underwent two scintigraphic examinations, the first to assess the biodistribution of the radiolabeled antibody and the second 2 weeks later to assess the specificity for TNF targeting and sensitivity for decreased inflammation after the administration of systemic corticosteroids. Each patient received a sub-therapeutic IV dose of 0.1 mg (740 MBq) of ^{99m}Tc-adalimumab prior to scintigraphy. The inflamed joints were clearly visualized at 4 hours and 24 hours after injection and the increase in uptake at 20 hours was 20–30%. Interestingly,

no uptake of ^{99m}Tc-adalimumab was seen in the normal joints. Furthermore, this radiopharmaceutical specifically targets TNFα in the arthritic joint and it can detect clinically relevant changes in disease activity.

In another study conducted by our group, the use of ^{99m}Tc-infliximab and -adalimumab for therapy decision-making and follow-up was studied in seven and 12 rheumatoid arthritis patients, respectively [174]. Scintigraphic examination was performed before and 3 months after the intra-articular/systemic therapy with infliximab or systemic therapy with adalimumab. Planar anterior and posterior images of the arthritic joints were acquired at 6 hours and 20 hours after the injection of 10 mCi ^{99m}Tc-infliximab or ^{99m}Tc-adalimumab. No differences in biodistribution were observed between the two radiopharmaceuticals. For both, a variable degree of joint uptake was observed and this did not always correlate with joint pain or swelling (target-to-background ratio range 1.00–3.99). This study concluded that ^{99m}Tc-infliximab showed fast whole-body clearance and high inflammatory area localization, with no uptake in normal tissue and no human antibody response [174]. These data were confirmed in a larger population study in which ^{99m}Tc-infliximab was used for therapy decision-making and follow-up [175].

These preliminary studies in humans show the specific targeting of inflamed joints by this radiopharmaceutical. Moreover, it also demonstrates that ^{99m}Tc-infliximab scintigraphy before therapy may make it possible to select candidates for and predict response to anti-TNFα therapy.

Sjögren syndrome

A recent study has described the use of the new somatostatin analog ^{99m}Tc-HYNIC-TOC for the diagnosis of disease activity in patients with rheumatoid arthritis and secondary Sjögren syndrome before and after treatment with infliximab. Results showed that inflamed parotid glands could be diagnosed with this radiopharmaceutical. Inflamed joints were also detected in patients with active rheumatoid arthritis [106]. Interestingly, after treatment with infliximab, normalization of the uptake in most inflamed joints was noted, but not in salivary glands, probably reflecting the different nature of the two diseases.

Type 1 diabetes mellitus

In a recent study, newly diagnosed patients with type 1 diabetes and treated with two doses of nicotinamide (25 or 50 mg/kg), were studied with ^{99m}Tc-IL-2 scintigraphy at diagnosis and after treatment. At the time of diagnosis there was no difference between the two groups in metabolic, immunological and scintigraphic parameters. After 1 year of treatment, however, patients positive on ^{99m}Tc-IL-2 scintigraphy showed a significantly lower daily insulin requirement, suggesting that nicotinamide in patients with persistent inflammation at the time of diagnosis is effective in protecting the residual β-cell mass present at diagnosis [176].

A significant accumulation of radiolabeled HIG has been observed in the pancreas of approximately 50% of newly diagnosed type 1 diabetic patients [177], probably as a consequence of the presence

of immune complexes or secondary to increased vascular permeability. This may be helpful in identifying those patients who may benefit from adjuvant immunotherapy at the time of diagnosis, with the aim of inducing clinical remission.

Sarcoidosis

Whole-body [^{18}F]FDG-PET scans are of value in identifying occult and reversible granulomas in patients with sarcoidosis. The metabolic activity measured with [^{18}F]FDG-PET may reflect the disease activity in sarcoidosis in quantitative terms. [^{18}F]FDG-PET also has a role in evaluating therapy; glucose uptake in the granulomas has been shown to decrease after corticosteroid therapy [178].

A recent study reported that somatostatin receptor scintigraphy using ^{99m}Tc-HYNIC-TOC in a patient with systemic sarcoidosis could detect pulmonary and extrapulmonary localizations of sarcoidosis. It was also possible to select the best therapeutic option for this patient. After treatment with infliximab, there was normalization of the scintigraphy scan and this correlated with improvement in the patient's clinical status [179].

References

1. Bonecchi R, Bianchi G, Panina Bordignon P et al. Differential expression of chemokine receptors and chemotactic responsiveness of type 1 T helper cells (Th1s) and Th2s. *J Exp Med* 1998;187:129–134.
2. Flanagan AM, Chambers TJ. Chronic inflammation. In: McGee JO'D, Isaacson PG, Wright NA (eds). *Oxford Textbook of Pathology*. Oxford: Oxford University Press, 1992, pp. 389–406.
3. Roitt I. *Essential Immunology*, 8th edn. Oxford: Blackwell Scientific Publications, 1994.
4. Peters AM, Jamar F. The importance of endothelium and interstitial fluid in nuclear medicine. *Eur J Nucl Med* 1998;25:801–815.
5. Reubi J, Mazzucchelli L, Laissue J. Intestinal vessels express a high density of somatostatin receptor in human inflammatory bowel disease. *Gastroenterology* 1994;106:951–959.
6. Wyllie AH, Kerr JF, Currie AR. Cell death: the significance of apoptosis. *Int Rev Cytol* 1980;68: 251–306.
7. Thompson CB. Apoptosis in the pathogenesis and treatment of disease. *Science* 1995;267: 1456–1462.
8. Palmer S, Burch L, David RD et al. The role of innate immunity in acute allograft rejection after lung

transplantation. *Am J Respir Crit Care Med* 2003;168: 628–632.

9. Muller-Quernheim J. Sarcoidosis: immunopathogenetic concepts and their clinical application. *Eur Repir J* 1998;12:716–738.

10. Mitchell DN, Scadding JG, Heard BE *et al.* Sarcoidosis: histopathological definition and clinical diagnosis. *J Clin Pathol* 1977;30:395–408.

11. Moller DR, Chen ES. Genetic basis of remitting sarcoidosis: triumph of the trimolecular complex? *Am J Respir Cell Mol Biol* 2002;27:391–395.

12. Agostini C, Adami F, Semenzato G. New pathogenetic insights into the sarcoid granuloma. *Curr Opin Rheumatol* 2000;12:71–76.

13. Borchers AT, Gershwin ME. Giant cell arteritis: a review of classification, pathophysiology, geoepidemiology and treatment. *Autoimm Rev* 2012;11: A544–554.

14. Glaudemans AWJM, Slart RHJA, Bozzao A *et al.* Molecular imaging in atherosclerosis. *Eur J Nucl Med Mol Imaging* 2010;37:2381–2397.

15. Lavender JP, Goldman JM, Arnot RN, Thakur ML. Kinetics of indium-111-labelled lymphocytes in normal subjects and in patients with Hodgkin's disease. *Br Med J* 1977;2:797–799.

16. Kaldany A, Hill T, Wentworth S *et al.* Trapping of peripheral blood lymphocytes in the pancreas of patients with acute-onset insulin-dependent diabetes mellitus. *Diabetes* 1982;31:463–466.

17. Pozzilli P, Pozzilli C, Pantano P, Negri Mandreani D, Cudworth AG. Tracking of indium-lll-oxine-labelled lymphocytes in autoimmune thyroid disease. *Clin Endocrinol (Oxf)* 1983;19:111–116.

18. Ten Berge RJM, Natarajan AT, Hardeman MR, van Royen EA, Schellekens P. Labelling with Indium-111 has detrimental effects on human lymphocytes: concise communication. *J Nucl Med* 1983; 24:615–620.

19. Signore A, Beales P, Sensi M, Zuccarini O, Pozzilli P. Labelling of lymphocytes with Indium-111-oxine: effect on cell surface phenotype and antibody-dependent cellular cytotoxicity. *Immunol Lett* 1983; 6:151–154.

20. Fischmann AJ, Rubin RH, Khaw BA *et al.* Detection of acute inflammation with 111In-labelled nonspecific polyclonal IgG. *Semin Nucl Med* 1988;18: 335–344.

21. Oyen WJG, van Horn JR, Claessens RAMJ *et al.* Diagnosis of bone, joint and joint prosthesis infections with indium-111-labelled human immunoglobulin G scintigraphy. *Radiology* 1992;182:195–199.

22. Kinne RW, Becker W, Schwab J *et al.* Comparison of 99mTc-labelled specific murine anti-CD4 monoclonal antibodies and nonspecific human immunoglobulins for imaging inflamed joints in rheumatoid arthritis. *Nucl Med Commun* 1993;14: 667–675.

23. Marcus C, Thakur ML, Huynh TV *et al.* Imaging rheumatic joint disease with anti-T lymphocyte antibody OKT-3. *Nucl Med Commun* 1994;15: 824–830.

24. Becker W, Goldenberg GM, Wolf F. The use of monoclonal antibodies and antibodies fragments in the imaging of infectious lesions. *Semin Nucl Med* 1994; 24:1–13.

25. Palestro CJ, Caprioli R, Love C *et al.* Rapid diagnosis of pedal osteomyelitis in diabetics with a technetium-99m-labeled monoclonal antigranulocyte antibody. *J Foot Ankle Surg* 2003;42:2–8.

26. Gratz S, Behr T, Herrmann A *et al.* Intraindividual comparison of ^{99m}Tc-labelled anti-SSEA-1 antigranulocyte antibody and ^{99m}Tc-HMPAO labelled white blood cells for the imaging of infection. *Eur J Nucl Med* 1998;25:386–393.

27. Gratz S, Raddatz D, Hagenah G, Behr T, Béhé M, Becker W. ^{99m}Tc-labelled antigranulocyte monoclonal antibody FAB' fragments versus echocardiography in the diagnosis of subacute infective endocarditis. *Int J Cardiol* 2000;75:75–84.

28. Barron B, Hanna C, Passalaqua AM, Lamki L, Wegener WA, Goldenberg DM. Rapid diagnostic imaging of acute, nonclassic appendicitis by leukoscintigraphy with sulesomab, a technetium 99m-labeled antigranulocyte antibody Fab' fragment. LeukoScan Appendicitis Clinical Trial Group. *Surgery* 1999;125:288–296.

29. Harwood SJ, Valdivia S, Hung GL, Quenzer RW. Use of Sulesomab, a radiolabeled antibody fragment, to detect osteomyelitis in diabetic patients with foot ulcers by leukoscintigraphy. *Clin Infect Dis* 1999;28:1200–1205.

30. Paul J, Anderson PJ. Tumor necrosis factor inhibitors: clinical implications of their different immunogenicity profiles. *Semin Arthritis Rheum* 2005;34 (Suppl):19–22.

31. Knight DM, Trinh H, Le J *et al.* Construction and initial characterization of a mouse-human chimeric anti-TNF antibody. *Mol Immunol* 1993;30: 1443–1453.

32. Rau R. Adalimumab (a fully human anti-tumour necrosis factor a monoclonal antibody) in the treatment of active rheumatoid arthritis: the initial results of five trials. *Ann Rheum Dis* 2002;61 (Suppl II):70–73.

33. Rituxan® (Rituximab), package insert. San Francisco: Genentech Inc; revised February 21, 2007.

34. Reff ME, Carner K, Chambers KS *et al.* Depletion of B cells *in vivo* by a chimeric mouse human monoclonal antibody to CD20. *Blood* 1994;83: 435–445.

35. Dorner T, Rumester G. The role of B-cells in rheumatoid arthritis: mechanisms and therapeutic targets. *Curr Opin Rheum* 2003;15:246–252.

36. Utset TO, Auger JA, Peace D et al. Modified anti-CD3 therapy in psoriatic arthritis: a phase I/II clinical trial. *J Rheumatol* 2002;29:1907–1913.

37. Alegre ML, Peterson LJ, Xu D et al. A non-activating "humanized" anti-CD3 monoclonal antibody retains immunosuppressive properties *in vivo*. *Transplantation* 1994;57:1537–1543.

38. Woodle ES, Xu D, Zivin RA et al. Phase I trial of a humanized, Fc receptor nonbinding OKT3 antibody, huOKT3gamma1(Ala-Ala) in the treatment of acute renal allograft rejection. *Transplantation* 1999;68:608–616.

39. Trajkovic V. Nuvion Protein Design Labs. *Curr Opin Invest Drugs* 2002;3:411–414.

40. Cole MS, Stellrecht KW, Shi JD et al. HuM291, a humanized anti-CD3 antibody, is immunosuppressive to T cells while exhibiting reduced mitogenicity *in vitro*. *Transplantation* 1999;68:563–571.

41. Chatenoud L, Ferran C, Reuter A et al. Systemic reaction to the anti-T cell mAb OKT3 in relation to serum levels of tumor necrosis factor and interferon-gamma. *N Engl J Med* 1989;320:1420–1421.

42. Pohlers D, Schmidt-Weber CB, Franch A et al. Differential clinical efficacy of anti-CD4 monoclonal antibodies in rat adjuvant arthritis is paralleled by differential influence on NF-kappaB binding activity and TNF-alpha secretion of T cells. *Arthritis Res* 2002;4:184–189.

43. Reddy MP, Kinney CAS, Chaikin MA et al. Elimination of Fc receptor-dependent effector functions of a modified IgG4 monoclonal antibody to human CD4. *J Immunol* 2000;164:1925–1933.

44. Wu C, Jagoda E, Brechbiel M et al. Biodistribution and catabolism of Ga-67-labeled anti-Tac dsFv fragment. *Bioconjugate Chem* 1997;8:365–369.

45. Kobayashi H, Yoo TM, Drumm D et al. Improved biodistribution of ^{125}I-labeled anti-Tac disulfide-stabilized Fv fragment by blocking its binding to the α subunit of the interleukin 2 receptor in the circulation with preinjected humanized anti-Tac IgG. *Cancer Res* 1997;57:1955–1961.

46. Zhang M, Yao Z, Zhang Z et al. The anti-CD25 monoclonal antibody 7G7/B6, armed with the α-Emitter [211]At, provides effective radioimmunotherapy for a murine model of leukemia. *Cancer Res* 2006;66:8227–8232.

47. Hartmann F, Horak EM, Garmestani K et al. Radioimmunotherapy of nude mice bearing a human interleukin 2 receptor alpha expressing lymphoma utilizing the alpha-emitting radionuclide-conjugated monoclonal antibody [212]Bi-anti-Tac. *Cancer Res* 1994;54:4362–4370.

48. Choi CW, Lang L, Lee JT et al. Biodistribution of [18]F- and ^{125}I-labeled anti-Tac disulfide-stabilized Fv fragments in nude mice with interleukin 2 alpha receptor-positive tumor xenografts. *Cancer Res* 1995;55:5323–5329.

49. Kwa HB, Verhoeven AH, Storm J, van Zandwijk N, Mooi W, Hilkens J. Radioimmunotherapy of small-cell lung cancer xenografts using ^{131}I-labelled anti-NCAM monoclonal antibody [123]C3. *Cancer Immunol Immunother* 1995;41:169–174.

50. Ornadel D, Ledermann JA, Eagle K et al. Biodistribution of a radiolabelled monoclonal antibody NY3D11 recognizing the neural cell adhesion molecule in tumour xenografts and patients with small-cell lung cancer. *Br J Cancer* 1998;77:103–109.

51. Papanastassiou V, Pizer BL, Coakham HB, Bullimore J, Zananiri T, Kemshead JT. Treatment of recurrent and cystic malignant gliomas by a single intracavity injection of ^{131}I monoclonal antibody: feasibility, pharmacokinetics and dosimetry. *Br J Cancer* 1993;67:144–151.

52. Hopkins K, Chandler C, Bullimore J, Sandeman D, Coakham H, Kemshead JT. A pilot study of the treatment of patients with recurrent malignant gliomas with intratumoral yttrium-90 radioimmunoconjugates. *Radiother Oncol* 1995;34:121–131.

53. Hosono MN, Hosono M, Mishra AK et al. Rhenium-188-labeled anti-neural cell adhesion molecule antibodies with 2-iminothiolane modification for targeting small-cell lung cancer. *Ann Nucl Med* 2000;14:173–179.

54. Arimura Y, Koda T, Kishi M, Kakinuma M. Mouse HLA-DPA homologue H2-Pα: a pseudogene that maps between H2-Pb and H2-Oα. *Immunogenetics* 1996;43:152–155.

55. Sønderstrup G, McDevitt HO. DR, DQ, and you: MHC alleles and autoimmunity. *J Clin Invest* 2001;107:795–796.

56. Malviya G, de Vries EFJ, Dierckx RA, Signore A. Synthesis and evaluation of ^{99m}Tc-labelled monoclonal antibody 1D09C3 for molecular imaging of major histocompatibility complex class II protein expression. *Mol Imaging Biol* 2011;13:930–939.

57. Otero DC, Rickert RC. CD19 Function in early and late B cell development. II. CD19 facilitates the Pro-B/Pre-B transition. *J Immunol* 2003;171:5921–5930.

58. Vervoordeldonk SF, Heikens J, Goedemans WT et al. ^{99m}Tc-CD19 monoclonal antibody is not useful for imaging of B cell non-Hodgkin's lymphoma. *Cancer Immunol Immunother* 1996;42:291–296.

59. Mitchell P, Lee FT, Hall C et al. Targeting primary human Ph[+] B-cell precursor leukemia-engrafted SCID mice using radiolabeled anti-CD19 monoclonal antibodies. *J Nucl Med* 2003;44:1105–1112.

60. Stamenkovic I, Seed B. CD19, the earliest differentiation antigen of the B cell lineage, bears three extracellular immunoglobulin-like domains and an Epstein-Barr virus-related cytoplasmic tail. *J Exp Med* 1988;168:1205–1210.

61. Tedder T F, Tuscano J, Sato S *et al*. CD22, a B lymphocyte-specific adhesion molecule that regulates antigen receptor signaling. *Annu Rev Immunol* 1997;15:481–504.

62. Cesano A, Gayko U. CD22 as a target of passive immunotherapy. *Semin Oncol* 2003;30:253–257.

63. Tedder TF, Poe JC, Haas KM. CD22: a multifunctional receptor that regulates B lymphocyte survival and signal transduction. *Adv Immunol* 2005;88: 1–50.

64. Steinfeld SD, Youinou P. Epratuzumab (humanised anti-CD22 antibody) in autoimmune diseases. *Expert Opin Biol Ther* 2006;6:943–949.

65. Leung SO, Goldenberg DM, Dion AS *et al*. Construction and characterization of a humanized, internalizing B cell (CD22)-specific, leukemia/ lymphoma antibody, LL2. *Mol Immunol* 1995;32: 1413–1427.

66. Castillo J, Winer E, Quesenberry P. Newer monoclonal antibodies for malignancies. *Exp Hematol* 2008;36:755–768.

67. Lamonica D, Czuczman M, Nabi H, Klippenstein D, Grossman Z. Radioimmunoscintigraphy (RIS) with bectumomab (Tc99m labeled IMMU-LL2, Lymphoscan) in the assessment of recurrent non-Hodgkin's lymphoma (NHL). *Cancer Biother Radiopharm* 2002; 17:689–697.

68. Sen J, Bossu P, Burakoff SJ, Abbas AK. T cell surface molecules regulating noncognate B lymphocyte activation. Role of CD2 and LFA-1. *J Immunol* 1992; 148:1037–1042.

69. Vacca A, Buchegger F, Carrel S, Mach JP. Imaging of human leukemic T-cell xenografts in nude mice by radiolabeled monoclonal antibodies and F(ab')2 fragments. *Cancer* 1988;61:58–67.

70. Langley RG, Papp K, Bissonnette R *et al*. Safety profile of intravenous and subcutaneous siplizumab, an anti-CD2 monoclonal antibody, for the treatment of plaque psoriasis: results of two randomized, double-blind, placebo-controlled studies. *Int J Dermatol* 2010;49:818–828.

71. Pruett TL, McGory RW, Wright FH, Pescovitz MD, Yang H, McClain JB. Safety profile, pharmacokinetics, and pharmacodynamics of siplizumab, a humanized anti-CD2 monoclonal antibody, in renal allograft recipients. *Transplant Proc* 2009;41: 3655–3661.

72. Spertini F, Stohl W, Ramesh N, Moody C, Geha RS. Induction of human T cell proliferation by a monoclonal antibody to CD5. *J Immunol* 1991;146: 47–52.

73. Calvo J, Places L, Padilla O *et al*. Interaction of recombinant and natural soluble CD5 forms with an alternative cell surface ligand. *Eur J Immunol* 1999;29:2119–2129.

74. Vallera DA, Schmidberger H, Buchsbaum DJ, Everson P, Snover DC, Blazar BR. Radiotherapy in mice with yttrium-90-labeled anti-Ly1 monoclonal antibody: therapy of established graft-versus-host disease induced across the major histocompatibility barrier. *Cancer Res* 1991;51:1891–1897.

75. Foss FM, Raubitscheck A, Mulshine JL *et al*. Phase I study of the pharmacokinetics of a radioimmunoconjugate, ^{90}Y-T101, in patients with CD5-expressing leukemia and lymphoma. *Clin Cancer Res* 1998;4:2691–2700.

76. Vallera DA, Elson M, Brechbiel MW *et al*. Preclinical studies targeting normal and leukemic hematopoietic cells with Yttrium-90-labeled anti-CD45 antibody *in vitro* and *in vivo* in nude mice. *Cancer Biother Radiopharm* 2003;18:133–145.

77. Glatting G, Müller M, Koop B *et al*. Anti-CD45 monoclonal antibody YAML568: A promising radioimmunoconjugate for targeted therapy of acute leukemia. *J Nucl Med* 2006;47:1335–1341.

78. Signore A, Corsetti F, Annovazzi A *et al*. Biological imaging for the diagnosis of inflammatory conditions. *Biodrugs* 2002;16:241–259.

79. Signore A, Procaccini E, Annovazzi A, van der Laken C, Mire-Sluis A, Chianelli M. The developing role of cytokines in imaging inflammation and infection. *Cytokine* 2000;12:1445–1454.

80. van der Laken CJ, Boerman OC, Oyen WJ *et al*. Specific targeting of infectious foci with radioiodinated human recombinant interleukin-1 in an experimental model. *Eur J Nucl Med* 1995;22: 1249–1255.

81. van der Laken CJ, Boerman OC, Oyen WJ *et al*. Different behaviour of radioiodinated human recombinant interleukin-1 and its receptor antagonist in an animal model of infection. *Eur J Nucl Med* 1996;23:1531–1535.

82. van der Laken CJ, Boerman OC, Oyen WJ, van de Ven MT, van der Meer JW, Corstens FH. Imaging of infection in rabbits with radioiodinated interleukin-1 (alpha and beta), its receptor antagonist and a chemotactic peptide: a comparative study. *Eur J Nucl Med* 1998;25:347–352.

83. Morgan DA, Ruscetti FW, Gallo RC. Selective *in vitro* growth factor of T lymphocytes from normal human bone marrow. *Science* 1976;193:1007–1009.

84. Smith KA. Interleukin-2: inception, impact and implications. *Science* 1988;240:1169–1176.

85. Semenzato, G., Zambello, R., Pizzolo, G. Interleukin-2 receptor expression in health and disease. In: Waxman J, Balkwill F (eds). *Interleukin-2*. Oxford: Blackwell Scientific Publications, 1992, pp. 78–105.

86. Robb RJ, Greene WC, Rusk CM. Low and high affinity receptors for IL2. *J Exp Med* 1984;160:1126–1146.

87. Koths K, Halenbech R. Pharmacokinetic studies on ^{35}S-labelled recombinant interleukin-2 in mice. In: Sorg C, Schimpl A (eds). *Cellular and Molecular Biology of Lymphokines*. Orlando, Academic Press Inc, 1985.

88. Robb RJ, Mayer PC, Garlick R. Retention of biological activity following radioiodination of human interleukin-2: comparison with biosyntetically labelled growth factor in receptor binding assay. *J Immunol Methods* 1985;81:15–30.

89. Gennuso R, Spigelman, MK, Vallabhajosula S *et al*. Systemic biodistribution of radioiodinated interleukin-2 in the rat. *J Biol Resp Mod* 1989;8: 375–384.

90. Signore A, Parman A, Pozzilli P, Andreani D, Beverley PCL. Detection of activated lymphocytes in endocrine pancreas of BB/W rats by injection of 123-iodine-labelled interleukin-2: an early sign of Type 1 diabetes. *Lancet* 1987;2:536–540.

91. Signore A, Chianelli M, Toscano A *et al*. A radiopharmaceutical for imaging areas of lymphocytic infiltration: ^{123}I-interleukin-2: labelling procedure and animal studies. *Nucl Med Commun* 1992;13: 713–722.

92. Abbs IC, Pratt JR, Dallman MJ, Sacks SH. Analysis of activated T cell infiltrates in rat renal allografts by gamma camera imaging after injection of 123-iodine-interleukin-2. *Transplant Immunol* 1993;1: 45–51.

93. Chianelli M, Mather SJ, Grossman A *et al*. ^{99m}Tc-interleukin-2 scintigraphy in normal subjects and in patients with autoimmune thyroid diseases: a feasibility study. *Eur J Nucl Med Mol Imaging* 2008; 35:2286–2293.

94. Signore A, Chianelli M, Annovazzi A *et al*. ^{123}I-labelled interleukin-2 scintigraphy for the *in vivo* assessment of intestinal mononuclear cell infiltration in Crohn's disease. *J Nucl Med* 2000;41: 242–249.

95. Signore A, Chianelli M, Annovazzi A *et al*. Imaging active lymphocytic infiltration in coeliac disease with ^{123}I-interleukin-2 and its response to diet. *Eur J Nucl Med* 2000;27:18–24.

96. Chianelli M, Parisella MG, Visalli N *et al*.; IMDIAB Study Group. Pancreatic scintigraphy with ^{99m}Tc-interleukin-2 at diagnosis of type 1 diabetes and after 1 year of nicotinamide therapy. *Diabetes Metab Res Rev* 2008;24:115–122.

97. Signore A, Picarelli A, Chianelli M *et al*. ^{123}I-Interleukin-2 scintigraphy: a new approach to assess disease activity in autoimmunity. *J Pediatr Endocrinol Metab* 1996;9:139–144.

98. Signore A, Annovazzi A, Barone R *et al*. ^{99m}Tc-interleukin-2 scintigraphy as a potential tool for evaluating tumor-infiltrating lymphocytes in melanoma lesions: a validation study. *J Nucl Med* 2004;45:1647–1652.

99. Rennen HJ, Boerman OC, Oyen WJ, Corstens FH. Kinetics of ^{99m}Tc-labeled interleukin-8 in experimental inflammation and infection. *J Nucl Med* 2003;44:1502–1509.

100. Rennen HJ, Boerman OC, Oyen WJ, van der Meer JW, Corstens FH. Specific and rapid scintigraphic detection of infection with ^{99m}Tc-labeled interleukin-8. *J Nucl Med* 2001;42:117–123.

101. van der Laken CJ, Boerman OC, Oyen WJ, van de Ven MT, van der Meer JW, Corstens FH. Radiolabeled interleukin-8: specific scintigraphic detection of infection within a few hours. *J Nucl Med* 2000; 41:463–469.

102. Signore A, Annovazzi A, Chianelli M *et al*. Peptide radiopharmaceuticals for diagnosis and therapy. *Eur J Nucl Med* 2001;28:1555–1565.

103. Van Hagen P, Markusse H, Lamberts S, Kwekkeboom DJ, Reubi JC, Krenning ESP. Somatostatin receptor imaging: The presence of somatostatin receptor in rheumatoid arthritis. *Arthritis Rheum* 1994;37: 1521–1527.

104. Oyen WJG, Boerman OC, Claessens RAMJ, van der Meer JWM, Corstens FHM. Is somatostatin receptor scintigraphy suited to detection of acute infection disease? *Nucl Med Commun* 1994;15:289–293.

105. Krenning EP, Kwekkeboom DJ, Pauwels S, Kvols LK, Reubi JC. Somatostatin receptor scintigraphy. *Nucl Med Annual* 1995:1–50.

106. Chianelli M, Martin Martin S, Signore A *et al*. Assessment of disease activity by ^{99m}Tc-EDDA/tricine-HYNIC-Tyr-octreotide scintigraphy in patients with secondary Sjogren syndrome before and after infliximab treatment. *Eur J Nucl Med* 2005;32 (Suppl 2):S61.

107. Blankenberg FG, Katsikis PD, Tait JF *et al*. *In vivo* detection and imaging of phosphatidylserine expression during programmed cell death. *Proc Natl Acad Sci USA* 1998;95:6349–6354.

108. Ohtsuki K, Akashi K, Aoka Y *et al*. Technetium-99m HYNIC-Annexin V: a potential radiopharmaceutical for the *in vivo* detection of apoptosis. *Eur J Nucl Med* 1999;26:1251–1258.

109. Post AM, Katsikis PD, Tait JF, Geaghan SM, Strauss HW, Blankenberg FG. Imaging cell death with radiolabeled annexin V in an experimental

model of rheumatoid arthritis. *J Nucl Med* 2002; 43:1359–1365.

110. Cagnin A, Myers R, Gunn RN *et al*. *In vivo* visualization of activated glia by [^{11}C] (R)-PK11195-PET following herpes encephalitis reveals projected neuronal damage beyond the primary focal lesion. *Brain* 2001;124:2014–2027.

111. Banati RB, Goerres GW, Myers R *et al*. [11C](R)-PK11195 positrion emission tomography imaging of activated microglia *in vivo* in Rasmussen's encephalitis. *Neurology* 1999;53:2199–2204.

112. Hammoud DA, Endres CJ, Chander AR *et al*. Imaging glial cell activation with [^{11}C]-R-PK11195 in patients with AIDS. *J Neurovirol* 2005;11:346–355.

113. Banati RB, Newcombe J, Gunn RN *et al*. The peripheral benzodiazepine binding site in the brain in multiple sclerosis: quantitative in vivo imaging of microglia as a measure of disease activity. *Brain* 2000;123:2321–2337.

114. Debruyne JC, Versijpt J, Van Laere, KJ *et al*. PET visualization of microglia in multiple sclerosis patients using [^{11}C]PK11195. *Eur J Neurol* 2003;10: 257–264.

115. Davies LP, Barlin GB, Selley ML. New imidzaol [1,2-b]pyridazine ligands for peripheral-type benzodiazepine receptors on mitochondria and monocytes. *Life Sci* 1995;57:381–386.

116. Hardwick MJ, Chen MK, Baidoo K, Pomper MG, Guilarte TR. *In vivo* imaging of peripheral benzodiazepine receptors in mouse lungs: a biomarker of inflammation. *Mol Imaging* 2005;4:432–438.

117. De Bois MHW, Pauwels EKJ, Breedveld FC. New agents for scintigraphy in rheumatoid arthritis. *Eur J Nucl Med* 1995;22:1339–1346.

118. Liberatore M, Clemente M, Iurilli A *et al*. Scintigraphic evaluation of disease activity in rheumatoid arthritis: a comparison of technetium-99m human non-specific immunoglobulins, leucocytes and albumin nanocolloids. *Eur J Nucl Med* 1992;19: 853–857.

119. Martins FP, Gutfilen B, de Souza SA *et al*. Monitoring rheumatoid arthritis synovitis with ^{99m}Tc-anti-CD3. *Br J Radiol* 2008;81:25–29.

120. Becker W, Emmrich F, Horneff G *et al*. Imaging rheumatoid arthritis specifically with technetium 99m CD4-specific (T-helper lymphocytes) antibodies. *Eur J Nucl Med* 1990;17:156–159.

121. Jamar F, Chapman PT, Harrison AA, Binns RM, Haskard DO, Peters AM. Inflammatory arthritis: imaging of endothelial cell activation with an indium-111-labelled F(ab')2 fragment of anti-E-selectin monoclonal antibody. *Radiology* 1995;194: 843–850.

122. Chapman PT, Jamar F, Keelan ETM *et al*. Use of monoclonal antibody against E-selectin for imaging endothelial activation in rheumatoid arthritis. *Arthritis Rheum* 1996;39:1371–1375.

123. Keelan ETM, Harrison AA, Chapman PT, Binns RM, Peters AM, Haskard DO. Imaging vascular endothelial activation: An approach using radiolabelled monoclonal antibodies against the endothelial cell adhesion molecule E-selectin. *J Nucl Med* 1994;35: 276–281.

124. Jamar F, Chapman PT, Manicourt DH, Glass DM, Haskard DO, Peters AM. A comparison between ^{111}In-anti-E-selectin mAb and ^{99}Tc^m-labelled human non-specific immunoglobulin in radionuclide imaging of rheumatoid arthritis. *Br J Radiol* 1997; 70:473–481.

125. Malviya G, D'Alessandria C, Bonanno E *et al*. Radiolabeled humanized anti-CD3 monoclonal antibody visilizumab for imaging human T-lymphocytes. *J Nucl Med* 2009;50:1683–1691.

126. Beckers C, Jeukens X, Ribbens C, Andre B, Marcellis S, Leclercq P. (18)F-FDG PET imaging of rheumatoid knee synovitis correlates with dynamic magnetic resonance and sonographic assessments as well as with the serum level of metalloproteinase-3. *Eur J Nucl Med* 2006;33:275–280.

127. Barrera P, van der Laken CJ, Boerman OC *et al*. Radiolabelled interleukin-1 receptor antagonist for detection of synovitis in patients with rheumatoid arthritis. *Rheumatology (Oxf)* 2000;39: 870–874.

128. Signore A, Parisella MG, Conti F *et al*. ^{99m}Tc-IL2 scintigraphy detects pre-clinical lymphocytic infiltration of salivary glands in patients with autoimmune disease. *Eur J Nucl Med* 2000;27:925.

129. Podolsky DK. Inflammatory bowel disease (I). *N Engl J Med* 1991;325:928–938.

130. Podolsky DK. Inflammatory bowel disease (II). *N Engl J Med* 1991;325:1008–1018.

131. Saverymuttu SH, Peters AM, Crofton ME *et al*. ^{111}Indium autologous granulocytes in the detection of inflammatory bowel disease. *Gut* 1985;26: 955–960.

132. Wheeler JG, Slack NF, Duncan A, Palmer H, Harvey RF. Tc-99m-nanocolloids in inflammatory bowel disease. *Nucl Med Commun* 1990;11:127–133.

133. Annovazzi A, Biancone L, Caviglia R *et al*. ^{99m}Tc-interleukin-2 and ^{99m}Tc-HMPAO granulocyte scintigraphy in patients with inactive Crohn's disease. *Eur J Nucl Med* 2003;30:374–382.

134. D'Alessandria C, Malviya G, Viscido A *et al*. Use of a 99m-technetium labeled anti-TNFα monoclonal antibody in Crohn's disease: *in vitro* and *in vivo* studies. *Q J Nucl Med Mol Imaging* 2007;51:1–9.

135. Weetman AP, McGregor AM. Autoimmune thyroid disease: developments in our understanding. *Endocrinol Rev* 1984;5:309–315.

136. DeGroot LJ, Quintans J. The causes of autoimmune thyroid disease. *Endocrinol Rev* 1989;10:537–562.

137. Postema PTE, Wijnggaarde R, Vandenbosch WA *et al.* Follow-up in (In-111-DTPA-D-Phe-1)octreotide scintigraphy in thyroidal and orbital Graves' disease. *J Nucl Med* 1995;95 (Suppl):203P.

138. Kahaly G, Diaz M, Hahn K, Beyer J, Bockisch A. Indium-111-pentetreotide scintigraphy in Graves' ophthalmopathy. *J Nucl Med* 1995;36:550–554.

139. Diaz M, Kahaly G, Mühlbach A, Bockisch A, Beyer J, Hahn K. Somatostatin receptor scintigraphy in endocrine orbitopathy. *Rofo* 1994;161:484–488.

140. Bohuslavizki KH, Oberwöhrmann S, Brenner W *et al.* ^{111}In-octreotide imaging in patients with long-standing Graves' ophthalmopathy. *Nucl Med Commun* 1995;16:912–916.

141. Bahn R, Heufelder A. Pathogenesis of Graves' ophthalmopathy. *N Engl J Med* 1993;329:1468–1475.

142. Hurley J. Orbitopathy after treatment of Graves' disease. *J Nucl Med* 1994;35:918–920.

143. Krassas GE, Dumas A, Pontikides N, Kaltsas T. Somatostatin receptor scintigraphy and octreotide treatment in patients with thyroid eye disease. *Clin Endocrinol* 1995;42:571–580.

144. Nocaudie M, Bailliez A, Itti E, Bauters C, Wemeau JL, Marchandise X. Somatostatin receptor scintigraphy to predict the clinical evolution and therapeutic response of thyroid-associated ophthalmopathy. *Eur J Nucl Med* 1999;26:511–517.

145. Makino S, Kunimoto K, Muraoka Y, Katagiri K, Tochino Y. Breeding of a non-obese, diabetic strain of mice. *Jikken Dobutsu* 1980;29:1–13.

146. Bottazzo GF, Dean BM, McNally JM, MacKay EH, Swift PGF, Gamble DR. *In situ* characterization of autoimmune phenomena and expression of HLA molecules in the pancreas in diabetic insulitis. *N Engl J Med* 1985;313:353–360.

147. Eisenbarth G. Type I diabetes: a chronic autoimmune disease. *N Engl J Med* 1986;314:1360–1367.

148. Lendrup R, Walker G, Cudworth AG *et al.* Islet-cell antibodies in diabetes mellitus. *Lancet* 1976;ii:1273–1276.

149. Dean BM, Becker F, McNally JM, Tarn AC, Schwartz G, Bottazzo GF. Insulin autoantibodies in the pre-diabetic period: correlation with islet cell antibodies and development of diabetes. *Diabetologia* 1986;29:339–342.

150. McCulloch DX, Claff LJ, Kahn SE *et al.* Subclinical beta-cell dysfunction is not always progressive among first-degree relatives of Type I diabetes: five years' follow-up of the Seattle study. *Diabetes* 1990;39:549–556.

151. Gallina DL, Pelletier D, Doherty P *et al.* ^{111}Indium-labelled lymphocytes do not image or label the pancreas of BB/W rats. *Diabetologia* 1985;28:143–147.

152. Somoza N, Vargas F, Roura-Mir C *et al.* Pancreas in recent onset insulin-dependent diabetes mellitus changes in HLA, adhesion molecules and autoantigens, restricted T cell receptor Vb usage, and cytokine profile. *J Immunol* 1994;153:1360–1377.

153. Kalliokoski T, Simell O, Haarparanta M *et al.* An autoradiographic study of [(18)F]FDG uptake to islets of Langerhans in NOD mouse. *Diabetes Res Clin Pract* 2005;70:217.

154. Iannuzzi MC, Rybicki BA, Teirstein AS. Sarcoidosis. *N Engl J Med* 2007;357:2153–2165.

155. Prager E, Wehrschuetz M, Bisail B *et al.* Comparison of ^{18}F-FDG and ^{67}Ga-citrate in sarcoidosis imaging. *Nuklearmedizin* 2008;47:18–23.

156. Basu S, Zhuang H, Torigian DA, Rosenbaum J, Chen W, Alavi A. Functional imaging of inflammatory diseases using nuclear medicine techniques. *Semin Nucl Med* 2009;39:124–145.

157. Okumura W, Iwasaki T, Toyama T *et al.* Usefulness of fasting ^{18}F-FDG PET in identification of cardiac sarcoidosis. *J Nucl Med* 2004;45:1989–1998.

158. Hain SF, Beggs AD. C-11 Methionine uptake in granulomatous disease. *Clin Nucl Med* 2004;29:585–586.

159. Yamada Y, Uchida Y, Tatsumi K *et al.* Fluorine-18-fluorodeoxyglucose and carbon-11-methionine evaluation of lymphadenopathy in sarcoidosis. *J Nucl Med* 1998;39:1160–1166.

160. Halter G, Buck AK, Schirrmeister H *et al.* [^{18}F]3-Deoxy-3' fluorothymidine positron emission tomography: alternative or diagnostic adjunct to 2-[^{18}F]-fluoro-2-deoxy-D-glucose positron emission tomography in the workup of suspicious central focal lesions? *J Thorac Cardiovasc Surg* 2004;127:1093–1099.

161. Miller A, Chan M, Wiik A. An approach to the diagnosis and management of systemic vasculitis. *Clin Exp Immun* 2010;160:143–160.

162. Fuchs M, Briel M, Daikeler T *et al.* The impact of ^{18}F-FDG PET on the management of patients with suspected large vessel vasculitis. *Eur J Nucl Med Mol Imaging* 2012;39:344–353.

163. Ohtsuki K, Hayase M, Akashi K, Kopiwoda S, Strauss HW. Detection of monocyte chemoattractant protein-1 receptor expression in experimental atherosclerotic lesions: an autoradiographic study. *Circulation* 2001;104:203–208.

164. Fayad ZA, Amirbekian V, Toussaint JF, Fuster V. Identification of interleukin-2 for imaging atherosclerotic inflammation. *Eur J Nucl Med Mol Imaging* 2006;33:111–116.

165. Annovazzi A, Bonanno E, Arca M *et al.* ^{99m}Tc-interleukin-2 scintigraphy for the *in vivo* imaging of

vulnerable atherosclerotic plaques. *Eur J Nucl Med Mol Imaging* 2006;33:117–126.

166. Elkind MS, Rundek T, Sciacca RR *et al.* Interleukin-2 levels are associated with carotid artery intima-media thickness. *Atherosclerosis* 2005;180:181–187.

167. Tawakol A, Migrino RQ, Bashian GG *et al. In vivo* ^{18}F-fluorodeoxyglucose positron emission tomography imaging provides a noninvasive measure of carotid plaque inflammation in patients. *J Am Coll Cardiol* 2006;48:1818–1824.

168. Rudd JH, Myers KS, Bansilal S *et al.* (18)Fluorodeoxyglucose positron emission tomography imaging of atherosclerotic plaque inflammation is highly reproducible: implications for atherosclerosis therapy trials. *J Am Coll Cardiol* 2007;50:892–896.

169. Rudd JH, Myers KS, Bansilal S *et al.* Atherosclerosis inflammation imaging with ^{18}F-FDG PET: carotid, iliac, and femoral uptake reproducibility, quantification methods, and recommendations. *J Nucl Med* 2008;49:871–878.

170. Tahara N, Kai H, Nakaura H *et al.* The prevalence of inflammation in carotid atherosclerosis: analysis with fluorodeoxyglucose-positron emission tomography. *Eur Heart J* 2007;28:2243–2248.

171. Conti F, Priori R, Chimenti MS *et al.* Successful treatment with intraarticular infliximab for resistant knee monarthritis in a patient with spondylarthropathy a role for scintigraphy with ^{99m}Tc-infliximab. *Arthritis Rheum* 2005;52:1224–1226.

172. Abrams MJ, Juweid M, ten Kate CI *et al.* Technetium-99m-human polyclonal IgG radiolabelled via the hydrazino nicotinamide derivative for imaging focal sites of infection in rats. *J Nucl Med* 1990;31:2022–2028.

173. Barrera P, Oyen WJG, Boerman OC, van Riel PLCM. Scintigraphic detection of tumour necrosis factor in patients with rheumatoid arthritis. *Ann Rheum Dis* 2003;62:825–828.

174. Annovazzi A, D'Alessandria C, Lenza A *et al.* Radiolabelled anti-TNF-α antibodies for therapy decision making and follow-up in rheumatoid arthritis. *Eur J Nucl Med* 2006;33 (Suppl 2):S146.

175. Conti F, Malviya G, Ceccarelli F *et al.* Role of scintigraphy with ^{99m}Tc-infliximab in predicting the response of intraarticular infliximab treatment in patients with refractory monoarthritis. *Eur J Nucl Med Mol Imaging* 2012;39:1339–1347.

176. Chianelli M, Parisella MG, Visalli N *et al.* Pancreatic scintigraphy with ^{99m}Tc-interleukin-2 at diagnosis of type 1 diabetes and after 1 year of nicotinamide therapy. *Diabetes Metab Res Rev* 2008;24:115–122.

177. Barone R, Procaccini E, Chianelli M *et al.*; IMDIAB Group. Prognostic relevance of pancreatic uptake of ^{99m}Tc-HIG in patients with type 1 diabetes. *Eur J Nucl Med* 1998;25:503–508.

178. Teirstein AS, Machac J, Almeida O, Lu P, Padilla ML, Iannuzzi MC. Results of 188 whole-body fluorodeoxyglucose positron emission tomography scans in 137 patients with sarcoidosis. *Chest* 2007;132:1949–1953.

179. Migliore A, Signore A, Capuano A *et al.* Relevance of ^{99m}Tc-HYNIC-tir-octreotide scintigraphy in a patient affected by sarcoidosis with lung and joints involvement and secondary Sjogren's syndrome treated with infliximab: Case report. *Eur Rev Med Pharmacol Sci* 2008;12:127–130.

Clinical cases

Case 1

A 16-year-old girl was admitted to hospital because of a long-lasting (>3 weeks) feeling of malaise, 15-kg weight loss, tiredness, earache and abdominal pain. The patient developed fever during her stay in hospital.

Her CRP was 14.1 mg/dL and WBC count was 11.9×10^9/L.

Chest X-ray, X-ray of the skeleton (for osteomyelitis), US of the abdomen, MRI of the abdomen and CT of the head were performed but no explanation for her complaints was found. Gastrointestinal endoscopy was performed because of her bowel complaints, but again without abnormal findings.

$[^{18}F]$FDG-PET/CT (Figure 17.8A) was performed because of fever of unknown origin. High uptake was found in the thoracic and (part of) the abdominal aorta. Uptake was also found in mediastinal, hilar and axillary lymph nodes. Arteritis with reactive lymph nodes was suggested as a diagnosis. To confirm this finding MRI arteriography (Figure 17.8B) was performed with normal findings.

Despite the negative findings on MRI, Takayasu's arteritis was diagnosed from the clinical and PET findings. The patient was treated with high doses of prednisone with good results.

Teaching points
• As reported in many published studies, $[^{18}F]$ FDG-PET/CT is of value in patients with fever of unknown origin.
• Nuclear imaging should be performed early in the diagnostic work-up of these patients.

Case 2

A 46-year-old female affected by Sjögren syndrome and rheumatoid arthritis. . She was receiving treatment with methotrexate and steroids, but was still suffering from pain in the joints. At the baseline study, taken when the patient was still on treatment (Figure 17.9A), 1 hour after the injection of 370 MBq of ^{99m}Tc-HYNIC-TOC, scintigraphy reveals pathological uptake of the radiopharmaceutical in both hands, consistent with active disease. Therapy with infliximab was then started.

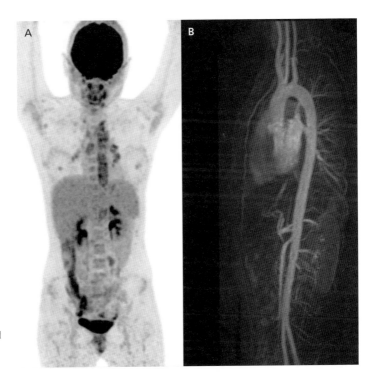

Figure 17.8 (A) $[^{18}F]$FDG-PET/CT and (B) MRI arteriography in a patient with fever of unexplained origin.

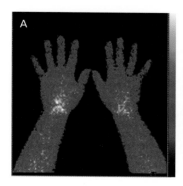
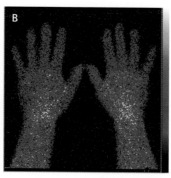

Figure 17.9 ^{99m}Tc-HYNIC-TOC images of the hands of a patient with rheumatoid arthritis (A) before and (B) after therapy with infliximab.

The scan taken 3 months after treatment with infliximab shows marked reduction of radiopharmaceutical uptake, concordant with reduction of symptoms (Figure 17.9B).

Teaching point

Radiolabeled somatostatin analogs, like ^{99m}Tc-HYNIC-TOC, are useful in the study of patients affected by rheumatoid arthritis and can contribute to the management of patients by selecting the appropriate treatment modality.

Case 3

A patient with Hashimoto's thyroiditis. The patient had presented with an enlarged thyroid with negative thyroid autoantibodies and high thyroid hormone levels.

Thyroid scintigraphy of the neck obtained 20 minutes after the injection of ^{99m}TcO$_4$ showed no uptake. There was suspicion of a possible thyrotoxicosis factitia. The patient underwent a ^{99m}Tc-IL-2 scan (Figure 17.10) and this revealed high uptake of the tracer in the thyroid, indicating thyroid infiltration by activated lymphocytes, consistent with hashitoxicosis.

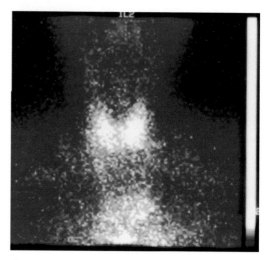

Figure 17.10 Anterior planar image of the neck 1 hour after injection of 5 mCi ^{99m}Tc-IL-2 scan in a patient with Hashimoto's thyroiditis.

Teaching point

Imaging with radiolabeled IL-2 may be used to confirm the autoimmune nature of diseases in dubious cases.

Index

Page references in *italic* refer to figures.
Page references in **bold** refer to tables.

Diagnostic Imaging of Infections and Inflammatory Diseases: A Multidisciplinary Approach, First Edition. Edited by Alberto Signore
and Ana María Quintero.
© 2014 John Wiley & Sons, Inc. Published 2014 by John Wiley & Sons, Inc.